Stanford Hospital Celebrates ~~WITHDRAWN~~ Year Ranking in the Top 10 of Hospitals Nationwide

Ranking on *U.S. News & World Report* Honor Roll based on quality, patient safety, and reputation

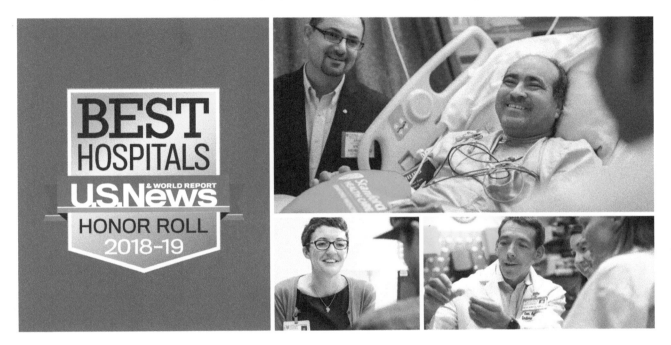

Stanford Hospital was just named to the Honor Roll of the top 1 percent of best hospitals in the country by *U.S. News & World Report*. The ranking, which reflects the hospital's spot among more than 4,500 hospitals surveyed, is based on outstanding performance across multiple areas of care, with factors such as quality, patient safety, and reputation.

This recognition is a tribute to our physicians, nurses, and staff for their world-class care of patients and their families.

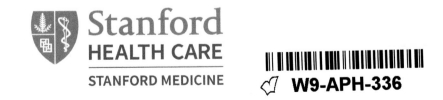

Stanford
HEALTH CARE
STANFORD MEDICINE

W9-APH-336

———————————— *Proudly ranked in 12 specialties* ————————————

Cancer • Cardiology & Heart Surgery • Diabetes & Endocrinology • Ear, Nose & Throat • Gastroenterology •
Geriatrics • Gynecology • Nephrology • Neurology & Neurosurgery • Orthopaedics • Pulmonology • Urology

U.S.News & WORLD REPORT

2019 EDITION

Best Hospitals

EXCLUSIVE RANKINGS

▶ Get **Expert Care** in Cancer, Cardiology, Neurology, Orthopedics and More

▶ The Best **Children's Hospitals**

Plus: The Top Hospitals in **Your State**

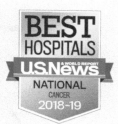
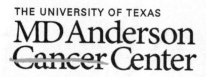

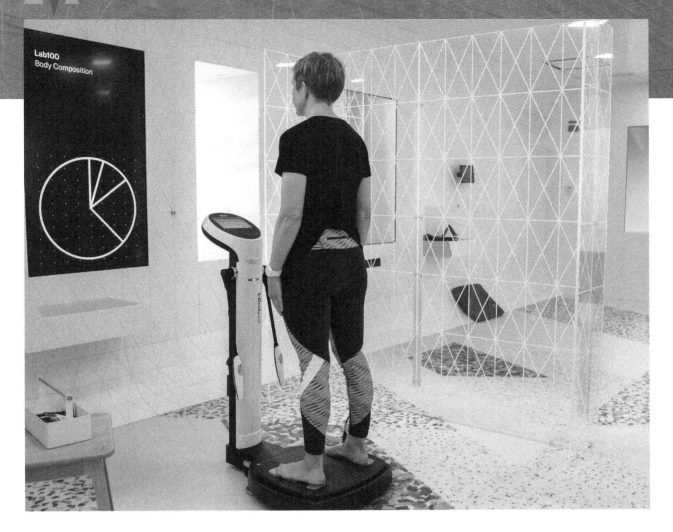

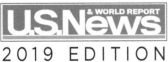

2019 EDITION

Best Hospitals

At Mount Sinai's new Lab100
KRISANNE JOHNSON FOR USN&WR

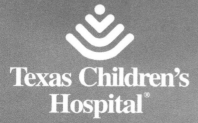
CONTENTS ▲▼▼

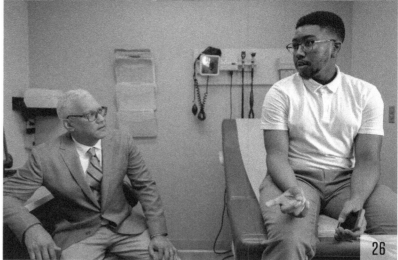

26

CONTENTS CONTINUED ON PAGE 4

66

FROM TOP: ELIAS WILLIAMS FOR USN&WR; ILLUSTRATION BY RANDY MORA FOR USN&WR
COVERS: GETTY IMAGES (2)

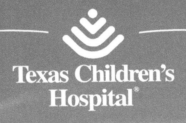

▲▼▲ CONTENTS

The U.S. News Rankings

BEST CHILDREN'S HOSPITALS
U.S.News
2018-19

156

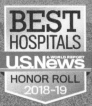

New York's top-ranked hospital since before phones were smart.

It's been 18 years.

NewYork-Presbyterian

Once again, ranked #1 in New York by *U.S. News & World Report.*

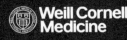 Weill Cornell Medicine | NewYork-Presbyterian | COLUMBIA

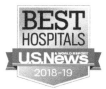

NUTRITION & LIFESTYLE

Best Diets

A look at some of the most popular and most researched diets, with reviews by a panel of health experts. Discover the top diets for weight loss, diabetes management and heart health, as well as the best plant-based and commercial diets.
usnews.com/bestdiets

Eat + Run

Doing what it takes to stay in shape can be tough to manage. We serve up expert advice daily.
usnews.com/eat-run

INSURANCE

Best Medicare Advantage Plans

State-by-state ratings of Medicare Advantage and Medicare Part D plans, plus tips on choosing one of these plans vs. original Medicare.
usnews.com/medicare

Health Insurance Guide

Your marketplace: a state-by-state guide. Plus answers to frequently asked questions.
usnews.com/healthinsurance

MEDICAL CARE

Health Care of Tomorrow

Health reform, technological innovation and big data are transforming hospitals and care delivery. U.S. News explores how the industry is adapting.
usnews.com/ healthcareoftomorrow

BEST HOSPITALS HONOR ROLL

A Visual Tour of the Top 20

See the best of the Best Hospitals – 20 medical centers that lead the pack in a host of specialties, procedures and conditions, excelling in both breadth and depth of care.
usnews.com/hospitalphototour

BEST HOSPITALS

In Specialties, Procedures & Conditions

We've evaluated more than 4,500 hospitals in up to nine common procedures and conditions, including hip replacement, knee replacement, heart bypass surgery, and COPD, as well as 16 medical specialties, including cancer care.
usnews.com/best-hospitals

SENIOR CARE

Best Nursing Homes

We've analyzed government data and published ratings of more than 15,000 facilities.
usnews.com/nursinghomes

PHARMACIST PICKS

Top Recommended Health Products

Which over-the-counter products do pharmacists prefer? Check out Top Recommended Health Products.
usnews.com/tophealthproducts

PHYSICIAN SEARCH TOOL

Doctor Finder

A searchable directory of more than 800,000 doctors. Patients can find and research doctors who have the training, certification, practical experience and hospital affiliation they want – and can see ratings based on other patients' experiences. With free registration, physicians can expand or update the profile patients see.
usnews.com/doctors

BEST HOSPITALS
2019 EDITION

Executive Committee Chairman and Editor-in-Chief Mortimer B. Zuckerman
Chairman Eric Gertler
Editor and Chief Content Officer Brian Kelly
Executive Editor Anne McGrath
Deputy Editor Lindsay Lyon
Managing Editor & Chief, Health Analysis Ben Harder
Art Director Rebecca Pajak
Director of Photography Avi Gupta
Contributing Editors Elizabeth Whitehead, Michael Morella
Associate Editor Lindsay Cates
Photography Editor Brett Ziegler
Assistant Photo Editor Lydia Chebbine
Contributors Ann Claire Carnahan, Stacey Colino, Avery Comarow, Geoff B. Dougherty, Lisa Esposito, K. Aleisha Fetters, Gaby Galvin, Elizabeth Gardner, Katherine Hobson, Beth Howard, Mary Brophy Marcus, Linda Marsa, Alison Murtagh, Courtney Rubin, Barbara Sadick, Steve Sternberg, Arlene Weintraub
Research Manager Myke Freeman

USNEWS.COM/HEALTH
Executive Editor Kimberly Castro
Managing Editors Liz Opsitnik, Katy Marquardt
Assistant Managing Editors Angela Haupt, Nathan Hellman
Senior Editors Dennis Kelly, Anna Medaris Miller
Editors Michael Schroeder, Whitney Wyckoff
Associate Editors Ray Frager, Ali Follman
Reporters Ruben Castaneda, Lisa Esposito
Research Manager Anna George
Analysts Zach Adams, Anwesha Majumder, Greta Martin

HEALTHCARE AND HOSPITAL DATA INSIGHTS
Vice President and General Manager, Healthcare & Insights Evan Jones
Product Director, Healthcare Anne Roberts
Product Director, Hospital Data Insights Laura Kovach
Manager, Marketing and Product Services Taylor Suggs
Product Manager, Healthcare Kayla Devon
SEO Analyst, Healthcare Jen McCallen
Associate, Hospital Data Insights Manny Plummer
Product Coordinator, Healthcare Lewam Dejen

TECHNOLOGY
Senior Director of Engineering Matt Kupferman
Senior Directors of Software Development Dan Brown, Jerome Gipe
Senior Systems Manager Cathy Cacho
Software Technical Lead Corey Hutton
Developers Jess Park, Marc Simon, Nicolas Soudee, Yasin Yaqoobi
Project Manager Derrick Stout
Quality Assurance Sandy Sathyanarayanan
Digital Production Michael A. Brooks (Manager); Michael Fingerhuth

President and Chief Executive Officer William D. Holiber

ADVERTISING AND MARKETING
Vice President, Advertising Linda Brancato
Vice President, Marketing and Advertising Strategy Alexandra Kalaf
Director, Integrated Media Solutions Peter Bowes
New York Advertising Director Heather Levine
Pacific Northwest Advertising Director Peter Teese
Midwest Advertising Director Paul Kissane
Health Care Advertising Director Colin Hamilton
Director of Education Advertising Shannon Tkach
Sales Manager Dan DeMonte
Senior Account Executive Ivy Zenati
Account Executives Julie Izzo, Eddie Kelly, Spencer Vastoler
Managing Editor, BrandFuse Jada Graves
Web Designer, BrandFuse Sara Hampt
Director of Programmatic, Data and Revenue Partnerships Joseph Hayden
Programmatic Account Manager Hector Guerra
Senior Manager of Ad Technology and Platforms Teron Samuel
Senior Manager, Sales Strategy Tina Lopez
Manager, Sales Strategy Gary DeNardis
Sales Planners Gina DeNatale, Jade-Ashley Thomas, Michael Zee
Director of Advertising Operations Cory Nesser
Senior Manager, Client Success Katina Sangare
Account Managers James Adeleye, Jennifer Fass, Katie Harper
Manager, Ad Operations Tessa Gluck
Senior Manager of Audience Development, Social Media Greg Hicks
Audience Development Specialists, Social Media David Oliver, Darian Somers, Megan Trimble
Director of Advertising Services Phyllis Panza
Business Operations Karolee Jarnecki
Administration Judy David, Anny Lasso, Carmen Caraballo
Vice President, Specialty Marketing Mark W. White
Director of Specialty Marketing Abbe Weintraub

Chief Operating Officer Karen S. Chevalier
Chief Product Officer Chad Smolinski
Chief Financial Officer Neil Maheshwari
Senior Vice President, Education, News/Opinion, Money Chris DiCosmo
Senior Vice President, Strategic Development and General Counsel Peter M. Dwoskin
Senior Vice President, Technology Yingjie Shu

Additional copies of U.S. News & World Report's Best Hospitals 2019 guidebook are available for purchase at (800) 836-6397 or online at usnews.com/hospitalbook. To order custom reprints, call (877) 652-5295 or email usnews@wrightsmedia.com. For all other permissions, email permissions@usnews.com.

A New
State of Health
for NEW JERSEY,
for the NATION,
for the WORLD

RWJBarnabas Health and Rutgers University launch the state's largest academic health system

With the partnership of RWJBarnabas Health and Rutgers University, it is the dawn of an incredible new era in health.

Jointly, RWJBarnabas Health and Rutgers University will operate a world-class academic health system dedicated to high-quality patient care, life changing research and clinical training of tomorrow's health care workforce. By partnering, these two higher education and health care industry leaders will improve access to care and reduce health disparities in New Jersey and across the nation.

At the center of all of this are the patients who will benefit from increased access to a world-class academic health system, clinical innovation, groundbreaking research and newly developed centers of excellence, as well as more providers that families need to manage their health and wellness.

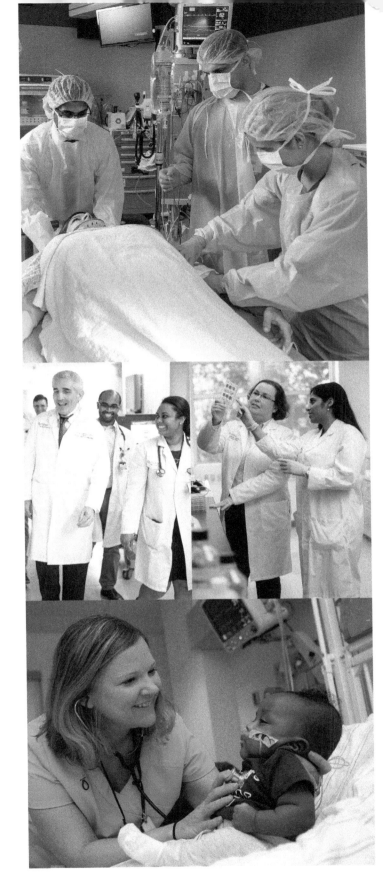

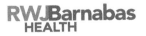

RUTGERS HEALTH   RWJBarnabas HEALTH

rutgersrwjbhtogether.org

UCSF Medical Center is ranked the
#1 Hospital in California

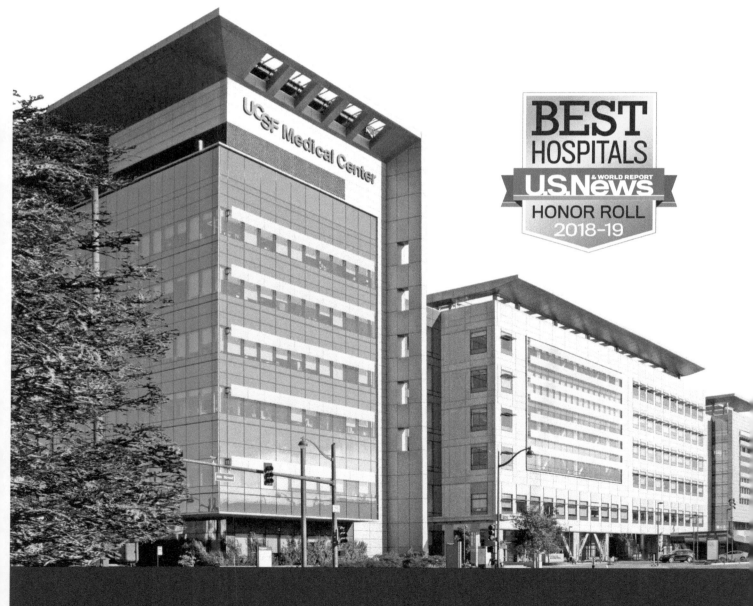

BEST
HOSPITALS
U.S.News & WORLD REPORT
HONOR ROLL
2018-19

UCSF Health

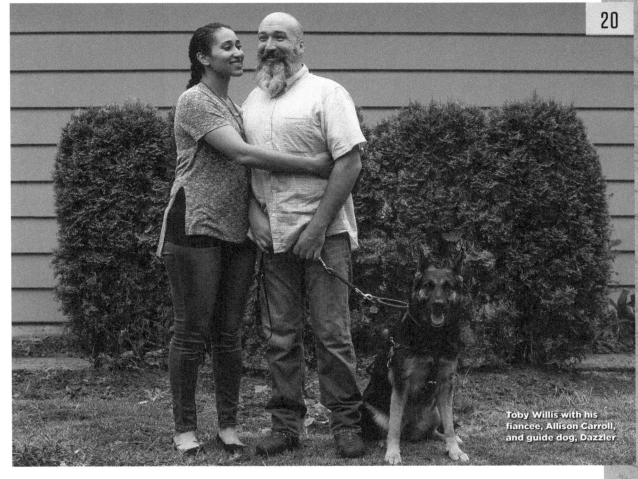

CHAPTER 1

20

Toby Willis with his fiancee, Allison Carroll, and guide dog, Dazzler

On Medicine's Front Lines

What Is Health, Precisely?

Researchers are out to prove that health is more than just the absence of disease

by **Katherine Hobson**

I was racing the clock. My task: Put nine small pegs into the equally small holes of a 3x3 grid, then take them out again. I was starting to sweat. The blood draw had been a breeze, the body composition assessment didn't faze me, and even a tough appraisal of my episodic memory went OK. But I had met my match in this test of dexterity, which declines with age and is key to many activities of daily living. And mine, I was learning, was not great.

I was in the beta version of Lab100, a slick hybrid clinic-research center that Mount Sinai Health System in New York

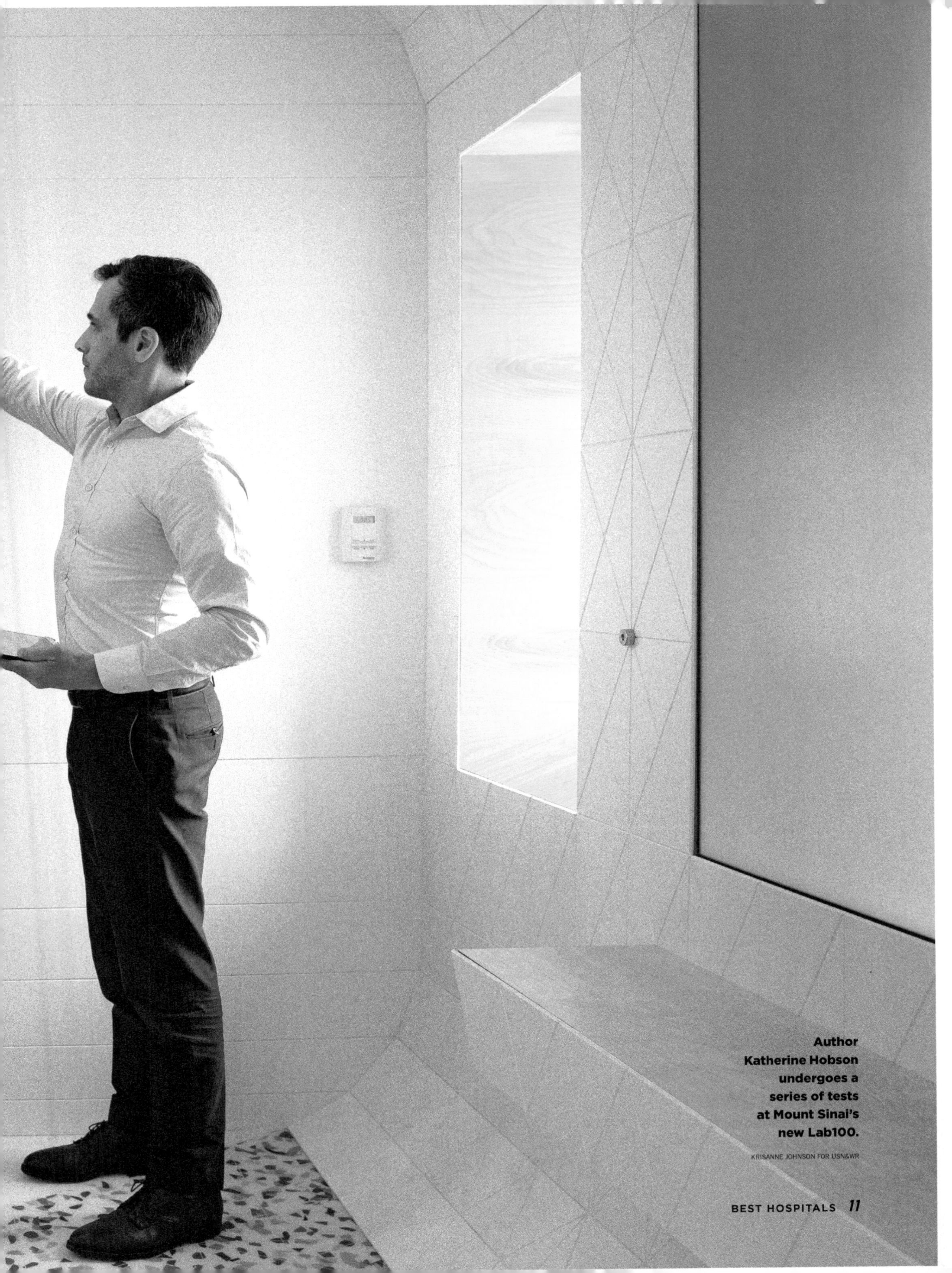

Author Katherine Hobson undergoes a series of tests at Mount Sinai's new Lab100.

KRISANNE JOHNSON FOR USN&WR

will officially open this year. By completing a one-hour assessment, I was gearing up to gain insights on my general health and how it's affected by my behavior and lifestyle. And with each detail I shared, I was also becoming a single data point in the emerging field of precision health. Lab100 joins several much larger efforts – including All of Us, from the National Institutes of Health, and Project Baseline, from Google's sister company Verily and partner institutions – in trying to develop a more nuanced picture of just how different health can look from you to me, as well as the quiet changes the body makes en route from wellness to disease.

Painting a total-continuum-of-health picture will require data – lots and lots of data. You've probably heard of precision medicine, which aims to better tailor treatments to a patient's individual characteristics. Think of precision health as the front end of that effort. The big idea behind these projects is that gathering information on genetics, biomarkers, and lifestyle and environmental factors from many thou-

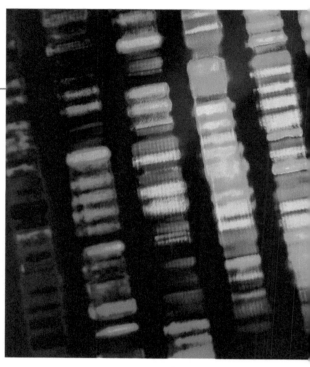

Decoding Your DNA

Not long ago, genetic testing was an expensive endeavor done strictly through the health care system. Nowadays, you can mail a saliva sample directly to companies, pay a few hundred dollars and get details on factors that may affect your disease risk. According to proponents, arming people with their genetic information helps them take charge of their health. But for most conditions, it's unclear whether learning about predisposition motivates behavior change. So before you spit in a test tube and put it in the mail, consider:

Why you want the test. Following a 2013 crackdown, the Food and Drug Administration has begun approving tests that offer genetic information to people without a physician's involvement, and has recently taken action to streamline the path to market. Through 23andMe, you can get screened for mutations you might pass on to your kids and for genetic variants linked to such conditions as age-related macular degeneration, Parkinson's disease, late-onset Alzheimer's disease, and some hereditary breast and ovarian cancers. Meantime, Veritas, Color

Genomics and some companies that sell their products through the online consumer genomics marketplace Helix require a doctor – in some cases your own, other times one that's assigned to you – to sign off on ordering tests that gauge your genetic risk of certain hereditary cancers, heart conditions and immune disorders, for example.

If health-risk information is what you're after, learn the limitations of the test you're considering, says Cecelia Bellcross, director of the genetic counseling training program at Emory University School of Medicine. Some harmful gene variants are highly predictive of future health, as with mutations in BRCA1 and BRCA2 genes for breast and ovarian cancer, and there are concrete ways to manage that risk. Others aren't nearly as prognostic. Think hard about how you'd feel if the results were negative, positive or uncertain, what action you might take afterward and how the results might affect your family members – who may get clues about their own genetic makeup from your results. Some companies include genetic counseling as part of their packages; if you need more input on the potential risks and benefits, talk to your doctor.

You won't get the full picture. Companies analyze your DNA to varying degrees, and the cost differs accordingly: Veritas, for example, charges $999 for whole-genome sequencing, the most extensive sequencing strategy. Color Genomics ($99-$349) fully sequences specific genes. Other companies, such as 23andMe ($199 for both health and ancestry information), use genotyping, which is more limited, to look for certain gene variants. Their BRCA1 and BRCA2 tests, for example, target three variants of more than 1,000

sands of volunteers will give researchers a trove of data that they can mine to discover better ways of spotting – and perhaps preventing – disease, while accounting for our unique differences even more precisely than before.

"What we're hoping to do is to go from a reactive approach, when we only encounter people when they're sick, to a more proactive, preventive approach," says Adrian Hernandez, a cardiologist and vice dean for clinical research at Duke University School of Medicine, a Project Baseline study site and partner. Hernandez compares the vision to how smartphone apps flag upcoming road congestion. "When you see a traffic jam down the road on a map, you have choices and can take alternate routes," he says. "We've got to get better in terms of saying, 'What's that person's risk over a 10-year or shorter period and what are the interventions that can dramatically change that risk?'"

Of course, finding and addressing conditions earlier isn't a new goal, nor is it always the case that doing so saves lives or

> ❝Make sure you understand the limitations of the test you're considering.❞

known to raise the risk of cancer. But – as the company makes clear in the results – testing negative for those variants doesn't mean a person lacks another harmful variant, and could lead to a false sense of security. Make sure you know how complete the test you're considering is.

Moreover, the most common diseases, including most cancers, are caused by a complex interplay of multiple genes and nongenetic factors. Genetic information may not add meaningfully to the risk details you can find from other sources. "All of this information needs to be put into the broader context of your health history, family history, environmental exposures and symptoms," says Amy McGuire, a bioethicist and lawyer at the Baylor

College of Medicine.

If testing turns up something you want to act on, first talk to your provider. Even negative results are worth discussing. As FDA Commissioner Scott Gottlieb noted last year, "Consider the consequences of a person who is told they're not at risk for coronary heart disease and incorrectly opts to forgo dietary changes or drugs that reduce their risk of heart attack and death." If your test wasn't done in a clinical setting, your results may need to be confirmed – and the cost may not be covered by insurance. And doctors might not know what to do with information that has a modest or uncertain impact on your health.

The results probably won't make you anxious. When consumer genetic tests first hit the market, there was concern that learning about disease risk would spur anxiety, especially for diseases with no clear prevention strategy. That hasn't panned out, says Timothy Caulfield, a professor of law and public health at the University of Alberta in Canada. A 2016 research review found no increase in depression or anxiety in people who received personalized DNA-based disease-risk estimates.

That's in the aggregate – some, of course, may stew more than others.

But results don't necessarily inspire behavior change. The same review found no significant effects of communicating DNA-based risk estimates on smoking cessation, diet, physical activity, alcohol use or sun-protection behaviors, for example. (Still, Francis Collins, National Institutes of Health director, has said he was inspired by direct-to-consumer genetic testing to lose 35 pounds after learning he is at higher risk of Type 2 diabetes.)

Not all of the claims are steeped in science. The FDA doesn't oversee the accuracy of gene-based tests that claim to predict your ideal diet, wine or romantic partner, which experts say have much less scientific backing than those that test for established genetic health risks. The bottom line: Some tests offer legitimate, actionable health information, says Megan Allyse, an assistant professor of biomedical ethics at the Mayo Clinic. Others offer interpretation based on less definitive science, or should be considered educational or "infotainment," she says. Eric Topol, a cardiologist, geneticist and researcher at the Scripps Translational Science Institute, sees the need in the marketplace for an independent evaluator to show whether the data and interpretation a company provides are accurate and useful. Until then: Proceed carefully. *–K. H.*

ON MEDICINE'S FRONT LINES

improves health, as the overscreening controversy surrounding certain cancer tests has shown. And while these ambitious efforts to collect and analyze data may pay off with new detection and prevention strategies, questions remain about whether they will outperform our current tools – and at what cost. Managing expectations about when precision health research will bear fruit is a chief concern of its proponents. "The human body is more complicated than we think," says Sanjiv Sam Gambhir, professor and chair of radiology at Stanford Medicine, another Project Baseline partner. "People want quicker solutions, but there are no quicker wins in health and disease."

But given that caution, let's imagine one precision health world that might emerge from these efforts, as envisioned by Gambhir and his colleagues in a recent Science Translational Medicine paper. Your disease risk would be estimated very

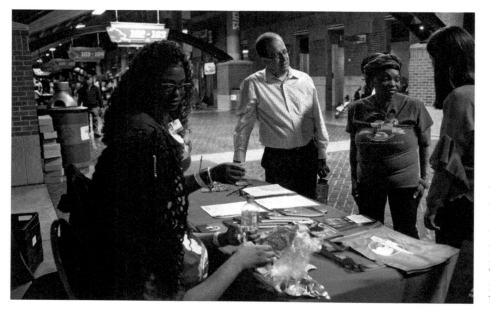

a health portal where data analytics suggest next steps, such as scheduling a doctor's visit, health coaching session, treatments or tests.

New gadgets have natural appeal, but Gambhir emphasizes that they must also be accurate and reliable. Moreover, the information they provide must be predictive, actionable and not prone to false alarms that prompt unnecessary and costly follow-up tests. That will all require a lot of research, data collection and machine learning. And some of the biomarkers these devices might detect – such as molecules in urine or breath that could indicate disease – simply haven't been discovered.

Several precision health efforts varying in size and scope are underway. The NIH's All of Us project, with $1.5 billion in authorized funding over 10 years, kicked off in May of 2018 with the ultimate goal of gathering genomic and other key information from 1 million Americans, allowing researchers to study that data to ask fundamental questions about health and disease. "We still don't understand how environmental and genetic and socioeconomic and behavioral factors combine to make one person healthy and another not healthy," says Eric Dishman, All of Us director. The project aims to develop improved treatments, yes, but also to discover new risk markers for disease and to give participants data to improve their health.

early in life – even before birth – using genetics and family history. Based on those results, you'd be tracked by specific devices that capture a range of continuous health data, including familiar indicators (e.g., blood pressure), new biomarkers, environmental factors (e.g., air quality) and behavioral ones (think sleep activity or exercise levels). Some of that information would come from the kinds of wearables you're used to (e.g., fitness trackers), but Gambhir foresees a whole new set of passive – but smart – monitors that would gather data without necessarily requiring individuals to strap them on daily.

Among the possibilities, some of which are being developed or studied: Sheets to monitor heart-and-lung function; toilets that analyze urine and stool for glucose and other biomarkers; mirrors that capture facial changes that might signal disease onset; a bra that detects early signs of breast cancer; and smartphones that spot usage patterns linked to anxiety. Those devices would "learn" your individual variation to differentiate between a random quirk and a potentially disturbing pattern. That information would feed into

All of Us director Eric Dishman attends a May launch and recruitment event in Detroit.

Through more than 270 planned study sites, All of Us aims to reach a more diverse group of people – in terms of race, ethnicity, income, age, sexual orientation and geography – than has historically been achieved in large, long-term, government-funded studies. (Because the project will still rely on a self-selecting group of volunteers, though, it may not truly represent the U.S. population as a whole.) As of mid-June 2018, All of Us had collected blood and urine samples from more than 34,000 people who also granted access to their electronic medical records. Soon participants will be able to provide researchers with information from their own wearable devices; the next step is to begin analyzing the genes of those who opt into that part of the pro-

"Help kids live their dreams, just like me"

AMY PURDY
PARALYMPIC MEDALIST, AUTHOR,
MOTIVATIONAL SPEAKER, AMPUTEE PATIENT

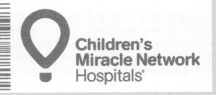

Children's
Miracle Network
Hospitals®

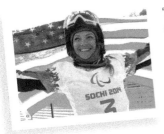

"As a kid, I wanted to explore every inch of the world — on a snowboard, when possible. But then I contracted bacterial meningitis. My kidneys shut down. My spleen burst. Both of my legs were amputated below the knees. Everyone told me I would never snowboard again. But, I didn't give up on my dreams. I medaled in the Paralympics. I'm a motivational speaker, published author, Dancing with the Stars runner up and training to compete in the next Paralympic Games. Help kids live their dreams – just like me."

PUT YOUR MONEY WHERE THE MIRACLES ARE.
Give Today to your children's hospital

CMNHospitals.org/Amy

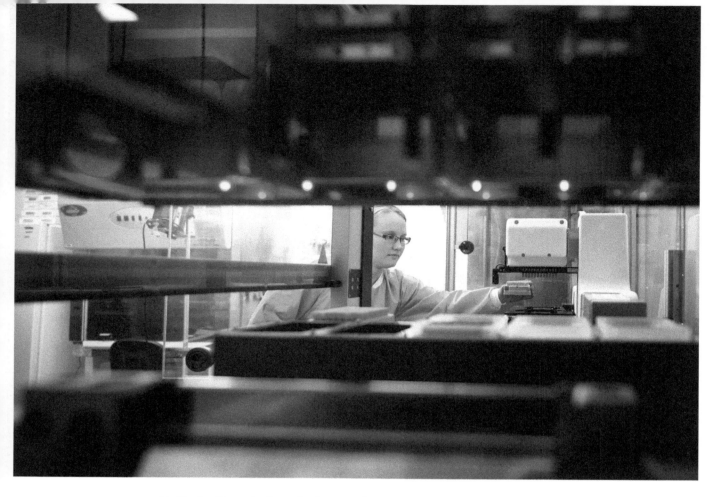

gram. (Achieving the project's goals of sequencing the genomes of participants will take time – for starters, it will require many more sequencing machines than are currently available in the U.S.)

Project Baseline is also trying to capture a more comprehensive picture of human health by recruiting 10,000 participants who visit sites at Duke, Stanford and elsewhere. Launched in 2017, the study is collecting information through health tests, wearables (such as a special watch equipped with sensors not available for sale to the public), and app-based health diaries. Researchers will comb those datasets to ideally discover new signals or insights that correlate to health or disease. Scarlet Shore, the initiative's project manager, says that Verily hopes the project will expand, either virtually or with more physical sites.

Not everyone is convinced that these large-scale data-gathering efforts will pay off with big

improvements in health. "The question I'd ask is, 'What hole is being filled? What are we attempting to solve here?'" says Nigel Paneth, a professor of epidemiology and biostatistics and of pediatrics and human development at Michigan State University's College of Human Medicine. There's already significant opportunity to change health outcomes by addressing societal issues, he says. In the U.S., for example, an individual's ZIP code may be as important as his or her genetic code for health. "Those with the lowest income and who

At Geisinger, MyCode lab technician Larissa Orzolek prepares DNA for testing.

were least educated were consistently least healthy," concluded a 2010 paper published in the American Journal of Public Health. Moreover, any new biomarkers would have to improve on the pretty high levels of risk prediction we get from factors such as body mass index, cholesterol and blood pressure, Paneth says. "Strong signals don't take a lot of data to reveal," says H. Gilbert Welch, a professor of medicine at the Dartmouth Institute for Health Policy and Clinical Practice.

As for the future vision of monitoring constant streams of data from healthy people? The more health information that's gathered, the more likely it is that things will pop up that are outside the "normal" range – even if they don't signal disease, Welch notes. (Gambhir counters that knowing a person's serial measurements over time will lower the chance of false positives, however.)

Leaders of these precision health projects must also wrestle with what data should be returned to research participants – and how. Consider genetic-risk information, which isn't usually assessed in healthy people without a specific reason, such as having a strong family history of certain cancers or other diseases.

The American College of Medical Genetics and Genomics, or ACMG, has a list of potentially harmful gene variants that, if discovered incidentally, it recommends people be told about, as they both carry significant risk of health problems and could potentially be mitigated. (Examples are variants tied to diseases including breast and ovarian cancers, the heart-rhythm disorder Long QT syndrome and aortic aneu-

"My children's hospital never gave up on me"

JOSH SUNDQUIST
AUTHOR, ATHLETE, MOTIVATIONAL SPEAKER,
FORMER CHILDREN'S HOSPITAL PATIENT

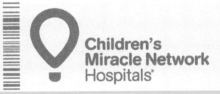

Children's
Miracle Network
Hospitals

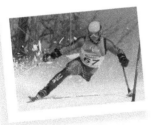

I was 9 when I lost my leg to bone cancer. I had a 50 percent chance to live. After chemotherapy treatments at my children's hospital and the amputation, I had beaten the odds. But would I ever be as active as I once was? Fast forward 20 years: I've competed in the Paralympics and now play on the U.S. Amputee Soccer Team. My successes are because of my children's hospital. They never gave up on me.

PUT YOUR MONEY WHERE THE MIRACLES ARE.
Give Today to your children's hospital

CMNHospitals.org/Josh

rysm.) Statistically, 1 to 2 percent of All of Us participants will have those variants, Dishman says, and a pilot project starting this year will help determine how best to return that information. That means figuring out how to provide genetic counseling or other health care to people who may not have a doctor, he says. Project Baseline, for its part, has a committee of experts working to determine what information should be shared.

Separate from those efforts, at Pennsylvania's Geisinger health system, the MyCode Community Health Initiative, a research project, has registered more than 200,000 participants since 2007 who've agreed to have their DNA sequenced. (Sequencing began in 2014.) The information is stored for research, but Geisinger has also notified nearly 600 participants so far whose sequencing turned up risk-carrying variants. Geisinger is taking a conservative approach based on ACMG's recommendations, says its executive vice president and chief scientific officer David H. Ledbetter. As more evidence on the role of additional genes emerges, he expects to have reportable information for 5 percent of participants in the next few years, and 10 percent in the next five to 10 years. That, he says, has "profound health implica-

Katherine Hobson sees how she measures up. (Details have been blurred for privacy.)

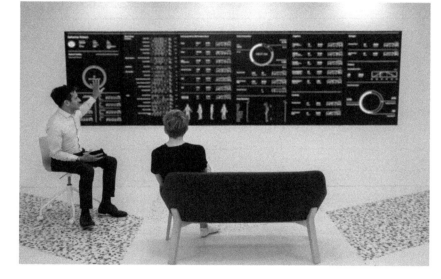

tions." (In May of 2018, Geisinger announced it will start a 1,000-person pilot project to incorporate DNA sequencing into standard clinical care.)

For now, most MyCode participants are like 75-year-old Philip Jewell, who signed up hoping researchers could ferret out useful information in his DNA. "I had throat and neck cancer. My daughter died of breast cancer. I did this not for ourselves, but to add to their studies. Maybe they can find something."

Lab100 won't return genetic information to its initial participants, though with consent, researchers can use that data. But participants will pay an as-yet-undetermined fee for feedback from their assessment, which is intended to complement

(not replace) usual health care visits and includes questionnaires on medical and family history, nutrition, physical activity and sleep. At each station, information is collected: bloodwork, body composition, the results of five different cognitive tests, grip strength, balance and dexterity metrics, among others. Patients sit down with a provider at the end of the hour – as I did – facing an array of screens to discuss what lifestyle steps they could take to improve health.

Additional information is gathered that isn't ready for prime time but feeds into research, says David Stark, who heads up Lab100. For example, the balance station collects data to see if a smart TV might someday passively collect those same insights. (Poor balance is linked to falls.) Videos of patients' dexterity tests may be correlated with their outcomes to see if tremors can be predicted or detected early. And overall outcomes will be tracked to see if this type of personalized assessment improves health.

It's not clear whether all this data-gathering will ultimately provide new knowledge about what lifestyle changes we should be making, or how to put them in motion. We already know many of the things we should be doing. A recent study confirmed the obvious: Avoiding smoking, maintaining a normal-range BMI, getting at least 30 minutes of daily physical activity, eating a high-quality diet and going easy on alcohol were associated with an extra 12 years of life for men and 14 for women. But Dishman says that even these known lifestyle factors need more nuanced research. "Exercise ends up being very effective for certain people and not for others," he says. "We're going to become more predictive about these things, so you can focus on the things that will matter for your body, depending on what it's been exposed to and your genetics."

Even when we know the route to health, the irritating reality remains: It's really hard to change our behavior. At Lab100, you learn how your test results stack up against people of similar age and gender, which might prod the competitive into action. Not only did I discover that my fine-motor skills are lacking, but my balance was comparatively average. That has motivated me to stand on one leg and close my eyes when I brush my teeth, but I don't know how long I'll keep it up or if improving my balance will boost my health. What is clear? Opportunities to amass heaps of data about ourselves will only expand. Whether that data flood will buoy our health remains to be seen. ●

"My children's hospital saved my life"

COURTNEY SIMMONS
STUDENT LEADER, FUTURE PEDIATRIC
ONCOLOGY NURSE, FORMER CHILDREN'S
HOSPITAL PATIENT

Children's Miracle Network Hospitals

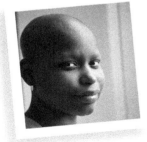

Before my 17th birthday, I lost my sister and my mom to cancer. Then I got it too. I had 30 weeks of chemotherapy and several surgeries to remove the tumor and repair my damaged bones. Thanks to my children's hospital, I'm cancer-free. They never gave up on me. I am now studying to be a pediatric oncology nurse and I started a Dance Marathon at my university to help my local children's hospital.

PUT YOUR MONEY WHERE THE MIRACLES ARE.
Give Today to your children's hospital

CMNHospitals.org/Courtney

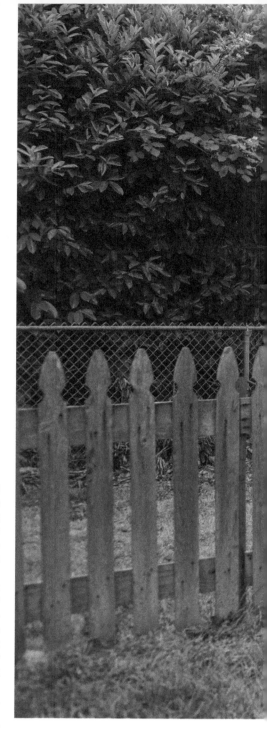

Rewriting the Faulty Code

Three treatments approved in 2017 have ushered in a new era of gene therapy

by **Arlene Weintraub**

By the time Toby Willis arrived at Children's Hospital Los Angeles in March 2018 to receive a first-of-its-kind gene therapy treatment, he had lost most of his eyesight to the inherited eye disease retinitis pigmentosa. Willis, 44, a software engineer for Expedia in Seattle, could only see shapes and shadows. He'd given up driving 20 years earlier, and while he could get along on foot with a cane and his seeing-eye dog, his remaining eyesight was deteriorating.

Then Willis learned from a geneticist that his disease was caused by a rare mutation in the gene RPE65 and that it could be treated with a new gene therapy surgically delivered into each eye. The therapy, called Luxturna, involves inserting a functional copy of RPE65 that takes over for the faulty gene, producing a protein vital for proper vision. While he wouldn't regain all his sight, doctors told him he might recoup enough to significantly improve his quality of life. He signed up right away for the new therapy at Children's Hospital LA – one of the first hospitals equipped to provide it.

"Almost immediately, everything appeared brighter. I could see a lot more contrast, lines and edges, and moving cars on the street," Willis says. The unwelcome bright flashes caused by his disease were greatly reduced, and his ability to navigate his surroundings in the dark improved. "I still need my dog to be safe, but the change has been dramatic for me."

Luxturna is one of just three gene therapies on the market, all of which were approved in 2017. It was a banner year for a technology that was nearly abandoned in 1999, after teenager Jesse Gelsinger died of an immune response during a clinical trial of a gene therapy to treat his rare metabolic disorder. But a handful of bold scientists stuck with the technology, fine-tuning methods of inserting healthy genes into the body to ideally correct diseases without causing toxic side effects. Their work led to Luxturna, as well as Kymriah to treat leukemia and Yescarta for lymphoma. There is still a risk of side effects: Some patients have experienced high fevers, confusion and other reactions, some life-threatening, to the cancer gene therapies, plus a loss of white blood cells, which must be replaced with regular plasma infusions. Luxturna has caused eye infections, increased eye pressure and retinal changes. The products are also pricey – Luxturna has a list price of $425,000 per eye, and the other two are similarly expensive. But many insurers are covering the treatments, recognizing the potential to cure patients with one-time procedures.

Those three products have ushered in a new age. Dozens of academic research centers and biotech companies are working intensely on gene therapies to treat many more cancer types, as well as a range of more common disorders, from heart failure and diabetes to Alzheimer's

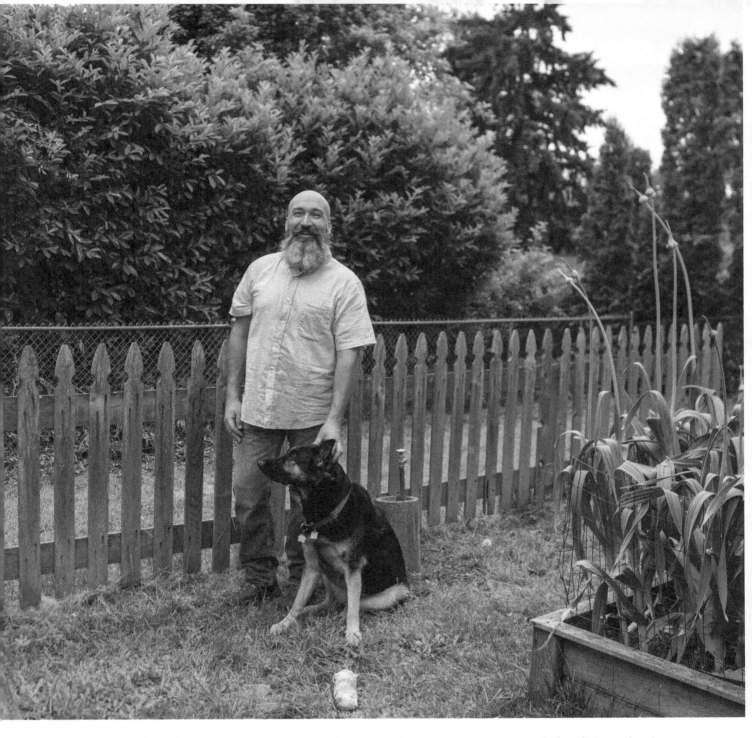

disease. Some of the therapies, like the two new blood-cancer treatments, entail removing immune cells from patients, modifying the cells' genes so the body can recognize and attack disease, and then reinjecting the cells into the bloodstream, unleashing a targeted assault. Others involve inserting a copy of a healthy gene that can take over vital functions from a faulty gene – the method by which Luxturna works.

There are some 1,200 human trials

TOBY WILLIS still relies on guide dog DAZZLER but calls changes to his vision "dramatic."

of gene therapies in progress worldwide. And pioneers in the field say this is only version 1.0 of a technology that could improve the outlook for millions of patients. "Genetic engineering is amazing. Soon we'll be able to hard-wire cells so they are smart enough to make sophisticated decisions," singling out diseased tissues for destruction but leaving healthy organs alone, for example, says Carl June, professor of immunotherapy at the University of Pennsylvania Perel-

man School of Medicine and an inventor of Kymriah.

Replacing Wayward Genes

At least 50 of the trials underway address diseases of the eye – an organ that's particularly well-suited to the technology. More than a dozen eye diseases can be blamed on bad genes that are inherited, including macular degeneration, a leading cause of blindness in people 50 and older. Plus the eye is a small organ that doesn't launch an overly aggressive immune system response to foreign invad-

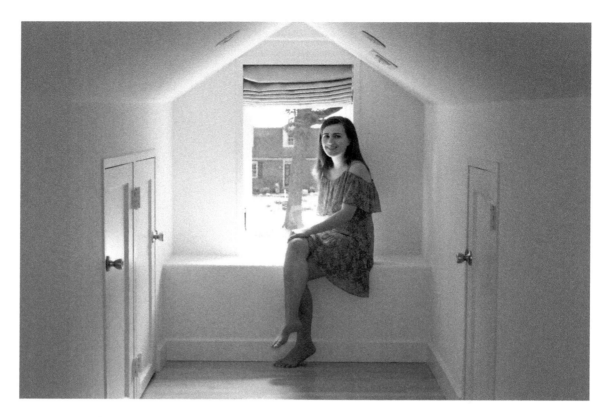

Before gene therapy, leukemia survivor RACHEL ELLIOTT had little hope for a cure.

ers. That's important, because new genes are introduced into the body using viruses that have been engineered to spread their therapeutic payloads in patients without themselves causing illness. The most popular family of viruses used for gene therapy, so-called adeno-associated viruses, initially raised the risk of immune responses like the one Gelsinger suffered. But they have been engineered over the last decade so that sort of reaction is less of a threat and to make them better at transporting good genes into precise locations.

In the case of Luxturna, the virus containing the therapeutic gene is placed in the retina, where the gene stays put, acting as a stunt double of sorts by pumping out a protein that a healthy RPE65 gene would normally make. A different treatment, called RGX-314, is now being developed to treat wet age-related macular degeneration. It uses an inserted piece of DNA that allows cells to continuously produce a therapeutic protein that stops blood vessels in the back of the eye from leaking – the cause of progressive blindness.

Although medicines that stop the leakage can themselves be injected directly into the eye many times a year, some ophthalmologists believe that setting the ongoing process in motion through gene therapy will ultimately be a better option for many patients. "It's not that much different from, say, a cataract surgery. We numb the eye, it's a painless procedure, and the patient goes home that day," says Jeffrey Heier, co-president and medical director at Ophthalmic Consultants of Boston, one of the sites conducting a phase one clinical trial of RGX-314. The therapy's developers

have early evidence that a single insertion of the gene results in continuous production of the therapeutic protein.

The idea of introducing therapeutic genes into the body is taking off in the treatment of blood disorders, too, including sickle cell disease, a hereditary condition that causes abnormal production of the oxygen-transporting protein hemoglobin. Scientists are testing a method of inserting a new gene that makes normal hemoglobin into stem cells taken from the blood of patients with the disorder. Then the cells are infused back into patients in hopes that the newly introduced gene will produce enough healthy hemoglobin to prevent the misshapen, or "sickled," cells from causing the inflammation, anemia and organ damage that are hallmarks of the disease.

Julie Kanter, associate professor at the Medical University of South Carolina, has treated a handful of sickle cell patients in an early stage trial of the therapy, called LentiGlobin, one of whom was cured, she says. Although the trial is designed for adults, Kanter envisions a day when the gene therapy will be performed in children with sickle cell disease, sparing them years of pain and life-threatening organ injuries. There is no effective treatment for the disease, and though it can be cured with a bone marrow transplant, fewer than 10 percent of patients are able to find a matching bone marrow donor. Gene therapy, she says, "could be transformative."

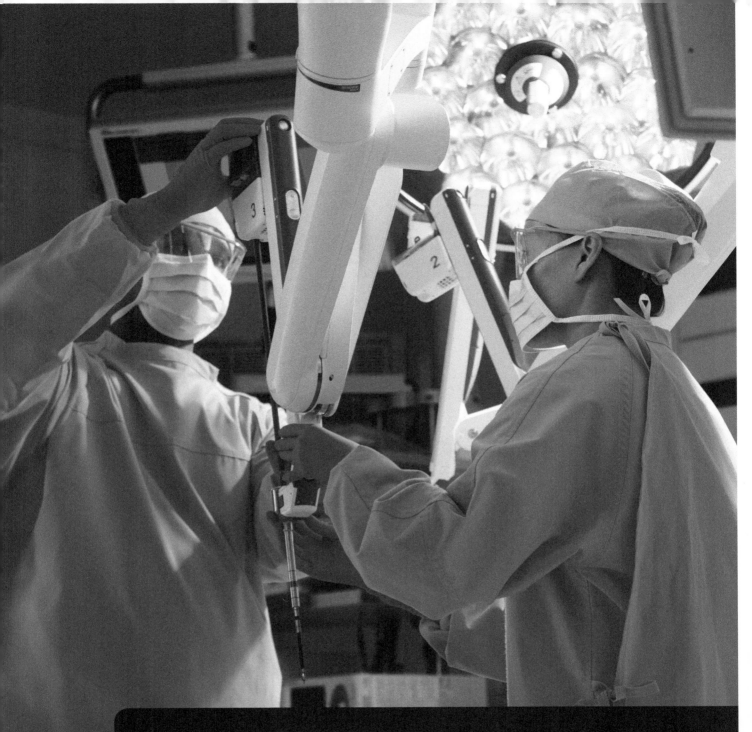

FOR SOME ELITE SOLDIERS,
THIS IS A PATH TO VICTORY.

As a surgeon and officer on the U.S. Army health care team, you'll work in cutting-edge facilities boasting the latest in surgical technology, like the da Vinci robotic surgical system, which allows doctors to perform less invasive laparoscopic surgery. Thanks to our Health Professions Scholarship Program, you may also be eligible to receive full tuition assistance, plus a monthly stipend of more than $2,200. But more importantly, you'll be protecting the Army's greatest assets: Soldiers and their families.

To see the benefits of being at the forefront of Army medicine call 800-431-6691 or visit healthcare.goarmy.com/ha84

U.S.ARMY

LentiGlobin is also in human trials to treat a severe form of beta thalassemia, which causes a chronic shortage of red blood cells and has only been treatable with frequent blood transfusions to date. During a recent trial of LentiGlobin in 13 patients, 12 were able to stop receiving the transfusions altogether.

Wielding "Molecular Scissors"

Other researchers are working with an emerging gene-editing technology known as CRISPR-Cas9. This technique, which could enter early-stage human clinical trials in the U.S. relatively soon, involves cutting out problematic DNA sequences with Cas9, an enzyme often described as molecular

Some 1,200 human gene therapy trials are underway.

scissors, thus creating a changed sequence at the break and often inserting new genetic material.

Scientists at CRISPR Therapeutics in Cambridge, Massachusetts, are using CRISPR to edit blood-forming stem cells so they continuously produce fetal hemoglobin – a protein that prevents symptoms of sickle cell but that the body normally stops producing in childhood. Similar techniques are now being developed to treat hemophilia, cystic fibrosis, HIV, severe combined immunodeficiency, or SCID, and more, says Matthew Porteus, a scientific co-founder of CRISPR Therapeutics and associate professor of pediatrics at Stanford University School of Medicine.

Gene editing isn't free of controversy. Some critics worry that the potential to edit out so-called germline mutations – genetic abnormalities in sperm, eggs or embryos – could theoretically result in changed traits being passed to future generations and could be used to delete undesirable but non-life-threatening traits like short stature. And in June 2018, the CRISPR world was shaken by two scientific studies reporting that some CRISPR-edited cells could spark the growth of cancerous tumors. Still, the recent successes have inspired other scientists to target some of the most prevalent diseases. A team at the Icahn School of Medicine at Mount Sinai in New York is planning a 2019 trial of a therapy that will introduce a gene into the coronary arteries that produces a calcium-regulating protein essential for improving heart function in patients with chronic heart failure. And scientists at Seattle Children's Research Institute are investigating the possibility of using CRISPR-Cas9 to introduce a gene that would halt the immune process that destroys insulin-producing cells in the pancreas, potentially providing a permanent solution for Type 1 diabetes.

A New Tack in Cancer Treatment

At age 11, Rachel Elliott survived a bout of acute lymphoblastic leukemia, or ALL, but seven years later, in 2015, her disease relapsed, and side effects from chemotherapy landed her in a medically induced coma for a month. When she relapsed again in 2016, she had few options for a cure. That is, until Elliott was accepted into a clinical trial of the gene therapy developed by Penn's Carl June.

Kymriah is a chimeric antigen receptor T cell, nicknamed CAR-T – a gene therapy made from immune cells taken directly from patients. The genes of the cells are altered in a lab so they recognize and target CD19, a protein marker that's prevalent on certain leukemia and lymphoma cells. Then the T cells are grown and infused back into patients, where they track down and kill leukemia cells. The treatment was approved in 2017 based on remarkable results from the pivotal clinical trial: 83 percent of patients with ALL who received the treatment went into remission within three months.

CAR-T treatments are now being developed to treat other blood cancers, including multiple myeloma, as well as solid tumors like glioblastoma, a deadly form of brain cancer. One major challenge is that many cancers either lack a clear marker like CD19, or they share markers with vital organs in the body, making it difficult to develop CAR-Ts that will kill cancer but leave healthy tissues alone. June and others are working to engineer gene therapies that will enable the creation of CAR-Ts that are smart enough to distinguish cancer cells from normal ones. "If a cancer cell has targets A, B and C, but the heart also has A, the CAR-T will only kill the cancer and it will spare your heart," June says. Penn scientists are now recruiting people with multiple myeloma, melanoma and one form of bone cancer into the first human trial in this country to test CRISPR-Cas9. They plan to use the DNA-snipping technique on the CAR-T cells in the lab to insert genes that will make them even better at pursuing their targets.

For now, the first generation of engineered T cells is already making a difference for patients like Elliott. She received two infusions of gene-altered T cells in December of 2016, after which her cancer disappeared. Now 21, she's studying at Virginia Commonwealth University School of Business, with dreams of working in the health care industry. "I hope to be part of making this therapy readily available to many more patients," Elliott says. "I truly believe gene therapy will become the pillar of all cancer treatments." ●

Cancer is smart…and relentless. At Dana-Farber, we are too. Each year, we conduct over 800 clinical trials

THINK LIKE

giving patients access to the latest advances. And, in partnership with Brigham and Women's Hospital

CANCER

and Boston Children's Hospital, we're mapping out the genetic weaknesses of 25,000+ tumors to create

TO BEAT

precision treatments that destroy cancer. These are just a few reasons why U.S. News & World Report

CANCER

has recognized us as a national leader in cancer for 18 years straight. It's also why, here, cancer is quickly losing ground.

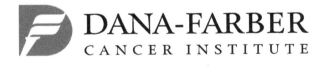

DANA-FARBER
CANCER INSTITUTE

In Search of More Organs

New techniques are allowing surgeons to transplant previously unusable livers and kidneys

by **Katherine Hobson**

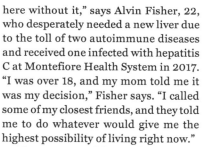

The statistics are grim: Nearly 115,000 Americans are awaiting an organ transplant, more than three times the number of transplants performed last year. The simplest way to increase the organ pool is for more people to become donors. But researchers and clinicians are narrowing the gap in other ways, too. They're exploring new techniques to keep organs functioning outside the body, making use of organs that were previously discarded, and coaxing the immune system to tolerate organs from donors who aren't compatible. Back in the lab, scientists are studying animal-to-human transplants, how to preserve organs for longer stretches and even how to print them out.

Some of the biggest advances are changing how organs are preserved outside the body. Historically they've been cooled to slow metabolism, and then raced to the recipient on ice before they deteriorate too much. But new devices can keep the organ at body temperature while maintaining a flow of oxygenated blood, medications and nutrients. In May of 2018, European scientists reported that using this technique with livers reduced rates of organ damage and increased the average preservation time, opening the possibility of longer-distance transplants.

Shekhar Kubal, surgical director of liver transplantation at Indiana University Health and an investigator on a separate trial of one of these devices, explains that keeping the organ warm allows physicians to "see how the liver will work in the patient without actually trying it out in the patient," for example. And that means it's possible to use organs that would otherwise be dismissed as too risky, he says.

In that European trial, the rate of discarded livers was half that of the usual on-ice approach. Eventually, those organs may be repaired or treated while on the machine – harmful fat could be removed from a liver, for example. This approach was first developed for lungs – a device was just approved in the U.S. that keeps lungs breathing outside of the body – and is used in other countries for the heart as well.

Transplant centers are also re-examining previously ineligible donors. Doctors at Johns Hopkins Medicine and Penn Medicine were the first to show the success of transplanting donated kidneys infected with hepatitis C into people who didn't have the virus, then treating them with new, highly effective antiviral medications. "I probably wouldn't be

here without it," says Alvin Fisher, 22, who desperately needed a new liver due to the toll of two autoimmune diseases and received one infected with hepatitis C at Montefiore Health System in 2017. "I was over 18, and my mom told me it was my decision," Fisher says. "I called some of my closest friends, and they told me to do whatever would give me the highest possibility of living right now."

After surgery, Fisher took two drugs to knock out the hepatitis C virus. It worked; he is virus-free and attending college at William Paterson University in New Jersey, not far from his home in Newark. Since then, Montefiore has done 11 additional hep C liver transplants, says Milan Kinkhabwala, chief of the division of transplantation at the Montefiore Einstein Center for Transplantation.

It's even now possible to use organs from HIV-positive donors. Transplanting organs from HIV-positive donors to HIV-positive recipients was pioneered, and shown to be successful, in South Africa

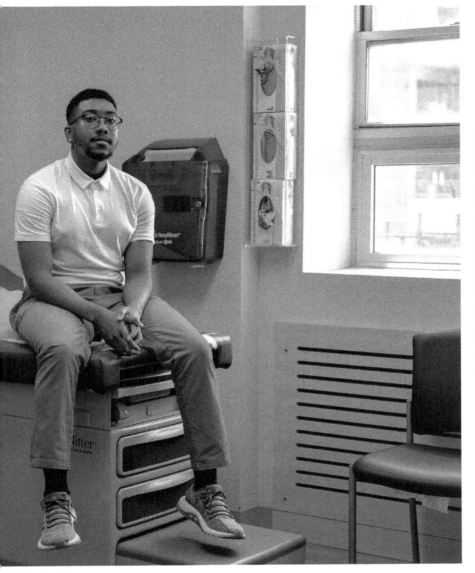

Alvin Fisher is virus-free after receiving a liver infected with hepatitis C at Montefiore.

but was illegal in the U.S. until 2013. Three years later, Johns Hopkins surgeons transplanted a liver and a kidney from a deceased HIV-positive donor to two HIV-positive recipients. The challenge now is getting the word out to hospitals and to potential donors that this is possible, says Dorry Segev, a transplant surgeon at Hopkins who led the transplant team.

At UCLA, meantime, surgeon Jeffrey Veale last year transplanted a kidney into a 69-year-old woman from a deceased young man who'd only had the kidney for two years – because he, too, had received it from a donor. The worry has been that an organ that has gone through two "death events" is too damaged to use again, but Veale says that depends on the circumstances. He has "regifted" kidneys two other times and believes the approach has potential to extend to livers and hearts.

Researchers are also working to sur-

mount the immunological differences that make donors and recipients incompatible. Some people who need a kidney have antibodies against certain proteins called HLA, which makes it difficult to find a suitable donor. But the recipient can be "desensitized" by having a procedure that removes antibodies from the blood and then getting a transfusion of new ones as the body also regenerates its own.

Somehow – the mechanism isn't clear – this prevents new anti-HLA antibodies from forming and staves off rejection. Segev led a study, published in The New England Journal of Medicine, showing that at 22 transplant centers, patients who underwent this desensitization process had higher survival rates than those who stayed on the waiting list or received a kidney from a deceased donor.

These advances are all at least in research trials, if not in wider clinical use.

Other scientists are looking at earlier-stage technologies, including using organs from other species.

Some pig tissues are already used in humans, and researchers are exploring whether pig organs might be, too. The idea is to use new gene-editing techniques (story, Page 20) to modify the antigens on the pig cell surfaces that humans react to, or to remove viruses from pig DNA that might cause infection in a human, says Devin Eckhoff, division director of transplantation at the University of Alabama–Birmingham. Studies in primates have shown promise, and Eckhoff estimates that a "limited" clinical trial might be two or three years away.

There's also interest in preserving organs for lengthier periods. A long-term deep freeze for cryogenic storage, as is used to preserve embryos and eggs, is technologically difficult for solid organs, says Mehmet Toner, a biomedical engineer at Massachusetts General Hospital. But a middle zone of cold temperatures might keep organs viable for weeks.

And then there's the promise of creating organs from scratch. "Bioprinting" uses special 3D printers to dispense "bioinks" full of cells, either within a scaffold made of water-based gels that will support their growth and interactions or into a small building block (similar to a gelatin mold), where they can grow and proliferate on their own without a scaffold. The approach depends on the tissue type, says Ibrahim Ozbolat, a tissue engineer at Pennsylvania State University.

The goal for bioprinting is to start with simpler, flatter tissues such as cartilage and skin, and progress to tubular structures like blood vessels, hollow organs such as stomachs or bladders, and eventually even to solid organs, says Anthony Atala, director of the Wake Forest Institute for Regenerative Medicine. Atala's lab has used a much more labor-intensive manual process to grow bladders that have been transplanted into people. Creating complex structures with blood vessels is difficult, and solid organs consist of many different types of cells, Ozbolat says. But scientists know that the tens of thousands of people in need of an organ, now and in the future, are depending on them. ●

The AI Advantage

Clinicians are getting smart new virtual partners to improve care

U.S. News & World Report interviewed **Keith Dreyer**, chief data science officer of Partners HealthCare and vice chairman of radiology at Massachusetts General Hospital and Brigham and Women's Hospital, to get his perspective on the extraordinary impact artificial intelligence will have on health care in coming years.

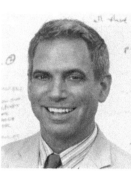

What exactly is artificial intelligence, and what will it mean to health care?

The formal term we use is data science. That includes artificial intelligence and machine learning – the science of getting computers to act without being programmed by humans. Currently, scientists can pick a specific type of machine-learning algorithm (basically a step-by-step mathematical process that tells a computer what to do) and then train it to handle a certain task. One such algorithm is called a neural network because it can learn and improve performance on its own like the human brain, but it can work much faster. Collectively, these powerful tools will one day help us find disease almost before a patient is symptomatic, treat it early, and achieve a higher survival rate with much less patient suffering and at far less cost.

How is AI being used now?

One key way is with diagnostic and imaging tools, like MRIs and CT and PET scans. Algorithms can be trained, for instance, to accurately measure all of the lymph nodes from a cancer patient's CT scan to see if they're changing size. It's a huge job that algorithms can do much more quickly than humans. The clinician can then take the results and decide whether a therapeutic regime is working or needs to be adjusted or changed. We now also use machine-learning tools in stroke detection and classification. We can train an algorithm to learn to assess thousands of data points covering the range of strokes and how each can be characterized. Over time, the algorithm learns how to read images with a high degree of accuracy. For example, the computer might say the patient had a hemorrhagic stroke. Then the neuroradiologist and neurologist will determine whether surgery or medication is needed to treat it.

Where else is data science having an impact?

Population health management is one area. You can look at electronic health records for many thousands of people and identify biomarkers or other data to make predictions, for example, about patients' likelihood of getting a disease. Patients with no prior history of diabetes, say, might have certain characteristics that put them on a path to the disease. So you could steer them to preventative care. Another area where AI can benefit patients is precision medicine. For example, it turns out diabetes has five or more types. With data science you can tease out a lot of information about how people with a specific type might react to different therapeutics and tailor treatments that will work best for each patient. Data science will also help in the laboratory in areas like pathology and genomics – anything that requires large amounts of data to be analyzed for discovery.

Should doctors and nurses be worried about their jobs?

You can't replace the comfort of human-to-human interaction, but in the near future doctors using AI will win out over those that don't in terms of delivering the best care. AI and machine learning will be critical in helping clinicians by aggregating and analyzing maybe thousands of data points for a particular patient (like lab results, genomics, imaging) to identify key conditions the doctor needs to manage, from pulmonary disease to congestive heart failure. So instead of clinicians being overwhelmed by data, they now have an AI partner to process and interpret the information and even advise them on treatment options.

How fast will these changes happen?

Incrementally. To put an algorithm into wide clinical practice, you have to collect and structure data to train the algorithm. Then you need to get FDA regulatory approval. Finally you need to figure out how to deploy that solution in clinical practice to providers using different electronic health records. And that's just one algorithm. We might eventually need thousands in radiology alone. For now, we focus on solving narrow problems like detecting lung or breast cancers. We're going to see big successes, but change won't seem dramatic at first. People in the field all say that in time we will no longer talk about artificial intelligence, but rather a smarter "something" – a smarter cellphone, a smarter CT scanner, a smarter stethoscope – or a smarter physician. •

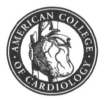

AMERICAN COLLEGE *of* CARDIOLOGY®

THE HEART OF QUALITY PATIENT CARE

The American College of Cardiology (ACC) is committed to supporting patients and health care providers by ensuring the right care is delivered to the right patient, every time.

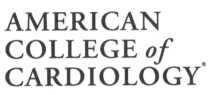

National Cardiovascular Data Registry (NCDR)
Utilizing real-world evidence to improve patient outcomes and achieve quality heart care

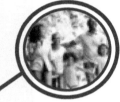

CardioSmart.org
Empowering patients and caregivers through education and interactive tools

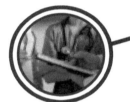

Clinical Tools
Providing practical solutions for health care providers to use at the point-of-care

National Quality Improvement Campaigns
Leveraging evidence-based best practices to improve patient outcomes

ACC Accreditation Services
Building communities of excellence by advancing the highest standards of quality patient care

Mobile Apps
Providing patients and the care team with decision-making tools

FOR CARDIOVASCULAR PROFESSIONALS, please visit *CVQuality.ACC.org* to learn more about ACC's Quality Improvement for Institutions program.

FOR PATIENTS AND CAREGIVERS, please visit *CardioSmart.org* to learn more about ACC's provider-directed heart health education and resources.

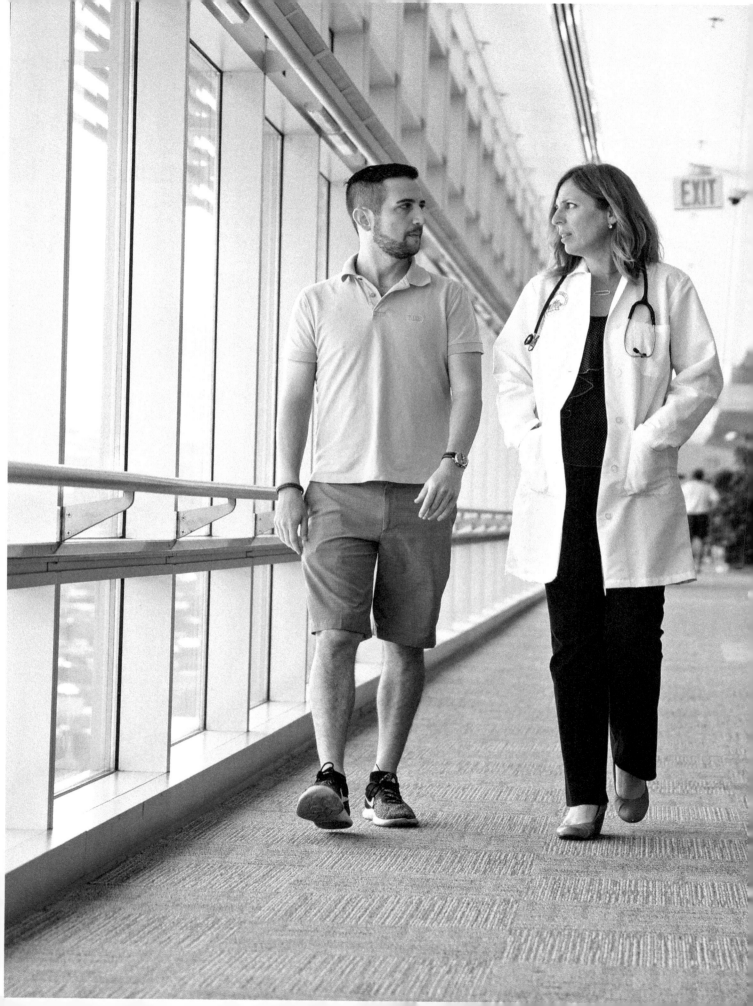

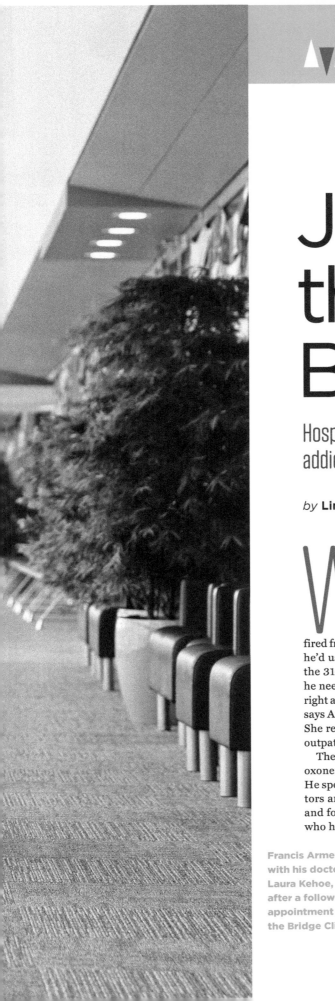

Joining the Opioid Battle

Hospitals are stepping up to address both addiction treatment and prevention

by **Linda Marsa**

When Francis Arment walked into the emergency room at Massachusetts General Hospital, he had hit "rock bottom." It was 3 a.m.; he'd been driving all over in search of an addiction treatment center. Earlier that day in 2017, he'd been fired from his insurance job when his boss discovered he'd stolen $40, which he'd used to buy black-market prescription opioids. But at Mass General, the 31-year-old Rhode Island resident found the supportive environment he needed to get well, mainly because he could enter a treatment program right away without having to get sober first. "The nurse was very empathetic," says Arment, who became hooked on Percocet pills a few years after college. She referred him to the hospital's Bridge Clinic, which enrolled him in an outpatient recovery program within hours.

The Bridge Clinic suited Arment because he was immediately put on Suboxone (buprenorphine) to stop withdrawal symptoms and curb cravings. He spent the next few months attending support groups, meeting with doctors and psychiatrists, and getting peer counseling from a recovery coach and former addict. "It was incredibly helpful to have someone to talk with who has been in my shoes," says Arment, who remains clean and manages the wire-transfer department at a bank's corporate office. The clinic "literally saved my life."

Even after patients like Arment have detoxed and been stabilized, they still need more help. But they and others in different stages of treatment often face lengthy waitlists for programs designed to sustain their recovery – at a time when they are particularly vulnerable to relapse or overdose – and

Francis Arment with his doctor, Laura Kehoe, after a follow-up appointment at the Bridge Clinic.

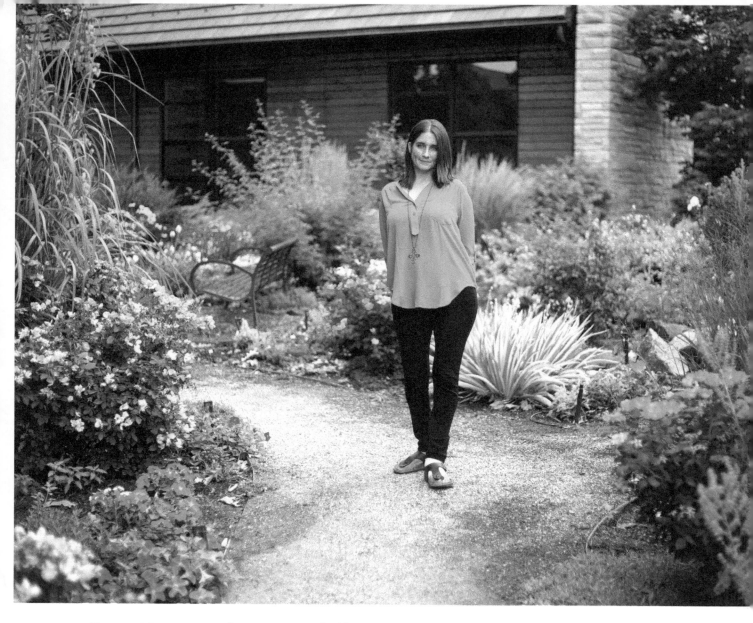

many such programs are so highly structured that people with active addiction can't meet the requirements, experts say. The Bridge Clinic, founded in 2016, is intended to fill that gap. It uses a flexible, immediate-access approach that welcomes walk-ins at any stage of illness or readiness, removing a barrier to treatment. No one is turned away.

The Bridge team also provides same-day access to medications. (Patients also get individualized medical care and other support services, including peer support, clothing and transportation assistance.) Although critics say using medication for the treatment of substance use disorders merely substitutes one addiction for another, it has become the standard of care because strong evidence indicates these medications are effective in helping prevent relapse and enable many people to return to normal functioning. "A lot of the work we do is simply treating people with respect and compassion and letting them start wherever they think they can," says Laura Kehoe, the clinic's medical director. "If we don't treat the acute craving and withdrawal, they'll self-treat and relapse. But no one is ever kicked out of this clinic for active drug use."

The Bridge Clinic is part of an innovative Mass General initia-

tive to identify people with substance use disorders, treat them and transition them to community programs for ongoing addiction care. It's just one way hospital systems nationwide are working to combat the opioid crisis, which kills more than 115 Americans through overdoses every day.

Still, hundreds of thousands of people who are desperate to quit lack the resources to get better. "There just aren't enough facilities – detox or opioid treatment programs – or enough beds in this country for patients with addictions," says neurologist Joanna Katzman, director of the University of New Mexico Pain Center. "There aren't enough outpatient centers that have methadone or buprenorphine for long-term aftercare and not enough trained doctors who can actually help those who are severely addicted."

Taking Pills Off the Streets
Several hospitals have launched aggressive programs to curb opioid prescriptions and reduce the number of pills flooding the black market. "Most people

who misuse opioids start out by getting them from the medicine cabinet of someone they know," says Margaret Jarvis, a psychiatrist and chief of addiction medicine for Pennsylvania's Geisinger health system.

The region around Geisinger has an opioid death rate that eclipses New York City's. Over the past three years, the health system has rolled out several initiatives that have reduced opioid prescriptions from 60,000 to 31,000 per month. Pharmacists and addiction specialists are embedded at 15 primary care and specialty sites across the system to ensure safe and appropriate prescribing of painkillers and to monitor addiction risks among patients. "To prevent addiction, we write opioid prescriptions for a brief period – maybe for seven to 14 days, rather than a 30-day supply," says Gerard Greskovic, director of Geisinger's ambulatory clinical pharmacy programs. The goal, he says, is to get patients off of opioids as soon as possible.

Utah's Intermountain Healthcare, which spans 22 hospitals and 170 clinics, has set an ambitious goal to achieve by the end of 2018: Cut the number of opioid pills prescribed for acute conditions by 40 percent (5 million pills annually) at its hospitals and community clinics through tracking of prescriptions and providing patients with other pain management methods, such as physical therapy.

Similarly, UCHealth University of Colorado Hospital launched a one-click tool in 2017 that allows busy ER docs to instantly see how many prescriptions a patient has filled at other locations. In the past three years, the hospital has trimmed the number of opioid prescriptions from about 20 percent of patients to about 8 percent. "Previously, it took three to five minutes and up to 35 clicks" to get into the system, versus about one second and one click now, says Jason Hoppe, an emergency medicine physician who helped integrate the statewide drug-monitoring program at UCHealth. (The program, used by most states, has been lauded by FDA Commissioner Scott Gottlieb.)

Treating the Youngest Casualties

Children's hospitals in hard-hit regions of the country – including Yale New Haven Children's Hospital, West Virginia's Cabell Huntington Hospital, and East Tennessee Children's Hospital in Knoxville – have created special programs for babies born drug dependent to mothers who used opioids or other drugs during pregnancy. They suffer from neonatal abstinence syndrome, or NAS, which involves trem-

ors, trouble sleeping and eating, and uncontrollable shaking and crying, among other problems. From 2004 to 2013, admission rates to U.S. neonatal intensive care units for NAS nearly quadrupled, and in 2012, nearly 22,000 babies were born drug dependent, according to the latest available statistics.

At the University of Vermont Medical Center in Burlington, the emphasis is on using medication to wean babies off of opioids, combined with parental bonding and empowerment. Parents are taught to administer methadone at home and

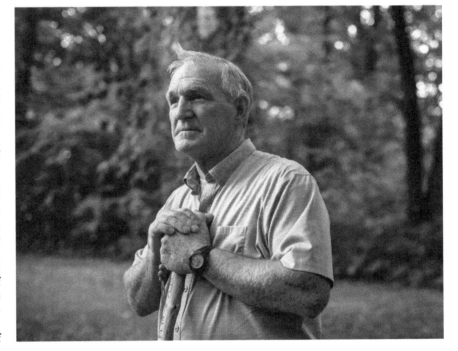

receive ongoing support through follow-up calls and regular office visits. As a partner organization in the CHARM Team (Children and Recovering Mothers) collaborative, UVM Medical Center treats parent and child using a multidisciplinary approach that includes the obstetrical team, social workers, public health nurses, and child and family services agencies. A major CHARM goal is to create a supportive atmosphere and relieve the stigma, shame and guilt that can prevent women from seeking help. "Most of these mothers want to do whatever is best for their babies," says Anne Johnston, a neonatologist and director of UVM Medical Center's Neonatal Abstinence Clinic. "We try to give them appropriate support and treat them medically – and create a community of recovery, which is so important for long-lasting sobriety."

When Skyler Browder, 28, gave birth to Cree in 2014, he weighed 4 pounds, 14 ounces and required a two-week stay at UVM Medical Center's NICU. There, he was given tiny doses of methadone to wean him off the drugs he'd absorbed in the womb. Browder, who had abused prescription opioids and graduated to heroin because it was cheaper and more acces-

Worried about the risks of treating his pain with medication, Greg McLaughlin found alternatives at Mayo Clinic.

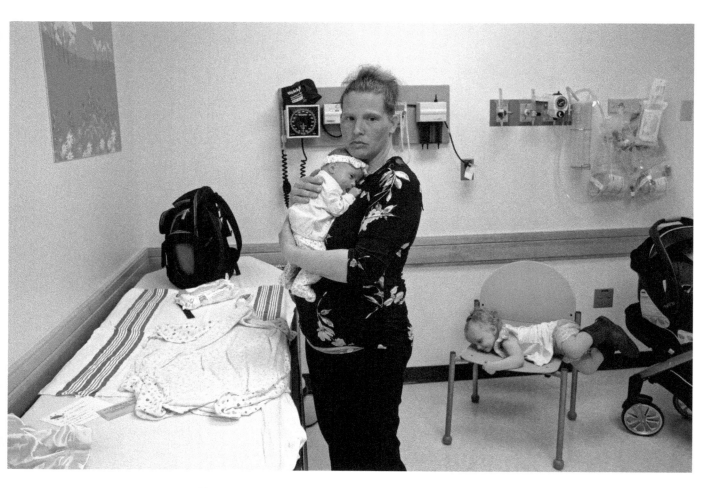

sible, detoxed before becoming pregnant. But she relapsed and was put on methadone to get her off street drugs. "I felt completely demoralized that I could potentially damage my child – I was a hot mess," Browder recalls. She was able to stay at the hospital for extended periods so she could bond with her baby, giving him the skin-to-skin contact that helped them both overcome their addictions. "Cree and I got clean together," says Browder, who remains sober and is working to finish college.

Offering Comprehensive Care

Some hospitals provide a full continuum of care to smooth the path to recovery. At UCHealth University of Colorado Hospital in Aurora, that path starts in the emergency department, where, with the help of its one-click tool, staff can see a patient's history of pain medication prescriptions and determine if the individual is high risk; should abuse be suspected, doctors can adjust their treatment plan accordingly, say by prescribing someone fewer pills and less often. "We want to identify

them before they switch to IV drug use," Hoppe says. "That's where they fall off the cliff."

Then, patients have several treatment options, based on their addiction severity. One is the Center for Dependency, Addiction and Rehabilitation, or CeDAR, the inpatient residential facility that treats adults and their families for up to 90 days and includes detox, therapy, 12-step groups and psychiatric care. Once in recovery, patients can transition to outpatient community programs that combine medication-based approaches with behavioral treatments to help them maintain sobriety.

Blair Hubbard, 37, needed intensive therapy to get clean after a 12-year opioid dependency. After having her wisdom teeth pulled as a high school senior, she was prescribed hydrocodone. She got hooked, eventually turning to OxyContin, then heroin. "I ran out of veins in my arms and started shooting up in my legs," Hubbard says. After passing out from an infection caused by her IV drug use, she was hospitalized for 10 weeks. Hubbard had sepsis. Open-heart surgery was needed when one of her valves became badly infected. A bright spot? Hubbard's life-threatening emergency connected her to a medical team that helped her get treatment, housing and medical insurance. "It was a blessing in disguise," says Hubbard, who still receives care for complications but has nonetheless earned her master's in

professional counseling and is now a behavioral health specialist helping people in recovery at CeDAR. "I was desperate to kick – and sick of this lifestyle."

Tapping Telemedicine to Help Rural Communities

In rural New Mexico – as in so many pockets of the U.S. – patients in impoverished, isolated communities are cut off from addiction specialists. But through the Project ECHO Pain and Opioid Management program, the UNM Health System is connecting doctors in rural communities with its Albuquerque-based team of pain specialists. During weekly teleconferences, as many as 20 medical teams in remote regions can discuss patient cases with specialists in Albuquerque – and learn from each other's experiences through this hub-and-spoke model. Say a primary care clinician from Sand Springs, Oklahoma, wants advice on how to switch a substance-abusing patient with multiple issues – severe facial pain, depression and PTSD – from high-dose opioids to withdrawal-blocking Suboxone. The (hub) team in Albuquerque can offer guidance while (spoke) doctors in nearby Oklahoma can point the physician to local resources that may benefit the patient, according to Katzman.

Since its inception a decade ago, ECHO Pain has helped greatly reduce the rate of overdose deaths in New Mexico, which had been among the highest in the nation. It's been adopted by the Indian Health Service and more than two dozen institutions nationwide. The Veterans Health Administration, the Army and the Navy now have ECHO hubs, and in 2016, the U.S. Department of Health and Human Services earmarked $9 million in grants to improve opioid addiction treatment in rural counties in Oklahoma, Colorado and Pennsylvania using the ECHO model. "Many local doctors don't have the time to keep up with what we know works for treating addiction," says Katzman, who launched ECHO Pain. "This model enables us to share evidence-based practices with them so everyone gets better care."

Adding Boot Camps for Pain Management

Many hospitals, including Stanford Health Care, Cleveland Clinic, Mayo Clinic and Johns Hopkins, have launched pain management boot camps that provide alternatives to painkill-

One Doctor's Addiction

This isn't a tidy story. It's complex. It's painful – sometimes ugly. This is the cautionary tale of how Daniel Logan, a rising emergency medicine physician, wound up with a syringe in his arm, setting in motion a 20-year addiction to opioids that nearly killed him. He wants to tell it because "I'm an example there's hope."

Rewind to the mid-80s, when the married father of five decided to open an urgent care clinic in partnership with the local hospital. A relatively novel concept then, these types of clinics were starting to take off, and Logan, in his 30s, went all in. Things seemed to be working out fine until the hospital decided to change course and the partnership dissolved. Soon, he was bankrupt, unemployed and awash with shame. "I was so angry," he says. "I felt guilty because I had let my family down."

While dismantling the remains of the business he'd opened with such optimism, he spotted the med box, stocked with drugs for patient care. Feeling powerless, he thought, "F--- it," two words, he says, that would become his mantra. "When that phrase would cross my mind, I knew I was in trouble." Then he grabbed a vial of Nubain, a potent opioid,

put a tourniquet on his arm, pushed the syringe plunger and was knocked out by a wave of warmth. An hour later, he came to, sprawled out on the bathroom floor. "It was frightening," he says. Four hours crawled by before he felt OK to navigate home – with the med box in hand.

Hidden habit. By the time Logan got a new job as an emergency medicine physician nearly a year later, he'd become expert at hiding his habit. "I could inject in the veins under my watchband," he says. "I didn't look impaired." In fact, he was excelling at work. Ascending, even. "During my active drug addiction, I was actually promoted to being chairman of my department," he says. But to avoid withdrawal during a 12-hour shift, he'd duck into the bathroom several times for a fix.

His successes didn't last. Logan recalls transforming from being affable to irritable. Productive to sluggish. His colleagues noticed and eventually confronted him. After admitting he had a problem, he was referred to an intensive four-month residential physician health program (most states offer these resources) for treatment. "My goal when I got there was to get out of there; do whatever I had to do to complete

ers for people suffering from chronic pain. These outpatient programs integrate traditional and complementary medicine techniques. The Mayo Clinic's intensive rehabilitation program, for instance, entails daily seven-hour sessions for three weeks. Part of the treatment is the schedule," says Wesley Gilliam, clinical director of Mayo's Pain Rehabilitation Center. "Many of our participants have been struggling with their addictions for so long that they've lost track of time and their whole

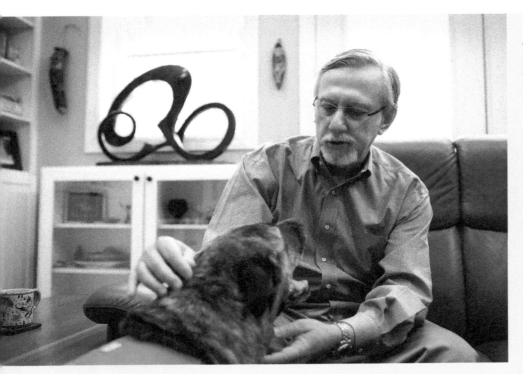

my four months and get back to work." Which he did. However, he chose not to divulge a secret he'd been trying to bury since childhood – that he had been sexually abused as a boy. The pain of those memories would flare up unpredictably. Opioids, he discovered, "were very soothing."

Turning point. He kept up this cycle – treatment followed by a return to work, then a relapse – for years, through several moves and divorce. Ultimately, when he was 50 and injecting into his femoral vein, he reached a crossroads. One day, while coming down from a night shift, he was stricken with fever, shaking, chills and severe dizziness. Septic from an injec-

Daniel Logan, at his home, overcame a decadeslong opioid addiction.

tion-related infection, he was admitted to intensive care and almost died. He'd developed "massive" blood clots in both legs. "I was truly a hopeless addict at that point," he says. He'd even stocked his car with a suicide kit – an injection of potassium.

Instead, Logan "finally gave up the secret I had been holding on to" in therapy. Only then, he says, could he commit to the arduous recovery process. Some research finds it can take eight years, on average, for people with substance use disorders to achieve one substance-free year. "The truth is, it's not easy. It's not like I'm cured," says Logan, now 65 and sober for 15 years. He avoids alcohol and takes great care when managing pain, for example.

These days, he lives in rural Gainesville, Florida, with his wife, Gladys, also in recovery, and their five rescue dogs. He has rebuilt relationships with his children. Although he no longer practices in the ER, he works in a specialty he knows about intimately, addiction medicine, and treats patients in an outpatient program. To give back, he and Gladys recently helped establish an addiction research and treatment center at the University of Kansas, his alma mater.

"This can happen to anyone. I've literally treated brain surgeons and rocket scientists," Logan says. "It isn't about how smart or brave you are – addiction is an equal-opportunity disorder." While doctors experience substance use disorders at a rate on par with the general public – and those in certain specialties, such as emergency medicine, appear to be particularly vulnerable – research suggests they are more likely to abuse prescription drugs.

Whenever Logan lectures a new group of medical students, he introduces himself two ways. First, as Dr. Daniel Logan, adjunct assistant professor of addiction medicine at the University of Florida College of Medicine. Then as Dan, recovering drug addict. They're shocked. He hopes it inspires them to "look at addicts differently" – as human beings who need help. *–Lindsay Lyon*

clock has been thrown off." Sessions include mindfulness meditation, yoga, cognitive behavioral therapy, physical and occupational therapy – even breathing exercises to ease the anxiety triggered by chronic pain.

Greg McLaughlin's experience was typical. After back surgery, the Minnesotan became reliant on pain pills and muscle relaxants. Because of a family history of addiction, he worried about his own risk. "The medications and the pain changed me completely,"

he says. He became increasingly isolated, spending his days in physical agony, struggling with depression and anxiety.

When his doctor suggested Mayo's pain clinic, he was skeptical but willing. Slowly, he stopped taking his meds and began moving again, doing physical therapy and cardio exercises, and yoga and deep-breathing when he felt anxious. "The tools I learned in rehab are an entirely different way of keeping the pain at bay," says McLaughlin, 65, who no longer takes drugs. "Chronic pain is now a small part of my life, which is full of purpose and amazing people." ●

A New Vision of Patient Care

Hospitals are taking ambitious steps to tackle community health problems

by **Beth Howard**

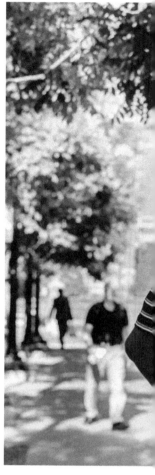

A job with Johns Hopkins Health System helped William Glover-Bey turn his life around.

William Glover-Bey, 61, of West Baltimore, started selling drugs at 13, began using soon after, and ended up spending more than 15 years incarcerated at different times. Only after joining Narcotics Anonymous in his 50s was he able to stay clean. But the prison record and spotty work history made it tough for him to find a job. "It's absolutely devastating to not know how to get back employed," he says. Then, in 2015, the father of five learned about an on-the-job adult internship training program with Johns Hopkins Health System. After two months, he landed a job in the hospital's environmental services department and recently he was promoted to be a community health worker. "I'm so grateful to be able to pay bills and take care of my family," he says.

Johns Hopkins' hiring program for ex-offenders exemplifies a growing trend: hospitals taking on the more fundamental needs of patients, from employment to housing, transportation, proper food and even legal aid. Research suggests that addressing these and other social and environmental factors may improve the health of traditionally vulnerable populations while cutting costs substantially. "Between 40 and 60 percent of an individual's health is determined by things that happen outside the doctor's office or hospital walls that, traditionally, health care has not touched," says Kate Sommerfeld, president of social determinants of health for ProMedica, a Toledo, Ohio-based health system serving northwest Ohio and southeast Michigan. Now, that's changing as hospitals nationwide are tackling some of the leading drivers of health in their communities:

The housing crunch. The average life expectancy of the chronically homeless is at least 27 years shorter than that of people in housing. "Without the basic stability of housing, it's virtually impossible to manage one's medical care or anything else, for that matter," says Stephen B. Brown, director of pre-

ventive emergency medicine for the University of Illinois Hospital & Health Sciences System in Chicago.

In 2015, when the system realized many of the most frequent – and costliest – users of emergency rooms were homeless, the organization along with the Center for Housing and Health, the lead agency of a network of supportive housing providers, established the Better Health Through Housing program. After the program's first 27 homeless patients were placed in permanent homes, the system saw a 42 percent drop in participants' health care costs and, over time, a 35 percent reduction in the use of the emergency department. A supportive case manager coordinates patients' medical care – getting them to appointments, for instance – and helps in other ways, such as negotiating disputes with landlords. Other hospital systems like St. Barnabas Hospital in the Bronx, New York, and Boston Medical Center have contributed or will be contributing to affordable housing initiatives.

Opening up job opportunities. Many employers reject applicants like Glover-Bey. But Johns Hopkins has welcomed hundreds of ex-offenders. The system considers the circumstances surrounding the conviction, such as the individual's age at the time

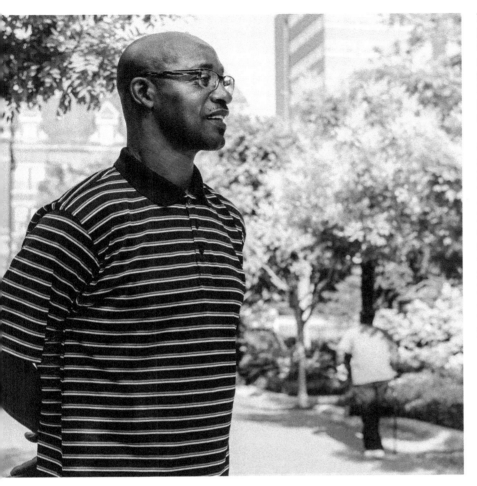

barriers. Grace Cottage Family Health & Hospital, a small critical access hospital in Townshend, Vermont, relies on a volunteer driver program to get patients to their appointments. At Taylor Regional Hospital in central Kentucky, two hospitality vans ferry patients to and from the dialysis, cancer and rehab centers.

Other transportation glitches can also erode care. Two years ago, Amy Friedman, the chief experience officer for Denver Health Medical Center, learned that an elderly pneumonia patient had waited hours for a ride home. Dismayed, Friedman approached the ride-sharing company Lyft about forming a partnership and got a foundation grant to pay for the trips. The hospital has now provided more than 3,700 Lyft rides to patients. Beginning in January 2019 the state will allow ride-sharing companies to be part of the Medicaid transportation program for patients. Other health care organizations are experimenting with similar arrangements, and both Lyft and Uber are rolling out ride reservation platforms and apps geared to health care organizations.

Combatting food insecurity. More than 12 percent of U.S. households have trouble putting food on the table or lack access to fresh fruits and vegetables. Yet poor diets are linked to chronic diseases such as diabetes, high blood pressure and heart disease. Now hospitals are stepping up to fill the need. "Using medicine to address chronic conditions only goes so far," says John Jay Shannon, CEO of the Cook County Health & Hospitals System in Chicago. The 1 in 4 patients in the system who screen positive for food insecurity are given prescriptions for fresh foods that they can "fill" at refrigerated food trucks. The hospital also offers nutrition counseling.

To address chronic health problems among vulnerable populations, Montefiore Medical Center in the Bronx uses patient health data to pinpoint city blocks with high obesity rates, then targets nearby bodegas for nutrition interventions. Staffers from Montefiore's Office of Community & Population Health encourage storekeepers to put healthier beverages like water at eye level and stock fresh produce, for instance. "Some don't realize they have a healthy sandwich on the menu or that nuts are healthy," says Liz Spurrell-Huss, senior project manager. Other institutions have implemented their own programs, including Arkansas Children's Hospital in Little Rock, which maintains its own on-site vegetable garden and donates produce to a local food pantry. The hospital also offers cooking classes taught by health educators.

of the crime, attempts at rehabilitation, and the job's duties – for instance, ensuring that the conviction isn't related to the position they're being considered for – before making an offer. "If you do not have household income, you can't go to the doctor and pay your copay, join a gym, or buy healthy produce," says Redonda Miller, president of Johns Hopkins Hospital. The system partners with community groups like Turnaround Tuesday, which trains job seekers and helps them with basics like proper attire and interviewing skills. The most recent study of ex-offenders in the hospital's workforce found they had the same turnover rate as those with no record in the first 30 months of employment.

Similarly, ProMedica has taken steps to improve the health of its community, including establishing a jobs program. Since 2015, it has hired people from low-income neighborhoods to order and stock food at the fresh food grocery it owns and operates, Sommerfeld says. It also recruits and trains people for health-related jobs like nursing assistants and helps staff a call center in office space it rents to a credit firm. Advocate Health Care, a major Midwestern health care provider, also operates a workforce program to train and hire unemployed or underemployed people in the Chicago area with funding from JPMorgan Chase & Co.

Finding transportation. Research shows that 3.6 million Americans go without medical care due to transportation

As hospitals continue looking for innovative ways to tackle often overlooked factors affecting health, administrators see another benefit of their efforts: "They show our patients we are invested with them," Shannon says. ●

The most awarded healthcare system in Texas

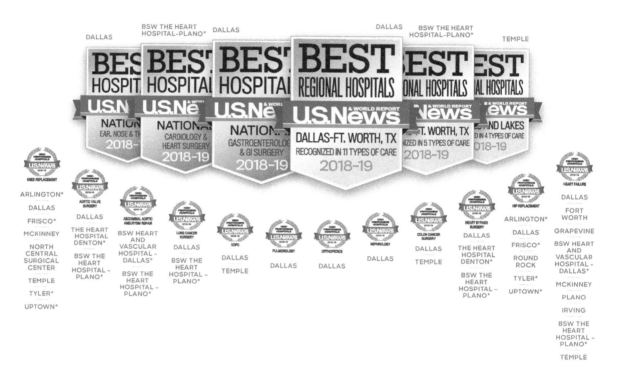

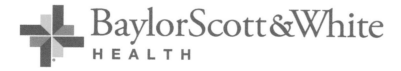

BaylorScott&White
HEALTH

GetBetterTexas.com

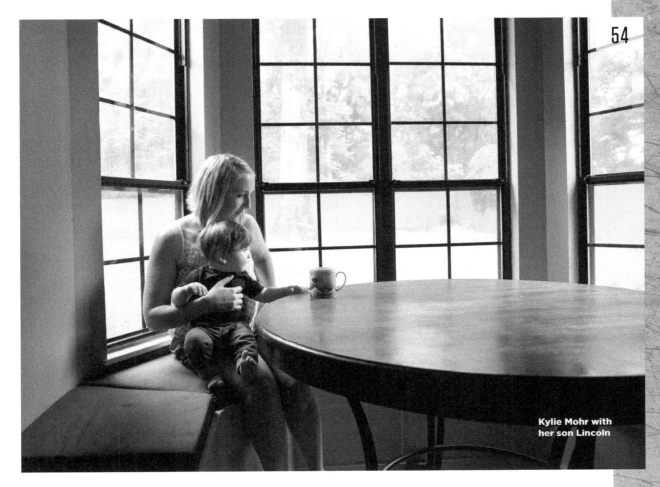

CHAPTER 2

54

Kylie Mohr with
her son Lincoln

Patient Power

Numbers That Really Count

A U.S. News investigation reveals why people facing surgery should ask how frequently surgeons perform their operations

by **Steve Sternberg**

When her son **Waylon was born with a severe** congenital heart defect, Tabitha Rainey trusted doctors to guide her to the best possible care. "You're thrown into this new world of things you don't fully understand," says Rainey, of Lexington, Kentucky. "You think your doctor knows everything. You go with what they're saying."

Waylon, now 6, was born with hypoplastic left heart syndrome, meaning his left ventricle – the heart's principal pumping chamber – was malformed and could not push blood throughout his body. Children born with this rare condition require complex reconstructive surgery beginning shortly after birth. Rainey's heart specialist referred the infant to Kentucky Children's Hospital for the first of three operations. He was a week old.

The results were far from what the family had hoped for. Following that first surgery, Waylon spent three months in intensive care, with infections, swelling and bleeding, Rainey says. He has permanent brain damage and cerebral palsy. While he was hospitalized, a doctor quietly advised Rainey that the pediatric heart surgery unit had been closed, coinciding with the reported deaths of two babies who had been operated on, and problems suffered by two others.

Kentucky Children's Hospital partnered with Cincinnati Children's Hospital Medical Center in 2016 to correct its deficiencies. The joint program has done more than 70 pediatric open-heart and other procedures since Kentucky Children's reopened its heart unit in August 2017. But Waylon had no time to wait. "We life-flighted him to Michigan," Rainey recalls. Doctors at the University of Michigan C.S. Mott Children's Hospital, which averages about 500 congenital heart procedures a year, took over his case. The family chose Mott because it was highly ranked by U.S. News, was closer to home than other leading hospitals, and had a proven heart transplant program in case Waylon's heart could not be saved. His reconstructive surgery was successful, and today his heart is stable.

Waylon's story surfaced during a U.S. News & World Report investigation of a practice that undermines patient safety in thousands of hospitals nationwide. Analyses of data from children's, adult and military hospitals revealed the same disturbing pattern: that surgeons in many hospitals perform complex and risky procedures in numbers too small to adequately hone their skills.

The procedures U.S. News has examined include congenital heart surgeries, joint replacement operations, and delicate and high-risk excisions of cancer of the esophagus, pancreas, rectum and lung. The critical takeaway for patients: You're likely to fare better if your surgeon routinely operates on patients like you. Surgeons who are consistently operating are always refining their decision-making, sharpening their techniques, and bracing for unexpected complications.

The results of the investigation have resonated with major medical institutions, too. Three leading health systems – Dartmouth-Hitchcock, Johns Hopkins Medicine and the University of Michigan – have all phased in minimum-volume standards for their hospitals and the surgeons they employ. They have also issued a "low-volume pledge" to encourage other health organizations to join them.

In 2018 The Leapfrog Group, a patient-safety organization comprised of purchasers of health care services – Boeing, Marriott and Walmart among them – also decided to stand behind minimum-volume standards. "Employers responded aggressively," says Leah Binder, Leapfrog's president and CEO. "As a result, Leapfrog began setting volume thresholds for hospitals and surgeons and holding hospitals accountable for meeting them." For instance, a hospital would have to perform 50 weight-loss operations in a year, and surgeons, 20. (Leapfrog has not addressed congenital heart surgery.)

Countless factors may influence how a patient responds to surgery, numerous studies show. These include everything from age to nutrition to coexisting health conditions to twists and turns of anatomy. But patients can control their choice of a surgeon or hospital. Rankings such as Best Hospitals and Best Children's Hospitals and the annual Leapfrog Hospital Survey, among many others, can help inform this decision. But patients can inquire, too, about how

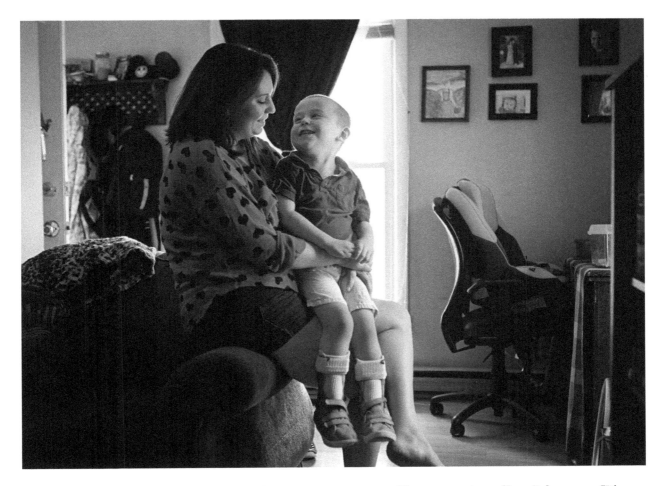

Tabitha Rainey's son Waylon had sucessful heart surgery at C.S. Mott Children's Hospital.

many hip replacements a surgeon has performed, for example.

"When I get a call from a friend or family member, and they're looking for a surgeon in Birmingham, Alabama – and I don't know anyone in the medical community there – I'd use relative volumes," says Robert M. Wachter, professor and chairman of medicine at the University of California–San Francisco and an expert on hospital performance. Absent more specific details about a surgeon or the surgery's outcomes, he says, volume may be the only useful quality marker you can get.

Asking surgeons about their procedure numbers answers two critical questions: Do they get enough practice to keep skills fresh? Does your chosen hospital have experienced surgical teams capable of responding if something goes wrong?

Some experts object to using volume as a proxy for surgical quality. Actual outcomes, such as complication and death rates, are superior, they say. "Some of the best performing hospitals are not necessarily the biggest," says John E. Mayer, Jr., pediatric heart surgeon at Boston Children's Hospital and a past president of The Society of Thoracic Surgeons, a professional group that uses clinical data to inform participating hospitals, surgeons and consumers about the quality of adult cardiac, congenital heart and general thoracic surgical care nationwide.

In addition, many hospitals and surgeons are reluctant to refer patients elsewhere, because surgery accounts for a sig-

nificant percentage of hospital revenue. "It's rare that you say, 'We'll stop doing something,' unless it's a money loser or you've had such obviously bad patient outcomes that there are malpractice lawsuits," Wachter says.

Nevertheless, a cascade of studies published over three decades has shown that volume matters. A study of more than 800,000 patients at about 1,500 hospitals published in 1979 found that death rates were 25 to 41 percent lower in hospitals where doctors did 200 procedures or more. The authors described their findings, published in the New England Journal of Medicine, as "clear evidence" that higher-volume hospitals are safer for patients undergoing a variety of procedures, including open-heart surgery, prostate surgery, vascular surgery and coronary-bypass surgery.

Still, little changed. In 2013, U.S. News began developing new ratings of hospital performance, focusing for the first time on a variety of procedures and conditions. An analysis of Medicare data for this project produced a startling finding. Thirty-six years after the NEJM study appeared, hospitals were still performing complex procedures in small numbers and patients were dying as a result.

It's not surprising that people continue choosing community hospitals close to home, especially when major academic centers can be chaotic, impersonal places. But low-volume hospitals pose risks even for patients requiring routine procedures

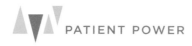

such as joint replacement surgery, the analysis showed. Knee replacement patients who had their surgery in the lowest-volume centers were nearly 70 percent likelier to die than patients treated at centers in the top quintile. For hip replacement patients, the risk was nearly 50 percent greater. Higher death rates extended to patients with certain chronic diseases as well. Patients treated for congestive heart failure and chronic obstructive pulmonary disease had a 20 percent increased risk of dying compared to those treated at high-volume centers.

John Birkmeyer, chief clinical officer of Sound Physicians, the national hospital-based physician practice, and formerly

executive vice president at Dartmouth-Hitchcock health system, used the U.S. News data to calculate that, in five procedures and conditions alone, more than 3,500 lives could be saved annually if patients in the lowest-volume tier were treated in hospitals with the highest volumes.

For more complex procedures, volume becomes even more important. A child's odds of surviving high-risk congenital heart surgery rise significantly if he or she is treated in a hospital with 250 such patients per year or more, U.S. News has found.

The evidence lies in The Society of Thoracic Surgeons' public reporting database, which displays star ratings for children's hos-

Need Surgery? Questions to Ask

Not every small hospital is a risky bet, and some big hospitals perform far fewer common procedures like joint replacement or heart bypass surgery than do some smaller hospitals. Ask your doctor the following questions to improve your odds of putting yourself – or a loved one – in good hands.

How many of the procedure you need does the surgeon perform in a year?
For a common procedure like heart bypass surgery, it's best to choose a surgeon who does at least 100 a year, says John Birkmeyer, chief clinical officer of Sound Physicians, a national physician practice, and an architect of The Leapfrog Group's volume standards for hospitals and surgeons. (Leapfrog is a patient-safety organization made up of purchasers of health care services.) For joint replacement, the American Association of Hip and Knee Surgeons requires that its members perform at least 50 hip and/or knee operations a year.

The average hospital does about 400 heart cases a year, Birkmeyer says, adding that it would be reasonable to choose a hospital that handles 200 to 300 annually. The volume may be different for less common proce-

dures. Pancreatectomies are so infrequent that a "high-volume" hospital may only perform 25.

In 2018, prompted by U.S. News reporting, Leapfrog introduced a Surgical Volume Standard into its annual hospital survey. To meet the standard, a hospital must disclose its total volumes for certain high-risk procedures and meet or exceed the Leapfrog minimums. Leapfrog also asks hospitals about whether they require surgeons to meet minimum standards to earn privileges to practice surgery at their institutions.

Leapfrog's Minimum-Surgical-Volume Standards

PROCEDURE	PER HOSPITAL	SURGEON
Bariatric surgery for weight loss	50	20
Esophageal resection for cancer	20	7
Lung resection for cancer	40	15
Pancreatic resection for cancer	20	10
Rectal cancer surgery	16	6
Carotid endarterectomy	20	10
Open abdominal aortic aneurysm repair	15	10
Mitral valve repair and replacement	40	20

The minimum procedure volumes for hospital and surgeon reflect either the annual total or an annual average over a two-year period.

What is the hospital's surgical infection rate? What is the surgeon's infection rate for the procedure?
A hospital with a high incidence of surgical-site infections or central-line

associated bloodstream infections could kill you or leave you with lifelong consequences. The information about infection rates is available on the government's Hospital Compare website: medicare.gov/hospitalcompare/search.html.

What are the hospital's and surgeon's success rates for the procedure and how do the rates compare with national benchmarks?
Increasingly, hospitals and medical registries track this information and provide doctors with reports on their performance. Doctors you're considering should be willing to share this information.

Is it wise to obtain my medical documents and images and seek a second opinion?
A second opinion is always in order before any operation, especially if it involves major surgery.

Do you really have the right to ask all these questions? You do indeed. In fact, you should be wary of a surgeon who puts you off or reacts defensively. "If they can't tell you, I wouldn't use them," says Leapfrog President and CEO Leah Binder. *-S.S.*

pitals and also publicly reports surgical volumes and outcomes for five categories of congenital heart procedures. Working with Matt Austin, assistant professor of anesthesiology and critical care medicine at Johns Hopkins' Armstrong Institute for Patient Safety and Quality, U.S. News examined publicly available data from 35 low- and medium-volume hospitals reflecting 4,000 of the more complex cases in the database and found that 104 of 395 observed deaths in those hospitals – 26 percent – might have been prevented had patients had their operations in high-volume centers. That's likely an undercount, Austin says, because the study was limited to hospitals that voluntarily participate in the reporting program.

For Jamie Dragon, of York, Maine, the evidence became

a call to action. In June of 2017, her daughter Harper, then 10, was diagnosed with a hole in the wall that divides the heart's upper chambers. Doctors said she would need surgery.

Dragon scoured the web for information and found a U.S. News report indicating that the nearest medical center, Barbara Bush Children's Hospital at Maine Medical Center in Portland, did not perform as well as Boston Children's Hospital, an hour south. Each year, surgeons at Boston Children's carry out an average of nearly 950 congenital heart surgeries, STS data indicate. Maine Medical Center's average is closer to 44. Dragon also worried about Maine Medical Center's overall congenital heart surgery mortality: 9 percent versus 3 percent at Boston Children's. Dragon decided to seek care in Boston.

Harper's surgery took place on Nov. 8, 2017. Within two weeks, she was back in school. Today, she's playing basketball and softball. "I couldn't be happier," Dragon says. "I feel fortunate that I had the time to do the research – and that STS made the information available." Maine Medical Center, for its part, recognized that its congenital heart surgery program wasn't producing the desired outcomes. The hospital initiated a "top-to-bottom" performance initiative, and in August 2018, STS upgraded Maine Medical Center from a one-star to a two-star facility, "in-line with the vast majority of congenital heart surgery programs that publicly report their outcomes," the hospital said in a statement. "We encourage other institutions to embrace this same level of transparency, which demonstrably can lead to better patient outcomes regardless of program volumes."

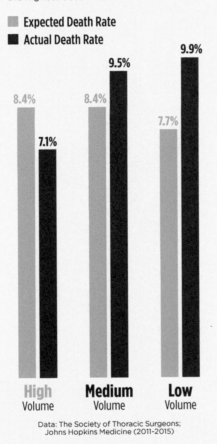

There's Safety in Numbers

Children's hospitals that care for the greatest number of children with complex congenital heart defects have significantly lower death rates than moderate- or low-volume hospitals. Even though patients in low-volume hospitals are expected to die at lower rates since they tend to have lower risk profiles, the hospitals still have the highest death rates.

■ Expected Death Rate
■ Actual Death Rate

High Volume: 8.4% / 7.1%
Medium Volume: 8.4% / 9.5%
Low Volume: 7.7% / 9.9%

Data: The Society of Thoracic Surgeons; Johns Hopkins Medicine (2011-2015)

In April 2018, U.S. News expanded its assessment of surgical volume to the Military Health System, a $50 billion network with 54 hospitals and 377 medical clinics, serving 1.4 million active-duty personnel, their families, and retirees. Military hospitals cater to a young, healthy population with an average age of 30 that rarely needs surgery. So military surgeons often have little to do. "You want to do more. In some cases, you're begging to do more," says Scott Steele, chair of the department of colorectal surgery at the Cleveland Clinic and a former Army surgeon with more than two decades of service, including deployments in Iraq and Afghanistan.

Working with Elizabeth Stedina, vice president of data analytics at the Dartmouth-Hitchcock Analytics Institute, U.S. News used data from every military hospital from 2012 to 2016. U.S. News then compared each hospital's volumes for 10 categories of procedures with Leapfrog safety standards. Twenty-two military hospitals failed to meet the standards for every procedure studied; 20 failed for many; and none achieved the thresholds for every procedure.

The findings raise critical questions for military personnel, who often have no option but to seek care in military hospitals. "Should surgeons who do less than three rectal cancers a year be doing them at all? No," says Steele, who reviewed U.S. News data showing that, in 2016 alone, surgeons performed three or fewer rectal cancer procedures at 25 military treatment facilities.

Monique Hassan shares Steele's concerns. Hassan, 41, is a former military surgeon and Army major who, in addition to regular deployments, launched a bariatric surgery program at Reynolds Army Health Clinic in Fort Sill, Oklahoma. At Fort Sill, Hassan did fewer than 20 bariatric procedures per year from 2013 to 2016, when she did just nine. During deployments, she did no bariatric surgery.

Hassan left the Army in June of 2017, when her commitment ended, because she feared that continuing would diminish her surgical proficiency. Today, she is completing a bariatric surgery fellowship at the Cleveland Clinic, one of the highest-volume programs in the world. There, she has done nearly 200 bariatric procedures, roughly four or five per week. To patients seeking bariatric surgery, she offers this advice: Choose a doctor who does more than 10 a month. "I know what can go wrong with bariatric surgery," she says, "if it's not done well." ●

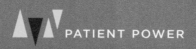
The Loneliness

Research suggests that
social isolation and feeling
lonely may rival obesity as a
threat to people's health

by **Barbara Sadick**

Ten years ago, following the deaths of her
parents and husband, Sally Hayward moved from
Florida, where she'd become increasingly isolated
and lonely, to Kenosha, Wisconsin, to be closer to her
brother. He put her to work picking up his grandchildren from
school, and she began to feel useful and connected. But as her
osteoarthritis and diabetic neuropathy worsened, she became
wheelchair-bound, stopped driving and retreated to her apartment in a complex for senior citizens with disabilities.

Hayward, 76, who had also been diagnosed with depression

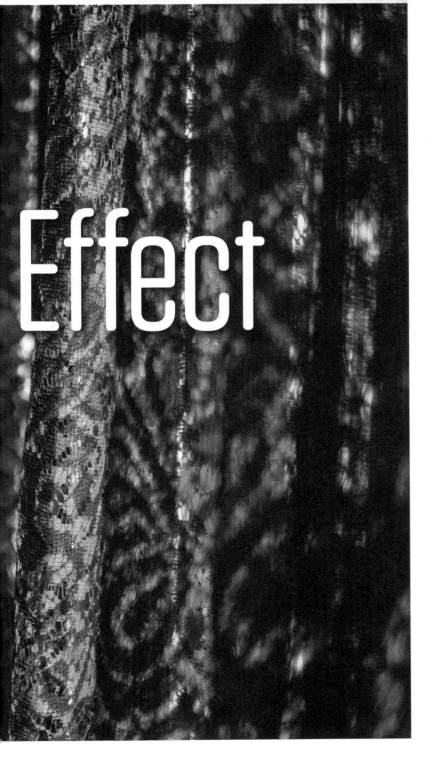

Effect

around the country by phone. Modeled on Well Connected, an initiative out of the San Francisco Bay Area, the program was affording people like Hayward telephone access to about 75 programs including support groups, general chat groups and various other educational subject groups run by specially trained volunteer participants.

These days, Hayward is leading weekly meditation and chat sessions. "Not only do I have new telephone friends," she says, "but I no longer feel constantly sad, lonely and useless."

Feeling sad, lonely and useless is more than just an emotional quagmire for millions of Americans. Researchers now contend that social isolation and loneliness may represent a greater public health hazard than obesity or a near pack-a-day smoking habit. And the problem is growing. An AARP loneliness study published in 2010 and now being updated reported that approximately 42.6 million U.S. adults ages 45 and older were suffering from loneliness. A 2018 Cigna survey indicates that Generation Z, adults between ages 18 and 22, may be the loneliest group of Americans. Additionally, census data reveal that more than one-fourth of Americans live alone and more than half are unmarried, with marriage rates and the number of children per household steadily declining.

It's clear that being alone and unhappy about it "are risk factors for early illness and death that need to be discussed more openly and for which solutions must continue to be developed," says Lisa Marsh Ryerson, president of the AARP Foundation.

Yet unlike heart disease, physical activity and smoking – which are national public health priorities – social isolation and loneliness have gotten relatively short shrift in this country, says Carla Perissinotto, a geriatrician at University of California-San Francisco. (The U.K., by contrast, recently appointed a minister of loneliness to lead a far-reaching initiative addressing the problem.) "Policy in this country doesn't support this kind of concern," Perissinotto says, "because many health care workers believe that social factors have nothing to do with medicine."

A social species. So why exactly is loneliness bad for health? Humans are a social species with an innate biological drive to connect, explains Dolores Malaspina, professor of psychiatry, neuroscience and genetics at the Icahn School of Medicine at Mount Sinai in New York. Human survival, she says, depends on connectedness, with feelings of loneliness serving as a biological signal to socialize. But the brain's wiring for socialization can malfunction, leading people to feel isolated and bereft. In fact, Malaspina says, evidence shows that

and bipolar disorder, found her mental health declining. She only left her apartment for medical appointments, spending most days alone. She lost her desire to do anything or meet anybody. She ate unhealthy food, rarely got dressed, and would only collect her mail at midnight when she was certain nobody in her building would be awake.

Then she got a lifeline. A staffer at Kenosha Area Family and Aging Services, an organization for which she had been volunteering, alerted Hayward to a virtual program being launched in her community that connects older adults

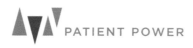
feelings of loneliness can begin in infancy, though treating the resulting depression "can restore the ability to connect and alter the brain's circuitry."

Julianne Holt-Lunstad, professor of psychology at Brigham Young University, says no age group is invulnerable to the effects of social isolation and loneliness. Her analysis of existing research finds that the health toll of loneliness is stronger for those under age 65 than for the older set, contrary to what stereotypes may suggest.

Social media may help explain why rates of so-cial isolation and loneliness are climbing among youth, as popular platforms blur the lines between appearing – and actually feeling – connected, says Joshua M. Smyth, a researcher in the department of biobehavioral health at Pennsylvania State University. On the other hand, social media interactions, texts, emails and photos from loved ones can improve self-esteem, quality of life and feelings of connected-ness, says Amy Gonzales, assistant professor in The Media School at Indiana University–Bloomington.

Holt-Lunstad and colleagues have found that those who are more socially connected have a 50 percent reduced risk of early death relative to those who are less socially connected. But studies show that meaningful, high-quality relationships have the greatest protective health effect. (Note: A person can have few social connections and not be lonely or have many connections and still be lonely.)

The fix. Despite the lack of a coordinated government response, private programs like Well Connected, which now reaches people in 38 states, are beginning to heighten aware-ness of and address America's loneliness problem (box). The UnLonely Project, a program led by Harvard Medical School internist Jeremy Nobel, is evaluating the use of creative arts to help participants explore their feelings about loneliness and bond with others by sharing their stories online and in person. The proj-ect includes the UnLonely Film Festival (unlonelyfilms.org), a collection of short films that deal with loneliness and have educational components. Additionally, the project partners with various senior centers, health systems, workplaces and schools to offer in-person programs that have shown promise in reducing isola-tion and improving health outcomes.

Hospitals and health systems may be best positioned to make a real dif-ference, both by shedding light on the problem and partnering with community organizations to offer solutions, Nobel says. But to date, few offer programs for the isolated and lonely. One that does: CareMore Health, a health care delivery system serving 150,000 Medicaid and Medicare patients in 10 states, helps Anthem Medicare Advantage patients reconnect socially through referrals to community centers and senior-focused fitness centers.

Becoming "unlonely." It's important to resist the pull of inertia and connect regu-larly with people who share similar interests, psycholo-gists stress. Social groups centered around activities, like walking clubs, exercise classes and community choirs, for exam-ple, can make it easier to engage with peers. Other avenues? Schedule a time each day to call a friend; take a class to learn something new; volunteer to deepen a sense of purpose. Lone-ly children and teens can make natural connections through school and community centers when encouraged to pursue interests such as chess, drama, art, running and other sports, says Rockville, Maryland, psychologist Mary Alvord.

When people give in to the urge to hide away, Alvord says, they lose the opportunity to gain encouragement and reinforce-ment in the world. Planning activities – and forcing yourself to follow through – is crucial. Feeling connected, she says, directly affects quality of life. ●

Reaching Out From Home

Sometimes it can be easier to start making connections if you can do so without venturing out. A few avenues:

Connect2Affect
Gauge your isolation level (and health risk) with a quick self-assessment and find services near you through this AARP Foundation initiative.
connect2affect.org

University Without Walls
Connects homebound seniors in classes by phone on everything from art and history to games. Run by the nonprofit DOROT.
dorotusa.org

Friendship Line
Feeling like you need a friend? The Institute on Aging operates a round-the-clock help hotline.
ioaging.org

My Life, My Stories
Share life memories with a vetted senior volunteer, who will transcribe, print and bind your story while providing connection and support.
mylifemystories.org

UnLonely Project
Combat loneliness through creative storytelling while gaining awareness of isolation's health risks through this program blending self-help with advocacy.
artandhealing.org

Well Connected
Tap at least 70 support and subject-interest groups by phone or computer through this program that connects more than 1,000 seniors nationwide each week.
covia.org/services/well-connected/

THIS IS THE SITE OF FRED AND
SUSAN'S HEART CONDITIONS.

THIS IS FRED AND SUSAN.

**THEY WON'T LET THEIR HEALTH
ISSUES DEFINE THEIR LIVES.**

Fred and Susan prefer to be known as a caring husband, loving
wife and partners in building their dream home. Thanks to the
heart experts at El Camino Hospital, they're back on track. With
sophisticated heart care like minimally invasive ablation therapy
for Fred and a pacemaker revision for Susan, we helped them get
back to enjoying retirement on their terms. At El Camino Hospital,
we believe in delivering care as dynamic as the people we serve.
People just like Fred and Susan.
Learn more at **elcaminohospital.org/stories**

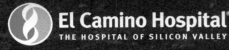
El Camino Hospital®
THE HOSPITAL OF SILICON VALLEY

Pain at the Prescription Counter

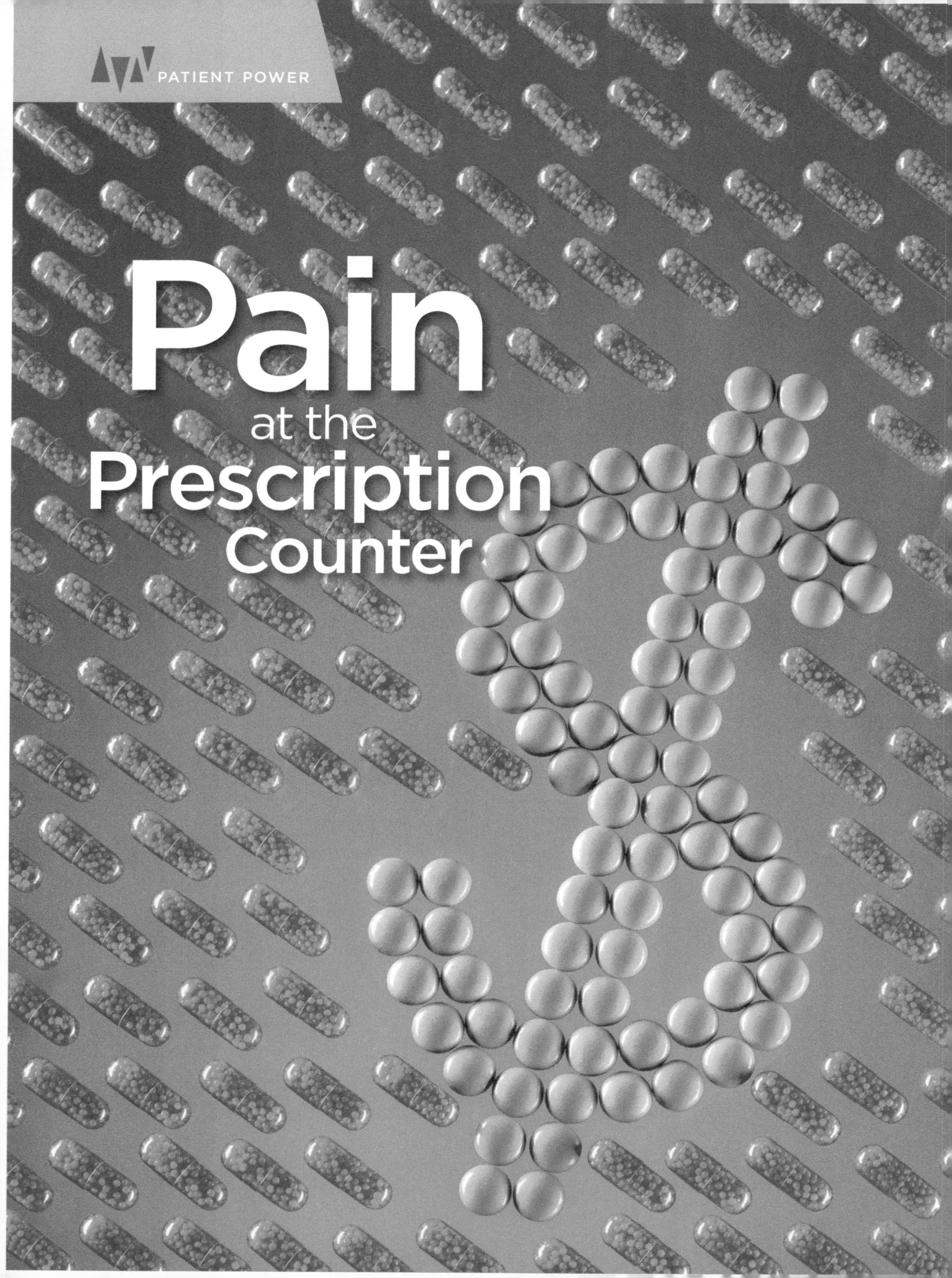

Even generic medications are often shockingly pricey. Here's what you can do to bring your drug costs down

by **Elizabeth Gardner**

Have you seen the cost of a prescription jump from $3 to $30 when your doctor changed your dosage? Were you ambushed by a $500 copay for a tube of steroidal skin cream? Are you carrying a $300 EpiPen – essential for emergency treatment of deadly allergic reactions – that used to cost $50? Have you discovered that your atorvastatin (generic Lipitor) costs less if you put away your insurance card and pay cash?

Welcome to the drug price maze! More and more, certain peculiarities of the pharmaceutical market are clashing with insurance arrangements that require patients to pay a bigger share for their prescriptions, leading to confusion and sticker shock. "When your insurer paid most of the cost and copays were minimal, no one complained as the prices skyrocketed," says physician Elisabeth Rosenthal, editor in chief of Kaiser Health News and author of "An American Sickness: How Healthcare Became Big Business and How You Can Take It Back." Now, she explains, "copays and deductibles are going up, and we're all feeling those prices in a way that has made everyone sit up and go, 'Whoa!'" There are ways for consumers to reduce what they pay for many drugs, but they must learn how to ask questions and where to look for answers.

Drug pricing has been relatively straightforward until recently, at least for consumers. Branded drugs, patented by their creators, cost a lot, but insurance picked up most of the bill. When the patents expired, manufacturers of generic drugs offered much cheaper versions, and typical copays dropped to just a few dollars. Pharmaceutical companies had an incentive to keep discovering new drugs, and the price burden for underwriting those discoveries was temporary and led to a steady flow of new, inexpensive generics.

It's still a straight path most of the time. Generic drugs accounted for 90 percent of the more than 5.8 billion U.S. prescriptions written in 2017, according to research firm IQVIA, and more than 97 percent of all prescriptions (both branded and generic) cost patients less than $50 out of pocket. Almost a third of prescriptions written in 2017 were free to the patient, because of regulations or insurance arrangements. (For example, the Affordable Care Act mandates no patient payment for all FDA-approved contraceptives and preventive medications, like cholesterol-lowering drugs and vaccines, and insurance plans may stop charging copays once patients have reached their deductible limit for the year.) "The vast majority of drugs are inexpensive and are one of the best values in the health care system," says Brigham and Women's Hospital's Aaron Kesselheim, associate professor of medicine at Harvard Medical School, who studies drug pricing.

But he notes that several factors distort the market for pharmaceuticals in general and generics in particular, and they can deliver extreme price blows to people whose prescriptions are in that expensive 3 percent, or to those whose insurance coverage, or lack of it, makes them responsible for a significant chunk of their medication costs. Those factors include:

No standard pricing. Retail pricing for prescription drugs is a black box, says Doug Hirsch, a former Facebook executive who co-founded GoodRx, a drug price comparison app and website, in 2011. He realized there was a need for such a service when he discovered that the cash cost for a month's supply of the ADHD medication Vyvanse, which wasn't covered by his insurance, could vary by as much as $150 depending on which pharmacy he went to. "I assumed the guy with the white coat had a master price list, but there isn't one," he says.

Most insurers rely on pharmacy benefit managers, or PBMs, to negotiate with drug companies, and those deals vary. If a pharmacist tells you that a drug isn't "on your formulary," Hirsch says, it means your insurer's PBM hasn't negotiated any savings on it and may not cover it. Sometimes you can make out by skipping your insurer entirely, using discounts available on price comparison websites or "doorbuster" specials offered by some pharmacies. Take the cholesterol drug atorvastatin, for example. In early June 2018, GoodRx showed that the cash price for a month's supply was $150 at Walgreens but a mere $17 at Costco ($7.84 with a GoodRx coupon). If you check your coverage, you may find that your copay at Walgreens is more than the cash price at Costco.

No competition. A three-month supply of 40-milligram capsules of the popular antidepressant fluoxetine (generic Prozac) costs as little as $10 at Walmart, according to GoodRx, and will rarely trigger more than the minimum copay at most pharmacies. But if your doctor ups your dosage to 60 mg, the cash price can hit $900 at many pharmacies, according to GoodRx, (though a store coupon can knock it down by more than one-quarter). Your insurance copay is likely to rise accordingly.

That's most likely because that particular dosage is available from only one or a small number of sources, Kesselheim says. "If there are eight manufacturers making a 40-mg version of a certain drug, but only one

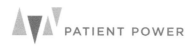

making a 60-mg version, then that manufacturer can charge whatever it wants." It takes four or more manufacturers of the same product for prices to go down significantly, according to his research. Patients can sometimes avoid the high-priced version by asking their doctors to prescribe a drug in its cheapest form (in the example above, by asking their doctor to prescribe a combination of 40-mg and 20-mg capsules), but that strategy requires knowledge. "Most physicians don't know anything about costs, or talk about them with their patients," Kesselheim says.

No price regulation. As a generic drug's price approaches rock bottom, manufacturers may lose interest and leave the field. The last one standing can jack up the price, and patients who need the drug have to pay. That's how the anti-parasite drug Daraprim went from $1 per pill several years ago to $750 in 2016. Martin Shkreli, who engineered that headline-grabbing increase while at the helm of Turing Pharmaceuticals, recently went to prison, though for securities fraud rather than price-gouging (still widely legal at this writing). But Daraprim still costs about $750 per pill (as of June 2018), leaving patients with life-threatening toxoplasmosis or other parasitic infections to either pay up or resort to less effective medications. This incident and others have prompted a flurry of state-level legislative activities – 357 bills in 47 states in the first five months of 2018 alone – directed at pricing and payment, according to the National Conference of State Legislatures.

No generics. Even if a product goes off patent, generic drug manufacturers may ignore it if it's hard to duplicate the branded version. Creams, ointments and inhaled medications are especially likely to be available only as branded products, Rosenthal says. In March of 2018, Kaiser Health News's "Bill of the Month" – a column that deciphers medical bills submitted by readers – featured a $1,500-per-month treatment for toenail fungus that drained the patient's health savings account without her knowledge when she relied on her insurer's mail-order pharmacy. "The dermatologist's office never told her it was expensive," Rosenthal says. "But it's the first thing you should ask." EpiPen supplier Mylan raised its price from about $100 to over $600 for a two-pack between 2007 and 2016. After public outcry and protests from lawmakers, the company started offering coupons and making a generic EpiPen.

You may be able to get your drug costs down with a few simple strategies. Jennifer Spare, of Hanover Park, Illinois, usually saves between $25 and $40 per prescription just by checking local pharmacies for the best prices. She usually skips large chains in favor of a small family-owned pharmacy. "They have the best pricing around, and they'll mail your prescription to you at no charge," she says. Spare has also saved as much as $60 just by asking the pharmacy for a discount. Comparison shopping is a little more complicated with electronic prescribing, where the doctor automatically sends the prescription to the patient's pharmacy of choice. Many states now require e-prescriptions for some or all medications. You might find it a pain to compare costs every time and request that the pharmacy in your electronic medical record be changed once you find the best price, but it should take your doctor under a minute to make the switch, says Los An-

> # Retail pricing of prescription drugs is a black box.

geles internist Sharon Orrange, a clinical associate professor of medicine at the University of Southern California's Keck School of Medicine. She often uses the GoodRx phone app to check local prices with patients before she writes a prescription.

Some patients look abroad to find deals. Consumers can sort through the many foreign sources of medication to find ones that are reputable at PharmacyChecker.com. The site verifies the credentials, contact information, product quality and pricing for foreign pharmacies, says Gabriel Levitt, president and co-founder. "It is technically against the law to import a medication, but as far as we know the government has never prosecuted anyone as long as it's for themselves or a family member." In a 2016 poll by the Kaiser Family Foundation, 8 percent of Americans said they had bought prescription drugs from another country. Rosenthal knows a U.S. asthma patient who buys his inhalers in Paris. With a $200 difference between the U.S. price and the French price, savings on two or three inhalers can cover his airfare.

Patients hit with big drug bills may have to choose between paying the rent or forgoing medications: a choice that can have dire ramifications. One study estimated the U.S. racks up $100 billion to $300 billion in avoidable health care costs annually from people not adhering to their regimen, and high costs accounted for 17 percent of those failures. In a 2016 survey by the Commonwealth Fund, 14 percent of insured Americans didn't fill a prescription or skimped on their dosage because of cost. For the uninsured, it was 33 percent.

Orrange, like all doctors, wants her patients to use their medications. If you're tempted to skimp or pass because of cost, she wants to know immediately – not three months later during a follow-up appointment. She's happy to go to bat with insurers, especially if her patient does much better on a branded drug than on its generic cousin, or if the insurer suddenly decides not to cover a drug that the patient has been taking for a long time. "Bring it up with me, and I'll help you find the best price," she says. "Both of us have a stake in you taking your medications."

If your doctor isn't as price-aware as Orrange (and most aren't), speak up. "Tell your physician about the price of your drugs," Kesselheim says. "It's possible there's another equally effective drug that might be cheaper." Rosenthal agrees. "Train your doctor," she says. "If all their patients ask how much their prescriptions will cost, they're going to have to know." ●

The American College of Cardiology's

Chest Pain – MI Registry™

Formerly the ACTION Registry®

Your Pathway to Achieve Quality Outcomes

The NCDR Chest Pain – MI Registry™ gives you all the high-quality benefits and features you've come to expect from the ACTION Registry, and is your pathway to delivering optimal heart care your patients count on.

Participating in the Chest Pain – MI Registry allows hospitals and health systems to:

- **Engage in quality improvement** efforts using interactive, real-time dashboards providing patient-level detail

- **Gain national and local recognition** through the Chest Pain – MI Registry Performance Achievement Awards program

- **Access the network of hospitals** ACC's Patient Navigator Program: Focus MI quality campaign, a MIPS Improvement Activity

- **Deliver guideline-driven treatments** to measure and improve AMI care

Learn how the Chest Pain – MI Registry can help your hospital meet its quality improvement goals at

ACC.org/ChestPainMIRegistry

The nation's **largest and most authoritative** quality improvement registry **with 1.5 million** patient records and **10+ years** of proven success.

Now with the option to include your unstable angina and low-risk chest pain patient populations

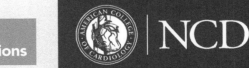

AMERICAN COLLEGE OF CARDIOLOGY | NCDR®

Advancing Quality. Improving Care.

©2018, American College of Cardiology N18768

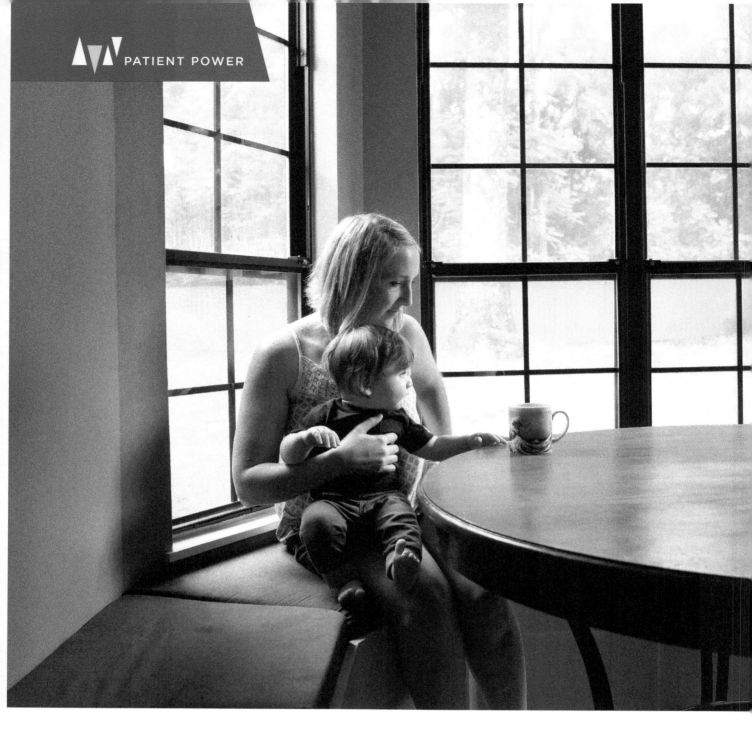

Dangerous Deliveries

Deaths and complications related to childbirth
are trending up. Here's what women need to know
to keep themselves and their newborns safe

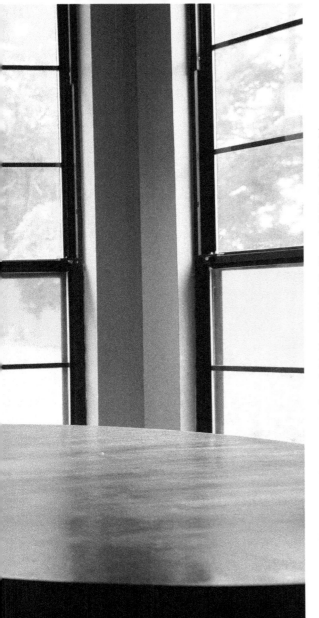

KYLIE MOHR spent
five days in intensive care
after LINCOLN was born.

by **Beth Howard**

J ust days after Kylie Mohr's September
2017 due date, her blood pressure rose and
labor was induced to hasten the birth. Over the
next 48 hours, Mohr's seemingly by-the-book
pregnancy turned into a cascade of life-threatening
complications. Her blood pressure suddenly spiked
out of control, leading to an emergency cesarean
section, hemorrhaging and kidney failure.

The 28-year-old Georgia Air National Guardsman

had to be transferred to a trauma center, and she spent five days
in intensive care before holding her healthy infant son Lincoln,
plus three more days in the hospital. Mohr continues to live with
the consequences of her traumatic birth experience, caused by
a form of pre-eclampsia, or high blood pressure associated with
pregnancy. She gets dialysis and is on the waiting list for a kidney
transplant. "Instead of being happy every time I see a pregnant
woman, I just want to say 'good luck,'" Mohr says.

Stories of birth-related deaths and near-fatal complications
have become alarmingly common. From 2000 to 2014, data
from 48 states plus the District of Columbia revealed a 27 percent increase in maternal mortality rates, from 18.8 deaths
per 100,000 births to 23.8. The rate of near misses rose even
faster, nearly tripling from 1993 to 2014. More than 50,000
women experienced severe complications related to childbirth
in 2014 – from blood pressure disorders like pre-eclampsia to
postpartum hemorrhage and pulmonary emboli that can choke
off blood to the heart and lungs.

These numbers contrast starkly with those in other indus-
trialized countries. While 26 of every 100,000 women die
of pregnancy-related causes in the U.S., there are just 9.2
deaths per 100,000 in the U.K., 7.8 in France, and 4.4 in
Sweden. "You would think in the U.S., where we have significant investment in health care and technology, that we
would rank very well on these measures," says Susan Garpiel,
co-leader of the Perinatal Patient Safety Initiative for Trinity
Health, a network of 94 hospitals in 22 states headquartered
in Michigan. "But we are really the only country, aside from
Afghanistan and Sudan, where the rate is actually rising."
Yet nearly two-thirds of perinatal deaths and complications
are preventable, experts say. Several factors are behind the
shocking numbers:

Chronic safety lapses. Needless harms often result
from a lack of implementation of standard procedures, notes
Barbara Levy, vice president of health policy at the American
College of Obstetricians and Gynecologists. Although there are
evidence-based guidelines on how to handle dangerous complications, not every obstetrician or hospital is up to date. Cases
of postpartum hemorrhage or eclampsia "are treatable with
the right setup," agrees Eugene Declercq, a professor of obstet-
rics and gynecology at Boston University School of Medicine
and assistant dean of the Boston University School of Public
Health. Hospitals should have a plan to handle emergencies,
have practiced the procedures in teams, and keep supplies like
needed medications on the floor, for example.

Pre-eclampsia offers a case study in what happens when
protocols are missing or inconsistent. The condition, sometimes signaled by swelling in the upper extremities, protein in
the urine, or severe headache along with high blood pressure,
is often diagnosed late and undertreated, setting the stage for
seizures and stroke. "Many OBs think most women die from
seizures," says Elliott Main, medical director of the California
Maternal Quality Care Collaborative, which has created tools
for better responding to maternal emergencies in the state.
But stroke is the real killer. Providers need to address both
potential harms – treating seizures with magnesium sulfate
and using hypertension medications to ward off stroke. Since

the risk of problems continues for several weeks after the baby is born, women should ideally be sent home with a blood pressure cuff and be instructed both to return for follow-up in seven to 10 days and to notify their doctor of severe headache, abdominal pain, or visual changes in the meantime.

Too many interventions. Many difficulties can be traced to a rise in cesarean sections and the early induction of labor, sometimes for the sake of convenience and without a medical reason. Induction can lower a baby's heart rate and in Mom lead to infection, increased bleeding after delivery, and the need for a C-section. Cesareans themselves – elective or not – are associated with blood clots, placenta problems,

Between 2008 and 2013, California **cut its fatality rate** in half.

postpartum bleeding, and even later rupture of the uterus, requiring an emergency hysterectomy.

Kat Butina, 39, a nurse in Latrobe, Pennsylvania, was 33 weeks pregnant with her fourth child in 2016 when she felt a sudden gush of blood and indescribable pain in her abdomen. Her uterus had ruptured. She nearly died as doctors worked to stop the bleeding and deliver her baby, who had lodged in her ribcage. "When they put me under for surgery, I didn't expect to wake up," she says.

Butina, who'd had three prior cesarean deliveries out of necessity, was suffering from two conditions associated with repeat C-sections that likely played a role: placenta previa, where the placenta covers the cervix, and placenta accreta, where it invades the uterine wall, greatly increasing the chances of catastrophic complications. Her baby daughter is healthy, but Butina suffered kidney damage and struggles with depression and post-traumatic stress disorder. "Some women look at a C-section as a shortcut, but it does have complications like any major surgery," Main says.

System failures. For many women, particularly minorities, access to pre- and postnatal care remains a problem. And that can have grave repercussions. "Black mothers are three to four times more likely to die than white mothers," Declercq says. Insensitivity to differences among races may play a role. For instance, providers may not be aware that the rate of pre-eclampsia and seizures in black women is much higher than it is in white women.

Another access issue is that nearly half of births are to women tapping Medicaid for pregnancy – and they are removed from the rolls by about 60 days postpartum. Yet 1 in 3 pregnancy-related deaths occurs between seven and 365 days after birth, Declercq says. That applies to some pregnancy-related cardiac conditions like cardiomyopathy, for example.

States have been lax about tracking pregnancy-related deaths and complications, which works against fixing the problems. "In Great Britain, maternal deaths are treated like homicides," says Marian MacDorman, a research professor at the Maryland Population Research Center at the University of Maryland. "There's an investigation into every single case." Yet maternal mortality review committees, which study maternal death cases, exist in only 34 states. Bills currently before Congress would expand the role of these agencies.

In response, ACOG and other professional, industry and patient groups have come together to develop patient-safety "bundles," evidence-based guidelines for handling emergencies. Blood products should be at the ready, for example, and blood loss should be measured to make sure moms receive the exact amount lost. Some 18 states now participate in a national effort to expand the bundles and promote the use of data to improve care. A recent study based on the experience in four of the states, representing more than 260,000 births, showed that implementing safety bundles for hemorrhage and hypertension decreased maternal complications by 20 percent, on average.

California has been a pioneer at establishing standard approaches to emergencies, "rather than everybody doing their own thing," Main says. Most California hospitals, as well as a growing number elsewhere, now have carts that can be rushed to the bedside during obstetric crises a la the crash carts that carry drugs and equipment used in emergency resuscitations. Hemorrhage carts contain medicines that squeeze the uterus and slow the flow of blood, instruments for repairing a tear, and balloons that can apply pressure to the inside walls of the uterus to help it contract and control bleeding, for instance. The result: Between 2008 and 2013, the state cut its maternal fatality rate in half.

Similar efforts are yielding benefits in pockets across the country. The University of Utah cut its obstetric hemorrhage rate by 30 percent after rolling out that safety bundle; both Trinity Health and Dignity Health, which has hospitals in California, Arizona and Nevada, rely on early-warning trigger systems – specific readings for heart rate, blood pressure, temperature and oxygen level, for instance – to identify problems early.

While the tide may be turning, Levy advises women to trust their instincts when they feel something is wrong and speak up. And it's wise to have an advocate. "We have some pretty good data," she says, "that women who have a champion – who have someone with them during their prenatal care and their birth experience and postpartum – have better outcomes." ●

Getting Great Care Via Video

Besides convenience, telemedicine offers a way to tap top experts from far away

by **Mary Brophy Marcus**

While telemedicine may sound 21st century-esque, it's actually been around for decades. From radio consultations between land-based doctors and seafarers in the early 1900s to NASA medical teams tracking the health of astronauts in space starting in the 1960s, doctors and patients have long been exploring new ways to connect when an office visit simply isn't possible.

Now, digital natives are expecting their health care to be served up more conveniently than the in-person scenarios their parents and grandparents accepted without question. As telemedicine continues to evolve, thanks to technological advances, consider these ways it could serve you or a loved one:

Avoid an avalanche – literally. For years, Cindy Kahler, mother of five, regularly drove hours through mountain passes to take her daughter to see specialists at Seattle Children's Hospital. In mild weather, the six-hour round-trip journey is long and exhausting, but in winter it can be downright treacherous. Once she turned back because of an avalanche risk.

But for the past year and a half, Kahler has been able to skip the long trips. Instead, 10-year-old Hadassah – who has special feeding needs due to cerebral palsy – has been seen via video either at one of

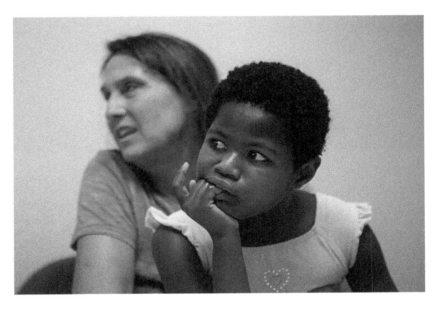

Cindy Kahler no longer faces six hours on the road to take daughter Hadassah to see the doctor.

the medical center's satellite offices about 17 miles from home, or, thanks to a new pilot program, in their home. During appointments, child psychologist Danielle Dolezal, head of Seattle Children's pediatric feeding program, beams in from Seattle. When they connect remotely, Dolezal can observe Hadassah sitting in a highchair as Kahler feeds her. A pediatric speech pathologist and a nutrition expert join in sometimes, too. "I'm watching, coaching – I'm a bug in their ear. It's like

we're FaceTiming," Dolezal says. "There's a camera on their end that I can manipulate and zoom in to see what she's doing with her mouth."

Seattle Children's serves a five-state region – Washington, Alaska, Montana, Wyoming and Idaho – that spans a huge landmass, much of it remote, says pediatric emergency physician Mark Lo, its medical director of telehealth and digital health. Nationwide, various telemedicine programs are helping people access expert specialty care that once may have seemed out of reach.

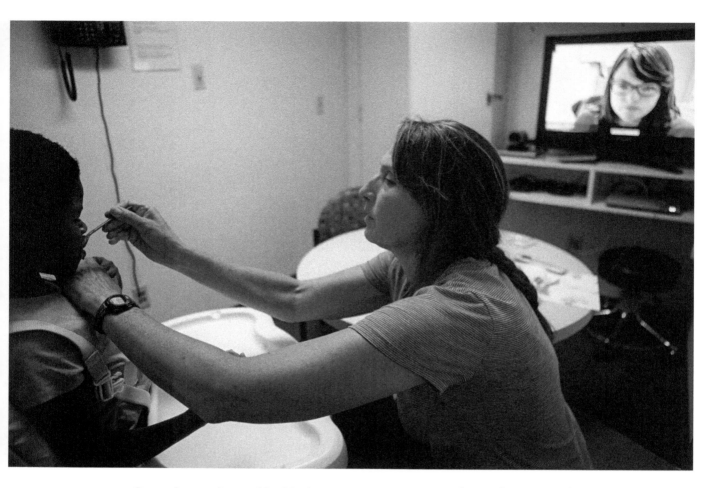

Kahler
feeds Hadassah
as Danielle
Dolezal of
Seattle Children's
consults.

See a doc on demand by kiosk.
Hit with a sinus infection or sore throat?
Self-service kiosks are appearing in pharmacies, office buildings and even YMCAs
around the country, enabling quick video
consults with doctors. In partnership
with New York-Presbyterian Hospital,
for instance, some Duane Reade drugstores in the
Empire State offer private kiosks outfitted with
medical devices that can give emergency medicine
physicians live details on a patient's health status.
Think: Thermometers that measure temperature
with the swipe of the forehead; a blood pressure cuff;
a pulse oximeter that gauges blood oxygen levels. The
$99 exams are conducted via high-definition video.
Prescriptions, if written, can be sent instantly to the
patient's preferred pharmacy. Other telemedicine-
kiosk initiatives operate similarly. Florida's BayCare
Health System, for example, has partnered with Pub-
lix to offer patients remote care via video at their
neighborhood grocery store.

Get after-hours care for a sick child. Nemours
Children's Health System – which serves pediatric
patients in Delaware, Florida, Georgia, New Jersey

and Pennsylvania – provides a 24/7 tele-urgent care
service, CareConnect. It entails a live video visit ($0
to $59 depending on a patient's insurance) acces-
sible on a desktop computer or via a free mobile
app. A pediatrician conducts a video exam and can
electronically prescribe medication. Users needn't
be Nemours patients to be seen, but must be in one
of the above states or Maryland to use the service – popular during flu season and for rashes, fevers, vomiting and more. "A lot
of times parents are trying to figure out, 'Do I really need to go
to the ER or not?'" says Carey Officer, operational vice president
of Nemours CareConnect. Surveys show the program has kept
25 percent of patients from ER care and 34 percent from urgent
care visits. When a child's condition is more serious, CareConnect guides parents to in-person emergency care.

Chat with your surgeon. Chris Toggweiler, 40, of Miami,
says a video visit with his Cleveland Clinic cardiac surgeon
weeks before his recent septal myectomy gave him peace of
mind. Toggweiler, who has hypertrophic cardiomyopathy – in
which heart muscles become abnormally thick – knew time
would be tight upon arrival in Cleveland, so one day on his
way to work, he dropped his daughter off at school, pulled into
a parking lot and dialed in for a scheduled video chat on his
smartphone. "It was nice to meet the surgeon who's going to

split you open. Just to ask some questions," Toggweiler says. Not only is telemedicine being used for virtual preop visits, but it's giving patients a more convenient way to have follow-up care after routine surgery as well. It is also being explored to aid patients and families throughout the entire surgery continuum, from providing nutrition counseling and helping smokers quit before surgery to training caregivers after loved ones have been discharged from the hospital, says Alex Cho, clinical lead for the Duke Telehealth Office.

Be treated at home. Technology has helped spur a "hospital at home" movement to monitor and treat patients who require care but don't necessarily need hospitalization. Duke HomeCare & Hospice is among those offering remote monitoring to patients receiving in-home skilled nursing care for several chronic conditions, Cho says. Brigham and Women's Hospital has its own Home Hospital program, giving select eligible patients admitted to the ER the option of returning home in lieu of a hospital stay to receive care. A remote wireless monitoring system is set up so doctors can constantly monitor the patient's heart rate and other key health measurements from afar. Patients can text or video chat with a doctor at any time, and, if a problem occurs, a doctor is available 24/7 for a home visit. Remote monitoring is supplemented by visits from providers who can perform bloodwork, X-rays and ultrasounds from the patient's bedside. Results of an initial small pilot study on the approach were published in early 2018 and revealed that it was more cost-effective than caring for similar patients in the hospital and that the patient experience and the quality of care were not appreciably diminished.

Access cancer expertise. Cancer patients living in more rural areas are likelier to die than those in more urban locations, data suggest. But through telemedicine and support from the National Cancer Institute, patients and their oncologists can tap into the expertise of an NCI-designated cancer center; the nation's 70 such centers are involved in hundreds of studies assessing the latest treatments.

UC Davis Health near Sacramento, for example, has formed the UC Davis Cancer Care Network, through which UC Davis cancer experts hold videoconferences with oncologists, pathologists, surgeons and other cancer experts in rural hospitals to review patient cases and, if deemed appropriate for those patients, alert them to clinical trials. Some hospitals, such as Roswell Park Comprehensive Cancer Center in Buffalo, New York, have recently created telemedicine programs in which their cancer experts can consult with both physicians and patients at partner community hospitals.

The NCI is also expanding its own telehealth initiatives. In December 2017, the NCI and the Federal Communications Commission announced a joint effort to bridge the gap in cancer care in Appalachia. They're studying how increasing broadband access in rural areas might "provide connections to cancer patients who have historically lacked them," says Bradford Hesse, chief of NCI's Health Communication and Informatics Research Branch.

Evidence suggests telemedicine can offer multiple benefits to patients. One study found that when people with cancer reported symptoms electronically to their providers, they saw greater boosts in their health-related quality of life than those in an unplugged control group, Hesse says. Another found that electronically connected patients were less likely to land in the emergency room and had greater survival rates than patients in the control group.

Getting mental health support. Telehealth is expanding counseling to more patients living with mental health issues from depression to addiction. Psychiatrist Jay H. Shore, director of telemedicine at the University of Colorado Anschutz Medical Campus depression center, oversees a team of nurse practitioners and psychiatrists who treat patients in Colorado and Alaska – some 3,000 miles away. "We see and

Now, digital natives are expecting their health care to be served up more conveniently.

treat patients who would not have access to psychiatric care without telemedicine, both in the rural clinics and even in the urban clinics," Shore says. A major perk of visiting with a patient virtually? You can get more insight seeing them in their world versus your clinical setting, he explains.

Beyond counseling, the mental health field is applying telemedicine in other ways. One project involves a collaboration between providers and patients with obsessive compulsive disorder, most of whom are newly discharged from an inpatient treatment program. Each pair works together to create an app that is customized to help the patient transition back to everyday life.

"The patient and therapist figure out together what's helpful. They focus on behavior reminders; they use humor; it's interactive," says Armen Arevian, who directs the Innovation Lab at UCLA's Semel Institute and Center for Health Services and Society and is an assistant professor in the school's department of psychiatry. Researchers are studying the role of the app in improving patients' symptoms. ●

A Dose of the Great Outdoors

Doctors are using their prescription pads to order a walk in the park

by **Beth Howard**

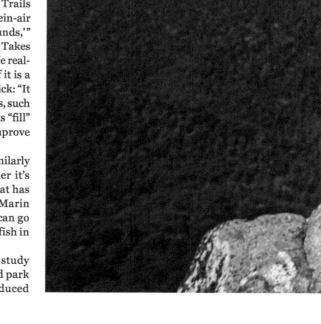

Everyone knows a walk in the woods is good for the body and the mind. Now, as data on the health perks accumulate, doctors are promoting or even prescribing time in nature.

"Hundreds of studies demonstrate that exposure to nature, and particularly outdoor exercise, is good for your health," says Sara Newman, director of the National Park Service Office of Public Health, which supports the National ParkRx initiative developed by a group of doctors and park agencies to encourage the use of natural spaces for purposes like losing weight, improving chronic health conditions, and lowering sky-high stress rates linked to depression and anxiety. That idea is also taking root at state, county and city park systems nationwide.

Health care professionals involved in New Mexico's Prescription Trails program actually pull out a prescription pad when recommending plein-air outings. "It's one thing to say 'go out and quit smoking and lose 20 pounds,'" says Charm Lindblad, executive director of New Mexico Health Care Takes On Diabetes, an advocacy organization, and of Prescription Trails. "We realized that the patient will take the recommendation more seriously if it is a prescription." A side benefit, says Albuquerque podiatrist Bill FitzPatrick: "It often starts a cascade of healthy activities – nutrition and other exercises, such as resistance training." About 50 percent of his participating patients "fill" their nature prescriptions, he says, and those with diabetes often improve their A1C levels, a measure of blood sugar control over time.

The Parks Prescription program in California's Marin County is similarly aimed at getting families active in natural areas close by, "whether it's just a beautiful space to be in nature and have a picnic or a place that has organized walks or fishing," says Tracey Hessel, a pediatrician at Marin Community Clinics. Visitors to McNears Beach Park in San Rafael can go for a stroll while enjoying breathtaking ocean views, for instance, or fish in the bay. Nearby parks offer Zumba classes and other activities.

Although data on the effectiveness of such programs is scant, a study by Marin County's public health division of 55 patients who received park prescriptions showed that 16 percent lost weight and 9 percent reduced

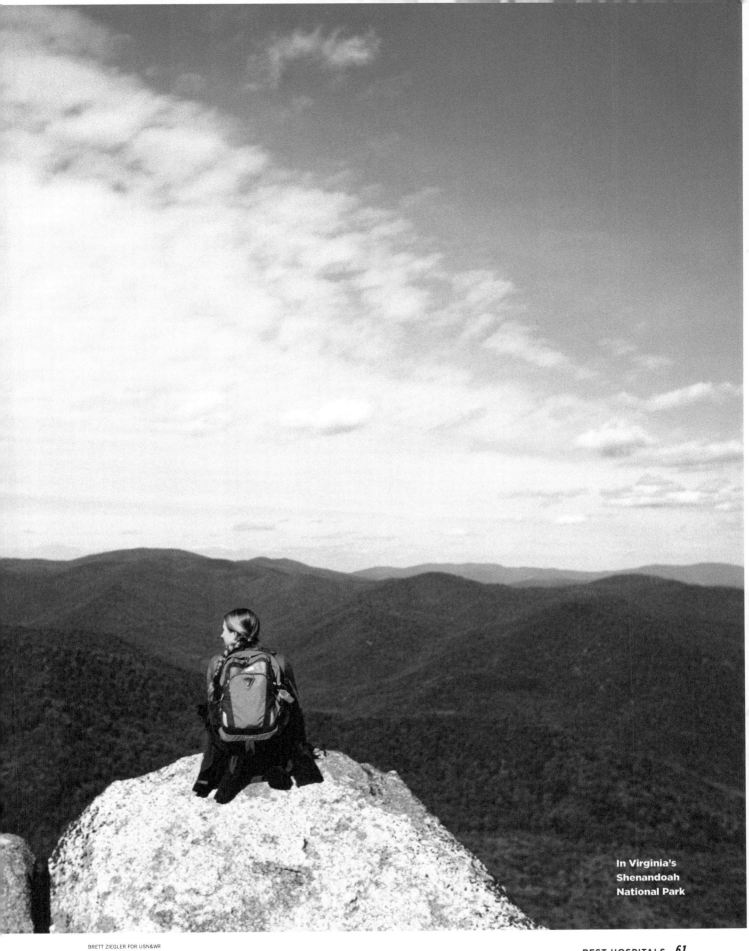

In Virginia's
Shenandoah
National Park

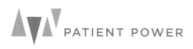
their blood pressure. In a pilot park prescription program sponsored by Humana in Plantation, Florida, older people who never went to the park reported an average of four more unhealthy days in the previous month than those who visited a park one to five times.

In fact, data on the benefits of connecting with nature go back decades. A 1984 study found that patients in hospital rooms with windows overlooking a natural scene had shorter hospital stays and required less pain medication than patients whose windows faced a brick wall. More recently,

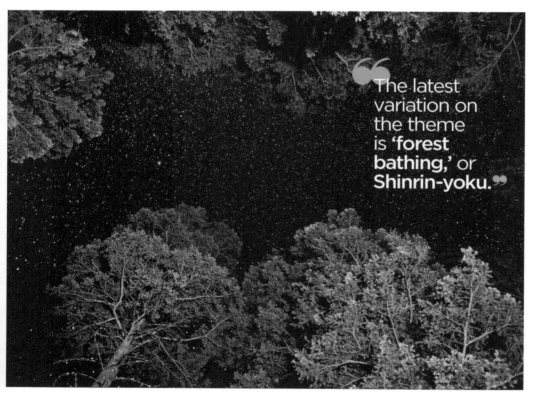

"The latest variation on the theme is 'forest bathing,' or Shinrin-yoku."

researchers from the University of Queensland in Australia showed that people who spent time in green spaces had lower rates of depression and high blood pressure. The combination of exercise and natural surroundings appears to be even more powerful. A 2007 study from the University of Essex in Great Britain found that a daily dose of walking outdoors could rival antidepressants for treating mild to moderate depression. Walking in a crowded shopping mall didn't have the same impact.

How green activity contributes to health outcomes isn't entirely clear. Regular exercise anywhere improves the cardiovascular system, lowers blood sugar and promotes a healthy weight. But when it's outdoors, it may take on more mean-

ing than, say, exercise in a gym or mall, increasing the chances that it becomes a habit. In addition, some experts theorize, volatile organic chemicals and exposure to the diverse microorganisms in nature, may aid cognition and mental well-being, respectively, and foster stronger immune responses in the skin and gut.

The latest variation on the theme is "forest bathing," or Shinrin-yoku. The idea is to simply spend time in a wooded setting and pay attention to what you see, smell, touch, feel and hear, akin to practices like mindfulness meditation, shown to lower levels of pain, depression and anxiety. The idea originated in Japan and appears to lower blood pressure and heart rate for at least as long as you are in the woods. Chemicals secreted by trees called phytoncides, which people inhale in a forested area, may help explain such effects. Phytoncides have been shown to improve immunity and lower levels of stress hormones like cortisol. "What I love about it is that, rather than walking through the forest and using the mind to identify all the plants and animals, one uses the senses to experience the forest," says Katherine Wagner-Reiss, 62, a retired Connecticut physician who gives forest tours at the New York Botanical Garden. She says these forays help to quiet her brain's chatter.

Diana Proemm, a certified therapeutic recreation specialist in San Antonio, can attest to the soothing power of nature. She's noticed a profound change in a young client with autism whom she has taken for nature walks over the last two years. "She's usually pacing the driveway when I come to pick her up," Proemm says. "When we get out on the trail, she quiets down and is at peace the whole time we are out there."

You don't have to go into the wilderness to get the effects. Some people find solace in practices like therapeutic horticulture – simply gardening or participating in plant-based activities. The Naples Botanical Garden in Florida partners with the Alzheimer's Support Network to offer a twice-monthly "Meet Me in the Garden" program for people with memory impairment and their caregivers. This experiential program provides a slow-paced "sensory" tour of the garden, which might involve stroking the soft stem of a chenille plant or smelling the evocative scent of a gardenia. "It's amazing to see how touching or smelling something can bring back memories," says Taylor Burnham, who coordinates the program. Data show that communing with plants helps improve sleep and reduce the anxiety and agitation common with dementia.

"We see ourselves as part of the solution," says the National Park Service's Newman. One big role for nature therapy, in fact, might be helping to prevent health problems in the first place. ●

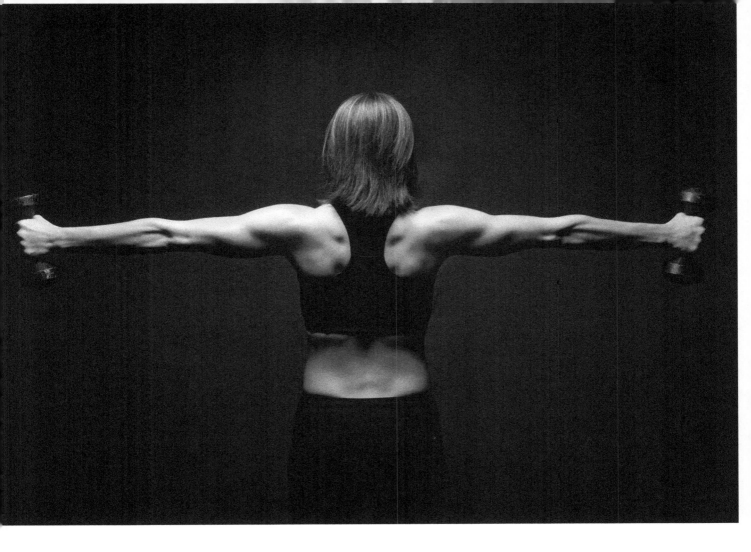

Muscle's Many Powers

Scientists are learning that resistance training confers much more than strength. It's key to your overall health

by **K. Aleisha Fetters**

Everyone knows that muscle moves you – that each time you blink, take a step, or cram your suitcase into an overhead bin, your muscles make it happen. But "what scientists are just now understanding," says Andy Galpin, director of the Biochemistry and Molecular Exercise Physiology Laboratory at California State University–Fullerton, "is just

how synonymous muscle health is with all health."

Recent research shows that the amount of muscle on your frame is a leading indicator of health and longevity with one 2017 study finding that lean muscle mass outperforms body mass index, or BMI, at gauging overall health. What's more, a 2015 study published in The Lancet suggests that grip strength – a widely recognized surrogate for total-body muscle strength and health – can more accurately predict our likelihood of death by heart disease than can blood pressure.

"We tend to compartmentalize the body as the muscular system and the

skeletal system and the cardiovascular system and the nervous system and the immune system, but the body is one system," Galpin says. "When one part gets healthier, everything gets healthier. And muscle is the one part over which you have the most direct control."

A Multitasking Organ

Muscle, which comprises roughly 40 percent of the body, is a massive endocrine organ, communicating via hormones to the liver, heart, brain and other endocrine glands to influence metabolic, hormonal and cardiovascular health. "I love to tease endocrinologists and tell them that diabetes is not a disease of the pancreas; it's a disease of the muscle," says Tim Church, adjunct professor of preventive medicine at Pennington Biomedical Research Center at Louisiana State University. "The biggest consumer of blood sugar in your body is skeletal muscle, so when you think about insulin resistance [a chronic condition in which the body does not properly process blood sugar], you have to understand it's happening at the muscle level."

By building muscle through resistance training, you increase the amount of tissue available to use and store glucose for energy. You also improve the ability of specialized proteins to deliver glucose to that muscle, per one review by Austrian and Yale scientists. They found that this enhances the body's ability to process glucose and to use fats and sugars for fuel, while combating abdominal fat and help-

suggests that muscle tissue accounts for approximately 20 percent of total daily caloric expenditure.

However, researchers are learning that muscle doesn't only process sugar and burn calories, it also builds. Muscle serves as the body's predominant amino acid reserve, supplying the materials needed for the body to produce wound-healing molecules, antibodies and other proteins that are important for sustaining health.

That may in large part explain why people with more muscle live longer and are better able to combat disease, says Arny A. Ferrando, a professor of geriatrics with the Center for Translational Research in Aging and Longevity at the University of Arkansas for Medical Sciences. He explains that muscle mass is a strong predictor of disease survivability, including cancer treatment outcomes. Muscle wasting is a common complication of cancer treatment, and contributes to a higher risk

coming an increasing health threat, even showing up at ages when muscle mass should be peaking. Meanwhile, the muscle that's left tends to be weaker. That's because so-called fast-twitch muscle fibers, those that contribute most to strength and power, are the first to go in young adults who let inactivity and poor nutrition set in. The ones that remain, the slow-twitch fibers more responsible for endurance, are more resistant to aging until later decades, says Christopher Travers, an exercise physiologist with Cleveland Clinic Sports Health.

Fortunately, science has made it easier than ever to build the muscle you need for optimal health. Here's your muscle health Rx:

▶ Strength train at least twice a week. Current guidelines from the Centers for Disease Control and Prevention prescribe at least two days per week of muscle-strengthening activities. Galpin recommends gradually increasing that weekly goal to three to five days as your technique and strength levels improve.

▶ Move through a full range of motion. When performing strength-training exercises, prioritize using resistance – think weights, bands or your own bodyweight – that you can control through a full range of motion. If you're doing a squat, say, that means sinking as low as you can without compromising your form. Doing so trains more muscle fibers and improves joint range of motion, Galpin says.

▶ Focus on compound exercises. "The body's muscles are like a symphony," says Jason Machowsky, an exercise physiologist and sports dietitian at the Hospital for Special Surgery in New York City. "There are different instruments at play, but it's them coming together that creates effective motion."

Compound movements, such as deadlifts, lunges, squats, presses and rows, achieve symphonic harmony by tapping multiple muscle groups and joints at once, while training the body to perform movements of everyday life. Bonus: Compound movements can burn more calories and build more muscle than can isolation exercises such as biceps curls.

When performing compound exercises, it's also important to remember that your body is a 3D object and meant to move in all planes of motion, Machowsky

> **1 in 3** adults **age 60 and older** suffers from severe muscle loss.

ing prevent or manage Type 2 diabetes.

That partly explains why, when Harvard T. H. Chan School of Public Health researchers followed 10,500 men over 12 years, they found that people who performed 20 minutes of resistance training per day gained less abdominal fat, a marker of overall health, than those who spent the same time frame doing cardio.

While aerobic exercise has long been prescribed to burn fat, current studies consistently demonstrate that resistance training, by building both the size and cellular health of muscle, leads to bigger reductions in body fat. After all, the biggest factor you can control when it comes to your basal metabolic rate – the number of calories your body burns each day to keep you alive – is your muscle mass, Church says. Evidence

of chemotherapy side effects and lower survival rates, research suggests.

"All of these fields are starting to turn their eyes heavily toward muscle and say, 'OK, muscle is a major priority,'" Galpin says. "If muscle is out of whack, the rest of our treatments and interventions become secondary to affecting the muscle issue."

Do You Have Enough?

Many of us don't. Sarcopenia, or age-related muscle loss, typically sets in after our 30th birthday. From age 50 on, people naturally lose 1 to 2 percent of their lean leg mass annually, and 1 in 3 adults 60 and older suffers from severe muscle loss, research suggests.

Thanks to our culture's embrace of sedentary lifestyles, muscle loss is be-

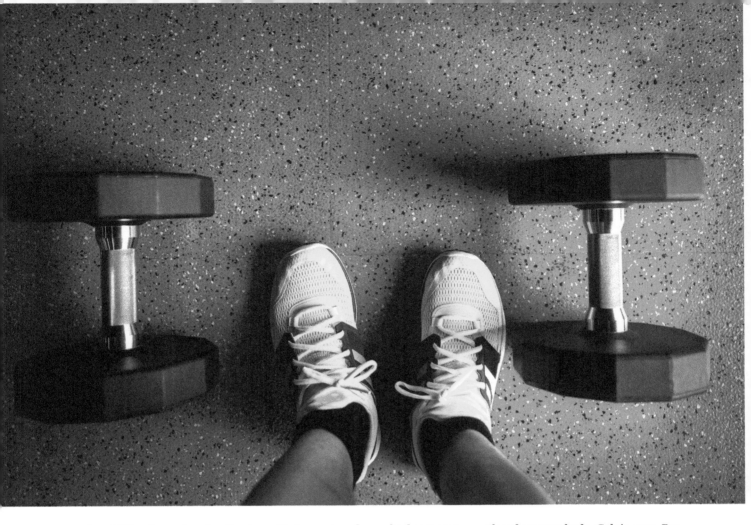

says. In addition to performing front-to-back exercises such as lunges, bench presses and rows, integrate side-to-side exercises such as lateral band walks, side lunges and shoulder raises. Lastly, incorporate rotational movements such as woodchops and rotational presses. You'll not only build more muscle, but also you'll build functional muscle that's prepared to support you through all of life's movement patterns.

▶ **Load up.** "One of the most common mistakes in resistance training is that the load, or weight moved, is too low," says exercise physiologist Abbie E. Smith-Ryan, director of the Applied Physiology Laboratory at the University of North Carolina–Chapel Hill. Resist the temptation to go easy. To build muscle, a repetition range of eight to 12 is generally a good place to start, she says. "You should pick a load that you cannot do for more than 10 to 12 reps."

▶ **Pump up the protein.** Skimping on protein is a surefire way to undercut your muscle goals, says Machowsky, explaining that every bout of strength training creates microscopic damage to the body's muscle cells. It's only by providing them nutrients, including protein, that they are able to repair and grow back stronger.

Currently, the recommended daily allowance of protein, which represents the minimum nutritional requirement, is 0.8 daily grams of protein per kilogram body weight, or about 55 grams for a 150-pound person. However, the latest science suggests that adults need up to double that amount to achieve optimal muscle health.

"Given that protein's amino acids are stored in the liver only temporarily, we have to pay attention to the timing if we are looking to maximize protein synthesis in the body," says Kelly Pritchett, assistant professor of sports nutrition at Central Washington University and spokesperson for the Academy of Nutrition and Dietetics. A 2018 review published in the Journal of the International Society of Sports Nutrition suggests that, for the best results, people should consume 0.4 to 0.55 grams of protein per kilogram of body weight four times per day. For a 150-pound adult, the recommendation works out to four meals of 27 to 37.5 grams of protein each.

▶ **Ramp up your routine.** As your muscles adapt to your workouts, it's critical to systematically increase the demand placed on your body, Galpin says. Progressive overload, as it's called, can be achieved by increasing exercise intensity, load lifted, number of reps and sets performed, or workout frequency. He recommends increasing how hard or much you work by no more than 5 to 10 percent per week to allow sufficient recovery.

▶ **Prioritize active recovery.** The hours and days in between each workout are meant to help your body repair and rebuild your muscles, with a given muscle group needing roughly 36 to 48 hours to fully recover after a hard workout. "But recovery is not just about waiting, it's about the things you do in that period to help your body recover," Machowsky says. He recommends prioritizing good sleep, balanced nutrition, as well as lower-effort movement. Research shows that low-intensity aerobic exercise such as cycling is an effective way to promote muscle strength and recovery after tough workouts. ●

....

K. Aleisha Fetters, MS, CSCS, is a freelance health journalist and certified strength and conditioning specialist. She is based in Chicago.

Food for Thought

Want to do your utmost to protect your brain from aging?
New research finds that what you eat may matter most

by **Courtney Rubin**

Everyone knows instinctively that food impacts the brain.
When you're depressed, you reach for chocolate; when you're
tired, you crave coffee. "But it seems to be taking forever to turn it
into science," says Lisa Mosconi, associate director of the Alzheimer's
Prevention Clinic at New York-Presbyterian / Weill Cornell Medical
Center and author of "Brain Food: The Surprising Science of Eating
for Cognitive Power."

Not anymore. A 2018 study Mosconi led suggests diet may be the No. 1
way to influence how your brain ages, compared to other lifestyle factors
such as exercise and intellectual-enrichment activities. And starting in your
40s or 50s – when Alzheimer's really begins – is also key, she says.

Fittingly, the brain is better protected than any other organ, thanks to
the blood-brain barrier, akin to little gates that open and close when the
brain needs a specific nutrient, such as vitamins B12 or C. If a nutrient is
essential, the brain has a gate (or receptor) for it; nutrients that are unnecessary or harmful, including cholesterol, are denied access, Mosconi
says. Historically, researchers have focused on specific nutrients when
making dietary recommendations, but no longer. "It's what you take in
total content, because there are interactions between everything," says
James Galvin, a neurologist and founding director of Florida Atlantic
University's Comprehensive Center for Brain Health. "You can't say, 'I'm
going to eat broccoli and everything will be fine.' It doesn't work like that."

So how can you eat to benefit your brain?

The simplest answer: Follow a diet that's already been shown to have
health benefits like the Mediterranean diet (whose data were recently
reanalyzed, though the findings remained the same). This plan is heavy
on fruit, vegetables, fish, legumes and whole grains, and light on dairy,
meat, poultry, saturated fat and processed foods, which are a cause
of inflammation, and thus, tissue breakdown and reduced brain
metabolism, hallmarks of cognitive decline. If the tissue
damage is sustained enough, microglia cells – the
brain's housekeepers – become activated and can
further harm the brain.

The Mediterranean diet serves up nutrients
– polyunsaturated fats, all the B vitamins – that
increase the survival of neurons in the lab and in
animal studies, Galvin explains. These nutrients

are not only building blocks for growth factors,
which encourage new neural cell growth, but also
help maintain cell membrane integrity and are
involved in sugar and protein transport and
gene expression. Two 2018 studies Mosconi
was part of found that people who ate a standard Western diet, high in processed food, fast
food, red meat and refined sugar but low in
fiber, showed a decline in brain metabolism of
about 3 percent per year while brain metabolism remained stable in the Mediterranean dieters. Western dieters also started the study
with 15 percent more amyloid plaques –
protein fragments associated with Alzheimer's – than the Mediterranean-
diet group. During the study, plaques
in the Western dieters increased by
about 2 percent yearly while the
Mediterranean dieters showed no
change in plaque buildup.

Another brain-friendly diet, called
MIND, prescribes less cheese and fish
than the Mediterranean diet and more
poultry, berries and green leafy vegetables. A 2015 study found that MIND
dieters who stuck with the plan for an
average of 4.5 years were at 53 percent
lower risk for Alzheimer's. While the
same study found that strict Mediterranean adherents were at 54
percent lower risk, people who
only moderately followed MIND
still saw a 35 percent lower risk. Loose-
ly following Mediterranean eating habits
conferred no risk reduction.

Mary Sano, director of the Alzheimer's
Disease Research Center at the Icahn School of
Medicine at Mount Sinai, cautions that there isn't

yet enough research on either diet to fully convince her of specific brain benefits. But you're unlikely to go wrong following a diet of unprocessed foods, she adds. Sano recommends keeping your weight in check versus attempting to eat for brain health. "There's some evidence that obesity has a whole set of risk factors," she says, "including potentially a cognitive one."

Before overhauling your eating plan, Rudolph Tanzi, a Harvard Medical School neurology professor and co-author of "The Healing Self" and "Super Genes," recommends first eating more fiber. The guideline is 14 grams per 1,000 calories, or roughly 25 grams per day for women and 38 per day for men. Fiber feeds the trillions of bacteria in your gut, and the gut microbiome controls the blood-brain barrier and profoundly affects the amount of those dementia-causing plaques. (The poor-quality gut microbiome in people consuming a Western diet also has been linked to obesity, coronary vascular disease, strokes, cancer and more.) How to get more fiber? Add whole grains, whole fruits and vegetables, and beans. Only after upping your fiber intake should you worry about consuming probiotics, Tanzi says. Probiotics add bacteria to the gut, but the new bacteria won't flourish without fiber. "You have to clean up the neighborhood first," says Tanzi, an author of several studies exploring how manipulating the gut microbiome impacts the brain. (He was also part of a team that figured out how to create mini-brains in petri dishes – small balls of translucent jelly full of firing human neurons – in which Alzheimer's can be replicated so drugs can be studied quickly and cheaply.) Look for a probiotic with bacteroidetes, actinobacteria and proteobacteria, he says.

Tanzi also suggests eating prebiotics – nondigestible carbohydrates that act as fertilizer for the gut bacteria. Good sources include Jerusalem artichokes, garlic, chicory, onions, asparagus, bananas, cabbage and leeks. Prebiotics can come in supplement form – many probiotics include them – but Mosconi cautions that supplements don't work as well as food. "There are so many nuances of nature you can't replicate," she says.

Another simple way to support your brain health, no matter what you eat: Drink more water – unfiltered tap, if safe and potable, or spring, both of which have necessary minerals and electrolytes. Many water filters remove key

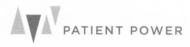

nutrients along with toxins and chemicals. (Purified water, distilled water, seltzer and club soda are fluids with no nutrients, Mosconi says.) Most people are walking around dehydrated, Mosconi explains. But the brain is 80 percent water and highly sensitive to dehydration, which can cause brain fog, fatigue and confusion. Eight glasses a day is a good benchmark, although everyone's needs are different. If you drink purified water, she advises taking mineral supplements to replace the missing – and vital – electrolytes.

It's never too late to start making changes, no matter how good or bad you think your genetic luck is. Gene expression can be influenced by myriad lifestyle factors, and what you eat is a powerful lever for switching hundreds of thousands of genes on and off. And that switch can be flipped fairly quickly, Tanzi says. It takes roughly 60 to 70 days, based on studies of mice. So what are you waiting for? ●

Weighing the Ketogenic Diet

The "keto" diet might seem like the newest thing to hit the weight-loss scene since sliced (whole-grain) bread. But it has actually been around for nearly a century – as a treatment for epilepsy.

Physicians first introduced the high-fat, low-carb eating approach in the 1920s after discovering that prolonged fasting (in which the body is forced to run off of its fat stores) reduced the frequency and intensity of seizures in epileptic patients, explains Dominic D'Agostino, an associate professor at the University of South Florida Morsani College of Medicine, who began studying ketogenic diets a decade ago as a way for the U.S. Navy to prevent seizures in underwater divers. While scientists still aren't sure exactly how the keto diet helps manage seizures, it may have other benefits, too, he says. The most popular purported perk: weight loss.

By following an extremely low-carb, high-fat diet, the body enters a state of ketosis. The liver converts fat into fatty acids and ketones, compounds the body can use for energy when it can't rely on carbs, says Eric C. Westman, director of the Duke Lifestyle Medicine Clinic. This fat includes body fat as well as dietary fat. (Hence the chorus of celebrity declarations that the diet has uncovered long-dormant abs.)

Appetite suppressant? What's more, ketones may send satiety signals to the brain, says Donald K. Layman, professor emeritus of food science and human nutrition at the University of Illinois–Urbana-Champaign. However, for ketone levels to be high enough to confer their purported weight-loss benefits, daily carb intake must be cut to about the amount in a single apple. (You read that right.) "The ketogenic diet is extremely restrictive and not sustainable for everyone," Layman says. D'Agostino adds that the

Don't Hold the Fat

A day's sample menu, served up by **Eric C. Westman,** director of the Duke Lifestyle Medicine Clinic

Breakfast
Two-egg omelet with cheese, spinach, mushrooms and tomato
Coffee (with cream)

Lunch
Lettuce-wrap bacon cheeseburger with tomato, avocado, mustard, ketchup (1-2 tsp)

Dinner
Salmon, sour cream & dill sauce, with asparagus

Dessert
Sugar-free Jell-O with a dollop of full-fat whipped cream

Snacks (if hungry)
• Full-fat string cheese
• Pepperoni, pork rinds with guacamole
• 1 serving of full-fat plain Greek yogurt with slivered almonds

original ketogenic diet required getting 85 to 90 percent of one's daily caloric intake from fat, 8 to 10 percent from protein, and as close to zero percent from carbs as possible. Current approaches have generally increased protein to about 100 to 120 grams or 20 to 30 percent of calories, but higher levels can hinder ketosis.

Ensuring ketosis involves diligent tracking of calories and macronutrients, and some followers opt to measure ketone levels with urine test strips. Because ketosis can influence how the body reacts to certain medications, anyone considering the diet should consult their doctor first, experts say. Also, without supervision by a registered dietitian, nutritional deficiencies are a real risk. Low energy levels and brain fog are common as the body adapts to using ketones for energy, and experts disagree over whether the body can perform optimally, especially during high-intensity exercise, when running on ketones. A panel of experts tied the diet in last place in U.S. News' 2018 Best Diets rankings (page 84), expressing concern over its emphasis on high-fat foods. Said one panelist: "This diet is fundamentally at odds with everything we know about long-term health."

Layman's research suggests the ketogenic diet is no more effective at spurring weight loss than similar-calorie diets that restrict daily carbs to less than 140 grams. He notes that the average American's consumption of carbohydrates, at roughly 300 grams per day, is more than double what the National Academy of Sciences states is consistent with good nutrition. And most of these carbs come from ultra-processed foods – think frozen pizza and soda – and added sugar. So, yeah, if you swear off carbs, you'll likely eat far fewer calories, he says. The result: You'll lose weight. *–K. Aleisha Fetters*

CHOSEN AGAIN
#1 HOSPITAL IN ORLANDO

Florida Hospital is recognized by *U.S. News & World* Report as one of Florida's best hospitals in 16 types of care.

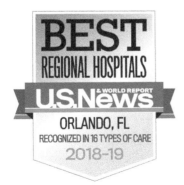

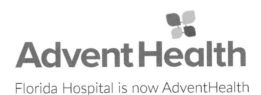

Florida Hospital is now AdventHealth

AdventHealth.com/USNews

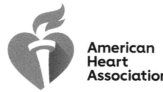

American Heart Association.

It's Time to Plan Ahead

Every 40 seconds, someone in America has a stroke or a heart attack.

Chances are it could be you or someone you love. That's why it's crucial to research the best options for receiving heart and stroke care before the time comes when you need it. Each year, the American Heart Association recognizes hospitals that demonstrate a high commitment to following guidelines that improve patient outcomes. Read more about the award categories and locate a participating hospital near you.

From 2005 to 2015 the annual death rate attributable to coronary heart disease declined 34.4 percent. The number of deaths declined 17.7 percent.

Currently, more than 2,500 hospitals participate in at least one American Heart Association quality initiative module. Many participate in two or more.

More than 7 million people have been treated through our hospital-based quality initiatives since the first one was launched in 2000.

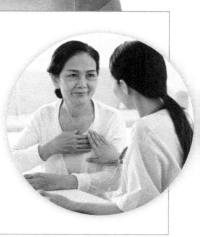

ISTOCK

Key to the Awards

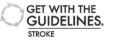 GET WITH THE **GUIDELINES.** STROKE

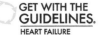 GET WITH THE **GUIDELINES.** HEART FAILURE

GET WITH THE **GUIDELINES.** RESUSCITATION

GET WITH THE **GUIDELINES.** AFIB

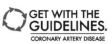 GET WITH THE **GUIDELINES.** CORONARY ARTERY DISEASE

Gold Achievement Ⓖ Ⓖ Ⓖ Ⓖ
These hospitals are recognized for two or more consecutive calendar years of 85% or higher adherence on all achievement measures applicable to each program.

Silver Achievement Ⓢ Ⓢ Ⓢ Ⓢ
These hospitals are recognized for one calendar year of 85% or higher adherence on all achievement measures applicable to each program.

Gold Plus Achievement Ⓖ⁺ Ⓖ⁺ Ⓖ⁺
These hospitals are recognized for two or more consecutive calendar years of 85% or higher adherence on all achievement measures applicable and 75% or higher adherence with additional select quality measures in heart failure, stroke and/or resuscitation.

Silver Plus Achievement Ⓢ⁺ Ⓢ⁺ Ⓢ⁺
These hospitals are recognized for one calendar year of 85% or higher adherence on all achievement measures applicable and 75% or higher adherence with additional select quality measures in heart failure, stroke, and/or resuscitation.

*These hospitals received Get With The Guidelines-Resuscitation awards for two or more patient populations.

Mission: Lifeline®
All Mission Lifeline awards used 2017 GWTG-CAD data.

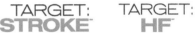 TARGET: STROKE™ TARGET: HF™

STEMI: Gold Receiving Ⓖ **or Referring** Ⓖ
These hospitals are recognized for two consecutive calendar years of 85% or higher composite adherence to all STEMI Receiving or Referring Center Performance Achievement indicators and 75% or higher compliance on each performance measure.

STEMI: Silver Receiving Ⓢ **or Referring** Ⓢ
These hospitals are recognized for one calendar year interval of 85% or higher composite adherence to all STEMI Receiving or Referring Center Performance Achievement indicators and 75% or higher compliance on each performance measure.

Target: Heart Failure ⒽⓇ **and Stroke Honor Roll** ⒽⓇ
These hospitals are recognized for at least three consecutive months of 50% or higher adherence to all relevant Target measures in addition to current Bronze, Silver or Gold Get With the Guidelines - Heart Failure or Stroke recognition status.

STEMI: Gold Plus Receving Ⓖ⁺ **or Silver Plus Receiving** Ⓢ⁺
Gold criteria plus recognized for 75% or higher achievement of First Door-to-Device time of 120 minutes or less for transferred STEMI patient for two or more consecutive years (gold plus) or one consecutive calendar year (silver plus).

NSTEMI: Gold Ⓖ **or Silver** Ⓢ
These hospitals are recognized for achieving 65% adherence to Dual Antiplatelet prescription at discharge and 75% or higher compliance on each of the other four performance measures for two consecutive calendar years (gold) or one consecutive calendar year (silver).

Honor Roll - Elite Plus Ⓔ⁺
These hospitals are recognized for at least a year of 75% or higher achievement of door-to-needle times within 60 minutes AND 50% achievement of door-to-needle times within 45 minutes in applicable stroke patients in addition to current Silver or Gold Get With The Guidelines - Stroke recognition status.

Honor Roll – Elite Ⓔ
These hospitals are recognized for at least a year of 75% or higher achievement of door-to-needle times within 60 minutes in applicable stroke patients in addition to current Silver or Gold Get With The Guidelines - Stroke recognition status.

Find Your Hospital Listed Alphabetically By State

For a searchable map of hospitals by region and across the U.S., visit heart.org/myhealthcare.

ALABAMA

Baptist Medical Center South, **Montgomery** ..... G+ HR
Brookwood Baptist Medical Center, **Birmingham** ..... G+ G+ E+
Coosa Valley Medical Center, **Sylacauga** ..... G+
Crestwood Medical Center, **Huntsville** ..... S G+ HR
Cullman Regional Medical Center, **Cullman** ..... S+ HR
Eliza Coffee Memorial Hospital, **Florence** ..... G+
Flowers Hospital, **Dothan** .....
Gadsden Regional Medical Center, **Gadsden** ..... G+ E
Grandview Medical Center, **Birmingham** ..... G+ G G+
Huntsville Hospital, **Huntsville** ..... G+ E
Marshall Medical Centers, **Guntersville** ..... S+
Mobile Infirmary, **Mobile** ..... G G G+ HR
Princeton Baptist Medical Center, **Birmingham** ..... G+ HR
Providence Hospital, **Mobile** .....
South Baldwin Regional Medical Center, **Foley** .....
Southeast Alabama Medical Center, **Dothan** ..... G+ HR
St. Vincent's Birmingham, **Birmingham** ..... G+
Thomas Hospital, **Fairhope** ..... S
UAB Hospital, **Birmingham** ..... G+ E
University of South Alabama Medical Center, **Mobile** ..... G+ HR G+ E+
Walker Baptist Medical Center, **Jasper** ..... G

ALASKA

Alaska Regional Hospital, **Anchorage** ..... G+ HR
Providence Alaska Medical Center, **Anchorage** ..... G+ E

ARIZONA

Abrazo Arrowhead Campus, **Glendale** ..... G+ E
Abrazo Central Campus, **Phoenix** ..... G+ HR
Abrazo West Campus, **Goodyear** ..... G+ HR
Banner Baywood Medical Center, **Mesa** ..... G+ E
Banner Boswell Medical Center, **Sun City** ..... G+ E
Banner Del E. Webb Medical Center, **Sun City West** ..... G+ E
Banner Desert Medical Center, **Mesa** ..... G+ E
Banner Estrella Medical Center, **Phoenix** ..... G+ E+
Banner Thunderbird Medical Center, **Glendale** ..... G+ E
Banner University Medical Center Phoenix, **Phoenix** ..... G+ E+
Banner University Medical Center Tucson, **Tucson** ..... G+ HR
Carondelet St. Mary's Hospital, **Tucson** ..... G+ E
Dignity Health-Chandler Regional Medical Center, **Chandler** ..... S+ G+ E+
Dignity Health-Mercy Gilbert Medical Center, **Gilbert** ..... G+ HR
HonorHealth Deer Valley Medical Center, **Phoenix** ..... G+ E+
HonorHealth John C. Lincoln Medical Center, **Phoenix** ..... G+ E+
HonorHealth Scottsdale Osborn Medical Center, **Scottsdale** ..... G+ E+
Mayo Clinic Hospital Arizona, **Phoenix** ..... S S+ HR G+ E+
Mountain Vista Medical Center, **Mesa** ..... G+ E
Phoenix VA Healthcare System, **Phoenix** ..... S+
Southern Arizona VA Health Care System, **Tucson** ..... G+
St. Joseph's Hospital and Medical Center, Barrow Neurological Institute, **Phoenix** ..... S+ HR G+ E+
The Carondelet Neurological Institute at St. Joseph's Hospital, **Tucson** ..... G+ E+
Tucson Medical Center, **Tucson** ..... G+ E
Yuma Regional Medical Center, **Yuma** ..... S+ E

ARKANSAS

Arkansas Heart Hospital, **Little Rock** ..... S+
Baptist Health Medical Center, **Little Rock** ..... G+ E+
Baptist Health Medical Center – Conway, **Conway** ..... S
CHI St. Vincent Hot Springs, **Hot Springs** ..... G+
CHI St. Vincent Infirmary, **Little Rock** ..... S+
Conway Regional Medical Center, **Conway** ..... S+
Five Rivers Medical Center, **Pocahontas** ..... S+ S
Forrest City Medical Center, **Forrest City** ..... S
Mercy Hospital Rogers, **Rogers** ..... G+ HR

Sparks Health System, **Fort Smith** ..... G+ HR
St. Bernards Medical Center, **Jonesboro** ..... G+
University of Arkansas for Medical Sciences, **Little Rock** ..... G+ E
Washington Regional Medical Center, **Fayetteville** ..... G+ E+

CALIFORNIA

Adventist Health Bakersfield, **Bakersfield** ..... G+ E G S
Adventist Health Glendale, **Glendale** ..... G+ E
Adventist Health Simi Valley, **Simi Valley** ..... G+ E
Adventist Health Ukiah Valley Medical Center, **Ukiah** ..... S+ HR
Adventist Health White Memorial, **Los Angeles** ..... G+ E+
Alameda Hospital, **Alameda** ..... G+ E+
Alta Bates Summit Medical Center-Summit Campus, **Oakland** ..... G+ E+
Arrowhead Regional Medical Center, **Colton** ..... G+ E
Bakersfield Heart and Surgical Hospital, **Bakersfield** ..... S
Bakersfield Memorial Hospital, **Bakersfield** ..... G+ E G
California Hospital Medical Center, **Los Angeles** ..... G+ E
California Pacific Medical Center, **San Francisco** ..... G+ E
Cedars Sinai Medical Center, **Los Angeles** ..... G+ E+
CHA Hollywood Presbyterian Medical Center, **Los Angeles** ..... G+ E+
Chino Valley Medical Center, **Chino** ..... S+
Citrus Valley Health Partners-Intercommunity Campus, **Covina** ..... G
Citrus Valley Health Partners-Queen of the Valley, **West Covina** ..... G+ E
Coast Plaza Hospital, **Norwalk** ..... S+
Community Hospital of the Monterey Peninsula, **Monterey** ..... G+ E+
Community Memorial Hospital, **Ventura** ..... G+ E+
Community Regional Medical Center, **Fresno** ..... G+ HR
Corona Regional Medical Center, **Corona** ..... G+ E+
Dameron Hospital, **Stockton** ..... S+
Desert Regional Medical Center, **Palm Springs** ..... G+ G+ G+ E+
Dignity Health dba St. Mary Medical Center, **Long Beach** ..... S
Dignity Health Dominican Hospital, **Santa Cruz** ..... G+ HR S+ E
Dignity Health Mercy General Hospital, **Sacramento** ..... G+ E
Dignity Health Mercy Hospital of Folsom, **Folsom** ..... G+ E+
Dignity Health Mercy Medical Center Merced, **Merced** ..... G+ E
Dignity Health Mercy Medical Center Redding, **Redding** ..... G+ E
Dignity Health Mercy San Juan Medical Center, **Carmichael** ..... G+ E+
Dignity Health Methodist Hospital of Sacramento, **Sacramento** ..... G+ E+
Dignity Health Northridge Hospital Medical Center, **Northridge** ..... G+ HR
Dignity Health Saint Francis Memorial Hospital, **San Francisco** ..... G+
Dignity Health Sequoia Hospital, **Redwood City** ..... G+ HR
Dignity Health St. Bernardine Medical Center, **San Bernardino** ..... G+ E+
Dignity Health St. John's Pleasant Valley Hospital, **Camarillo** ..... G+ E
Dignity Health St. John's Regional Medical Center, **Oxnard** ..... G+ E
Dignity Health St. Joseph's Medical Center, **Stockton** ..... G+ E S
Dignity Health St. Mary's Medical Center, **San Francisco** ..... G+
Dignity Health Woodland Memorial Hospital, **Woodland** ..... G+ E+
Dignity Health: Mercy Hospitals of Bakersfield, **Bakersfield** ..... G+
Doctors Hospital of Manteca, **Manteca** ..... G+
Doctors Medical Center, **Modesto** ..... G+ G+ E+ G+ S
El Camino Hospital, **Mountain View** ..... G+ E+
Enloe Medical Center, **Chico** ..... G+ E+
Fountain Valley Regional Hospital and Medical Center, **Fountain Valley** ..... G+ G+ E G+
Garfield Medical Center, **Monterey Park** ..... G+ E
Good Samaritan Hospital, **Los Angeles** ..... S+ E+
Good Samaritan Hospital, **San Jose** ..... G+ E+
Henry Mayo Newhall Hospital, **Valencia** ..... G+ HR
Hoag Memorial Hospital Presbyterian & Hoag Hospital Irvine, **Newport Beach and Irvine** ..... G+ G+ E
Huntington Hospital, **Pasadena** ..... G+ E
John F. Kennedy Memorial Hospital, **Indio** ..... G+
John Muir Medical Center – Concord, **Concord** ..... G+ G+ E+
John Muir Medical Center – Walnut Creek, **Walnut Creek** ..... G+ G+ E+
Kaiser Foundation Hospital – Antioch, **Antioch** ..... G+ E+
Kaiser Foundation Hospital – Fremont, **Fremont** ..... S G+ E+

American Heart Association.

*These hospitals received Get With The Guidelines-Resuscitation awards for two or more patient populations.

Kaiser Foundation Hospital – Fresno, **Fresno** .... G+ E+
Kaiser Foundation Hospital – Manteca, **Manteca**.......................... G
Kaiser Foundation Hospital – Modesto, **Modesto** .... S G+ E+
Kaiser Foundation Hospital – Oakland, **Oakland**.......................... S G+ E
Kaiser Foundation Hospital – Redwood City, **Redwood City** .... G+ E+
Kaiser Foundation Hospital – Richmond, **Richmond** .... G+ E+
Kaiser Foundation Hospital – Roseville, **Roseville**.......................... G+ E+
Kaiser Foundation Hospital – Sacramento, **Sacramento** .... G+ E+
Kaiser Foundation Hospital – San Francisco, **San Francisco** .... S G+ E+
Kaiser Foundation Hospital – San Jose, **San Jose** .... G+ E+
Kaiser Foundation Hospital – San Leandro, **San Leandro** .... G G+ E+
Kaiser Foundation Hospital – San Rafael, **San Rafael** .... G+ E+
Kaiser Foundation Hospital – Santa Clara, **Santa Clara** .... G G+ E+
Kaiser Foundation Hospital – Santa Rosa, **Santa Rosa** .... G+ E+
Kaiser Foundation Hospital – South Sacramento, **Sacramento**.......... G+ E+
Kaiser Foundation Hospital – South San Francisco, **South San Francisco** S G+ E+
Kaiser Foundation Hospital – Vacaville, **Vacaville**.......................... G+ E+
Kaiser Foundation Hospital – Vallejo, **Vallejo** .... S G+ E+
Kaiser Foundation Hospital – Walnut Creek, **Walnut Creek** .... G+ E+
Kaiser Foundation Hospital – West Los Angeles, **Los Angeles**.......... S+ E+
Kaiser Foundation Hospital – Zion Medical Center, **San Diego** .... G+ E+
Kaiser Foundation Hospital Orange County, **Anaheim and Irvine**.......... G+ E
Kaiser Permanente Baldwin Park Medical Center, **Baldwin Park** .... G+ G+ E+
Kaiser Permanente Downey Medical Center, **Downey** .... G+ E+
Kaiser Permanente Fontana Medical Center, **Fontana** .... G+ E+
Kaiser Permanente Moreno Valley Medical Center, **Moreno Valley**.......... G+ E+
Kaiser Permanente Ontario Medical Center, **Ontario** .... G+ E+
Kaiser Permanente Panorama City Medical Center, **Panorama City**.......... G+ E+
Kaiser Permanente Riverside Medical Center, **Riverside** .... G+ E+
Kaiser Permanente South Bay Medical Center, **Harbor City** .... G+ E+
Kaiser Permanente Woodland Hills Medical Center, **Woodland Hills** .... G+ E+
Kaiser Permanente - Los Angeles Medical Center, **Los Angeles** .... G+ E+
Kaweah Delta Health Care District, **Visalia** .... G+ HR
Keck Hospital of USC, **Los Angeles** .... S
Kern Medical, **Bakersfield** .... S
Loma Linda University Children's Hospital, **Loma Linda** .... S *
Loma Linda University Medical Center, **Loma Linda** .... S
Loma Linda University Medical Center – Murrieta, **Murrieta**.......... G+ HR
Long Beach Memorial, **Long Beach** .... G+ G+ E
Los Alamitos Medical Center, **Los Alamitos**.......... G+ HR G+ E+
Los Robles Hospital & Medical Center, **Thousand Oaks** .... G G+ E+
Lucile Packard Children's Hospital at Stanford, **Palo Alto** .... S *
Marin General Hospital, **Greenbrae** .... G+ E+
Methodist Hospital of Southern California, **Arcadia** .... G+ E
Mills-Peninsula Medical Center, **Burlingame** .... G+ HR
Mission Hospital Regional Medical Center, **Mission Viejo** .... S+ E+
NorthBay Healthcare Group, **Fairfield** .... G+ HR
O'Connor Hospital, **San Jose** .... G+ E
Orange County Global Medical Center, **Santa Ana** .... S+ E+
Oroville Hospital, **Oroville** .... G+ HR
Palmdale Regional Medical Center, **Palmdale** .... G+ E+
PIH Health Hospital – Whittier, **Whittier** .... G+ HR
Placentia-Linda Hospital, **Placentia** .... G+
Pomona Valley Hospital Medical Center, **Pomona** .... G+ G+ E+
Providence Holy Cross Medical Center, **Mission Hills** .... G+ HR
Providence Little Company of Mary Medical Center San Pedro, **San Pedro** .... G+ E
Providence Little Company of Mary Medical Center Torrance, **Torrance** .... G+ E+
Providence Saint John's Health Center, **Santa Monica** .... G+ E+
Providence Saint Joseph Medical Center, **Burbank** .... G+ E+
Providence Tarzana Medical Center, **Tarzana** .... G+ E+
Redlands Community Hospital, **Redlands** .... S G+ HR
Regional Medical Center of San Jose, **San Jose** .... G+ HR
Rideout Memorial Hospital, **Marysville** .... G+ E+
Riverside Community Hospital, **Riverside** .... G+ HR
Riverside University Health System-Medical Center, **Moreno Valley** .... G+ E+
Ronald Reagan UCLA Medical Center, **Los Angeles** .... G+ HR
Saddleback Memorial Medical Center, **Laguna Hills** .... G+ E+
Salinas Valley Memorial Healthcare System, **Salinas**.......... G+ HR G+ HR
San Antonio Regional Hospital, **Upland** .... G+ HR
San Joaquin General Hospital, **French Camp** .... G+ E+
San Ramon Regional Medical Center LLC, **San Ramon**.......... G+ G+ E
Santa Barbara Cottage Hospital, **Santa Barbara** .... S+ E+

Scripps Green Hospital, **La Jolla** .... G+
Scripps Memorial Hospital Encinitas, **Encinitas**.......................... G+ E
Scripps Memorial Hospital La Jolla, **La Jolla** .... G+ E+
Scripps Mercy Hospital, **San Diego and Chula Vista** .... G+ E
Seton Medical Center, **Daly City** .... G+ HR
Sharp Chula Vista Medical Center, **Chula Vista** .... G+ E+
Sharp Grossmont Hospital, **La Mesa** .... G+ E+
Sharp Memorial Hospital, **San Diego** .... G+ E
Sherman Oaks Hospital, **Sherman Oaks** .... G+ E+
Sierra Nevada Memorial Hospital, **Grass Valley**.......................... G+
Sierra Vista Regional Medical Center, **San Luis Obispo** .... G+
Southwest Healthcare Systems: Inland Valley Medical Center &
    Rancho Springs Medical Center, **Wildomar and Murrieta** .... G+ HR
St. Jude Medical Center, **Fullerton** .... G+ E+
St. Louise Regional Hospital, **Gilroy** .... G+ E
Stanford Health Care, **Stanford** .... HR
Sutter Health Eden Medical Center, **Castro Valley** .... G+ E+
Sutter Health Memorial Medical Center, **Modesto** .... G+ E
Sutter Medical Center Sacramento, **Sacramento** .... G+ HR
Sutter Novato Community Hospital, **Novato** .... S+ E+
Sutter Santa Rosa Regional Hospital, **Santa Rosa** .... G+ E+
Temecula Valley Hospital, **Temecula**.......................... G+ E
Torrance Memorial Medical Center, **Torrance**.......... G+ HR G G+ E G+
Tri-City Medical Center, **Oceanside** .... G+ HR G+ E G S
Twin Cities Community Hospital, **Templeton** .... G+
UC Davis Medical Center, **Sacramento** .... G+ HR
UC San Diego Health-Jacobs Medical Center, **La Jolla** .... S+ E+
UC San Diego Health-UC San Diego Medical Center, **San Diego** .... G+ E+
UCLA Santa Monica Medical Center, **Santa Monica** .... G+ HR
University of California Irvine Medical Center, **Orange**.......... G+ HR G+ E+
University of California San Francisco (UCSF) Medical Center,
    San Francisco .... G+ E+
USC Norris Cancer Hospital, **Los Angeles** .... S+
USC Verdugo Hills Hospital, **Glendale** .... G+
Ventura County Medical Center/Santa Paula Hospital, **Ventura** .... G+
Verity St. Francis Medical Center, **Lynwood** .... G+ E
Washington Hospital Healthcare System, **Fremont** .... G+ E+
Watsonville Community Hospital, **Watsonville** .... S

COLORADO

Avista Adventist Hospital, **Louisville**.......................... S+
Boulder Community Health Foothills Hospital, **Boulder**.......................... G+ E+
Castle Rock Adventist Hospital, **Castle Rock** .... S+
Denver Health Medical Center, **Denver** .... S
Littleton Adventist Hospital, **Littleton** .... G+ E+
North Suburban Medical Center, **Thornton** .... G+ E+
Parker Adventist Hospital, **Parker** .... G+ E+
Parkview Medical Center, **Pueblo** .... S+ E+
Penrose Hospital, **Colorado Springs** .... G G+ E
Platte Valley Medical Center, **Brighton** .... G+ E
Porter Adventist Hospital-Centura Health, **Denver**.......................... G+ E+
Presbyterian/St. Luke's Medical Center, **Denver** .... G+
Rose Medical Center, **Denver** .... G+ E
SCL Health-Good Samaritan Medical Center, **Lafayette** .... G+ E+
SCL Health-Lutheran Medical Center, **Wheat Ridge**.......................... G+ E+
SCL Health-Saint Joseph Hospital, **Denver** .... S+ HR
SCL Health-St. Mary's Medical Center, **Grand Junction** .... G+ E
Sky Ridge Medical Center, **Lone Tree** .... S+ E+
St. Anthony Hospital, **Lakewood** .... S+ HR G+ E+ G
St. Anthony North Hospital, **Westminster**.......... S+ HR G+ E+
St. Francis Medical Center, **Colorado Springs** .... G+ HR
Swedish Medical Center, **Englewood**.......................... S+ HR
The Medical Center of Aurora, **Aurora** .... G+ E
UCHealth Medical Center of the Rockies, **Loveland** .... G HR G+ E+
UCHealth Memorial Hospital Central, **Colorado Springs** .... S+ G+ E+
UCHealth Poudre Valley Hospital, **Fort Collins** .... G+ HR G+ E+
UCHealth University of Colorado Hospital, **Aurora**.......... S G+ HR G+ E+

CONNECTICUT

Bridgeport Hospital, **Bridgeport** .... G+ E
Connecticut Children's Medical Center, **Hartford**.......................... S

 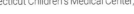

American Heart Association.

© 2018 American Heart Association

(CONNECTICUT CONTINUED)

Danbury Hospital, Part of the Western Connecticut Health Network, **Danbury** ...... S+ S+
Eastern Connecticut Health Network, Manchester and Rockville, **Manchester** ...... G HR
Greenwich Hospital, **Greenwich** ...... G G+ E+
Hartford Hospital, **Hartford** ...... G+ E+ S
Lawrence + Memorial Hospital, **New London** ...... S+ E+
MidState Medical Center, **Meriden** ...... G+ E+
Norwalk Hospital, **Norwalk** ...... S+ HR
Saint Francis Hospital and Medical Center, **Hartford** ...... G+ HR S+
St. Vincent's Medical Center, **Bridgeport** ...... G+ HR G+ E
Stamford Hospital, **Stamford** ...... G+ E G
The Hospital of Central Connecticut, **New Britain** ...... G+ E+ G+
UCONN Health / John Dempsey Hospital, **Farmington** ...... G+ HR G+ E G
Waterbury Hospital, **Waterbury** ...... G+ S
Yale-New Haven Hospital, **New Haven** ...... G+ E

DELAWARE

Bayhealth Medical Center Milford Memorial, **Milford** ...... S+
Bayhealth Medical Center-Kent General Hospital, **Dover** ...... G+ S+ HR S
Beebe Healthcare, **Lewes** ...... G+ G+
Christiana Care Health Services, Inc., **Newark** ...... G+ G+ E+ G
Nanticoke Memorial Hospital, **Seaford** ...... G+ G+ HR
Saint Francis Hospital, **Wilmington** ...... HR

DISTRICT OF COLUMBIA

Howard University Hospital ...... G+ HR
MedStar Georgetown University Hospital ...... S+ HR
MedStar Washington Hospital Center ...... G+ E
Providence Hospital ...... G+
Sibley Memorial Hospital ...... G+ E
The George Washington University Hospital ...... G+ E

FLORIDA

Arnold Palmer Hospital for Children, **Orlando** ...... G+ S+
Aventura Hospital and Medical Center, **Aventura** ...... G+ E+
Baptist Hospital of Miami, **Miami** ...... G+ E+
Baptist Medical Center – Beaches (Baptist Health), **Jacksonville Beach** ...... G+ E
Baptist Medical Center – Jacksonville (Baptist Health), **Jacksonville** ...... G+ E+
Baptist Medical Center – South (Baptist Health), **Jacksonville** ...... G+ E+
Bay Medical Center-Sacred Heart Health System, **Panama City** ...... S+ E S+
Bayfront Health Punta Gorda, **Punta Gorda** ...... S+
Bayfront Health St. Petersburg, **St. Petersburg** ...... G+ E+
Boca Raton Regional Hospital, **Boca Raton** ...... G+ E+
Brandon Regional Hospital, **Brandon** ...... G+ E+
Broward Health Coral Springs, **Coral Springs** ...... G+ E+
Broward Health Medical Center, **Fort Lauderdale** ...... G+ E+
Broward Health North, **Pompano Beach** ...... S+
Cape Canaveral Hospital, **Cocoa Beach** ...... S+
Cape Coral Hospital, **Cape Coral** ...... G+ E+
Capital Regional Medical Center, **Tallahassee** ...... G+ E
Cleveland Clinic Florida, **Weston** ...... G+ E
Coral Gables Hospital, **Miami** ...... G+
Delray Medical Center, **Delray Beach** ...... G+ E+
Doctors Hospital of Sarasota, **Sarasota** ...... G+ S
Dr. P. Phillips Hospital, **Orlando** ...... G+ E+
Englewood Community Hospital, **Englewood** ...... G+ HR G+ E+
Flagler Hospital, Inc., **Saint Augustine** ...... G
Florida Hospital Altamonte, **Altamonte Springs** ...... G+ E+
Florida Hospital Apopka, **Apopka** ...... G+
Florida Hospital Celebration Health, **Celebration** ...... G+ E+
Florida Hospital Dade City, **Dade City** ...... S+ HR
Florida Hospital DeLand, **DeLand** ...... G+ E+
Florida Hospital East Orlando, **Orlando** ...... G+ HR
Florida Hospital Fish Memorial, **Orange City** ...... G+ E+
Florida Hospital Flagler, **Palm Coast** ...... G+ E+
Florida Hospital Kissimmee, **Kissimmee** ...... G+ E+
Florida Hospital Memorial Medical Center, **Daytona Beach** ...... G+ E+
Florida Hospital New Smyrna, **New Smyrna Beach** ...... G+ E+
Florida Hospital North Pinellas, **Tarpon Springs** ...... G+

Florida Hospital Orlando, **Orlando** ...... G+ E+
Florida Hospital Tampa, **Tampa** ...... G+ E+
Florida Hospital Wesley Chapel, **Wesley Chapel** ...... G+ E
Florida Hospital Zephyrhills, **Zephyrhills** ...... G+ E G
FLORIDA MEDICAL CENTER a campus of North Shore, **Fort Lauderdale** ...... G+ E+
Fort Walton Beach Medical Center, **Fort Walton Beach** ...... G+ HR
Good Samaritan Medical Center, **West Palm Beach** ...... G+ E+
Gulf Coast Medical Center, **Fort Myers** ...... G+ E+
Halifax Health, **Daytona Beach** ...... G+ E+
Health Park Medical Center, **Fort Myers** ...... G+ E+
Hialeah Hospital, **Hialeah** ...... G+
Holmes Regional Medical Center, **Melbourne** ...... G+ HR
Holy Cross Hospital, **Fort Lauderdale** ...... G+ HR G+ G+
Indian River Medical Center, **Vero Beach** ...... G+ HR G+ E
Jackson Memorial Hospital, **Miami** ...... G+ E+
Jackson North Medical Center, **North Miami Beach** ...... G+ E+
James A. Haley Veterans' Hospital, **Tampa** ...... S+
JFK Medical Center, **Atlantis** ...... S+ E+
Jupiter Medical Center, **Jupiter** ...... G+
Lakeland Regional Health, **Lakeland** ...... G+ HR
Lakewood Ranch Medical Center, **Bradenton** ...... G+ E S
Largo Medical Center, **Largo** ...... G S+ HR G+ E G
Lee Memorial Hospital, **Fort Myers** ...... G+ E+
Manatee Memorial Hospital, **Bradenton** ...... G+ E G
Mease Countryside Hospital, **Safety Harbor** ...... G+ E S
Mease Dunedin Hospital, **Dunedin** ...... G+ E
Memorial Hospital, **Jacksonville** ...... S+ G+ E+
Memorial Hospital Pembroke, **Pembroke Pines** ...... G+
Memorial Hospital West, **Pembroke Pines** ...... G+ E+
Memorial Regional Hospital, **Hollywood** ...... G+ E+
Mercy Hospital, **Miami** ...... G+ HR
Morton Plant Hospital, **Clearwater** ...... G+ E
Morton Plant North Bay Hospital, **New Port Richey** ...... G+ S
Mount Sinai Medical Center, **Miami Beach** ...... S+ HR G+ E+
Munroe Regional Medical Center, **Ocala** ...... S+ HR
NCH Healthcare System, **Naples** ...... G+ E+
Nicklaus Children's Hospital, **Miami** ...... G+ *
North Florida Regional Medical Center, **Gainesville** ...... G+ E+
North Shore Medical Center, **Miami** ...... G+ E+
Northside Hospital and Tampa Bay Heart Institute, **St. Petersburg** ...... G+ HR G+ E+ G+
Ocala Health, **Ocala** ...... G+ E+
Orange Park Medical Center, **Orange Park** ...... G G G+ G+ E+ G
Orlando Regional Medical Center, **Orlando** ...... G+ E+
Osceola Regional Medical Center, **Kissimmee** ...... G+ E+
Palm Bay Hospital, **Palm Bay** ...... S+
Palm Beach Gardens Medical Center, **Palm Beach Gardens** ...... G+ HR G+ E+
Palmetto General Hospital, **Hialeah** ...... G+ G+ E+
Palms of Pasadena Hospital, **South Pasadena** ...... G+ E+ G
Physicians Regional Healthcare System, **Naples** ...... G+ E+
Sacred Heart Health System, **Pensacola** ...... S+ HR G+ HR
Sarasota Memorial Health Care System, **Sarasota** ...... G+ HR G+ E+
South Florida Baptist Hospital, **Plant City** ...... G+ E+
South Seminole Hospital, **Longwood** ...... S+ HR
St. Anthony's Hospital, **St. Petersburg** ...... G+ E G
St. Joseph's Hospital, **Tampa** ...... G+ E
St. Joseph's Hospital – North, **Lutz** ...... G+ E G
St. Joseph's Hospital – South, **Riverview** ...... G+ E+
St. Mary's Medical Center, **West Palm Beach** ...... G+ E+
St. Vincent's Medical Center Riverside, **Jacksonville** ...... G+ HR
St. Vincent's Medical Center Southside, **Jacksonville** ...... G+ HR E+
Tallahassee Memorial HealthCare, **Tallahassee** ...... G+ E
Tampa Community Hospital, **Tampa** ...... G+ E+
Tampa General Hospital, **Tampa** ...... G+ E+
UF Health Shands Hospital, **Gainesville** ...... G+ HR
University of Miami Hospital, **Miami** ...... G+ E+
Venice Regional Bayfront Health, **Venice** ...... G+ E+
Wellington Regional Medical Center, **Wellington** ...... G+ HR
West Boca Medical Center, **Boca Raton** ...... G+ HR G+ E+
West Florida Hospital, **Pensacola** ...... G+ E+
West Kendall Baptist Hospital, **Miami** ...... G+ HR
Westside Regional Medical Center, **Plantation** ...... S+ E+

© 2018 American Heart Association

American Heart Association.

*These hospitals received Get With The Guidelines-Resuscitation awards for two or more patient populations.

Winter Haven Hospital, **Winter Haven** .... S+ E
Winter Park Memorial Hospital, **Winter Park** .... G+ E
Wuesthoff Medical Center Rockledge, **Rockledge** .... G+ E+

GEORGIA

AU Medical Center, **Augusta** .... G+ E+
Candler Hospital, **Savannah** ....
Cartersville Medical Center, **Cartersville** .... G+ HR
Coliseum Medical Centers, **Macon** .... G HR
DeKalb Medical, **Decatur** .... G+ HR
Dekalb Medical Hillandale, **Lithonia** .... G+
Doctors Hospital Augusta, **Augusta** .... G+ E+
Eastside Medical Center, **Snellville** .... S+ E
Emory Johns Creek Hospital, **Duluth** .... S+ E G G
Emory Saint Joseph's Hospital, **Atlanta** .... G+ E G S
Emory University Hospital, **Atlanta** .... G+ E+ G S
Emory University Hospital Midtown, **Atlanta** .... G+ HR S S
Fairview Park Hospital, **Dublin** .... G+
Floyd Medical Center, **Rome** .... G HR G+ E+
Grady Health System, **Atlanta** .... G+ HR E+ G
Gwinnett Medical Center, **Lawrenceville** .... G+ E+ G+ S
Hamilton Medical Center, **Dalton** .... G HR
Meadows Regional Medical Center, **Vidalia** .... G HR
Medical Center Navicent Health, **Macon** .... G+ E+
Memorial Health University Medical Center, **Savannah** ..... G+ HR G+ E
Midtown Medical Center, **Columbus** .... G+ E+
Northeast Georgia Medical Center, **Gainesville** .... G+ E+
Northeast Georgia Medical Center Braselton, **Braselton** ...... S+ HR
Northside Hospital Atlanta, **Atlanta** .... G+ G+ E+ G S
Northside Hospital Cherokee, **Canton** .... G+ G+ E+ G S
Northside Hospital Forsyth, **Cumming** .... HR G G E+ G G
Phoebe Putney Memorial Hospital, **Albany** .... G+ E
Piedmont Athens Regional Medical Center, **Athens** .... G+ E+
Piedmont Fayette Hospital, **Fayetteville** .... G+ E+
Piedmont Henry Hospital, **Stockbridge** .... G+ E
Piedmont Hospital, **Atlanta** .... G+ E
Piedmont Newnan Hospital, **Newnan** .... G+ E
Piedmont Rockdale Hospital, **Conyers** .... G+ HR
Polk Medical Center, **Cedartown** .... G+ HR
Redmond Regional Medical Center, **Rome** .... G+ HR G+ E+
South Georgia Medical Center, **Valdosta** .... G G+ E+
Southern Regional Medical Center, **Riverdale** .... S+ E+ S S
St. Francis Hospital, Inc., **Columbus** .... G+ E+
St. Joseph's Hospital, **Savannah** .... G+ E
St. Mary's Health Care System, **Athens** .... G G+ HR
Tanner Medical Center/Carrollton, **Carrollton** .... S+
Tanner Medical Center/Villa Rica, **Villa Rica** ....
University Hospital, **Augusta** .... G+ S+ E
WellStar Atlanta Medical Center, **Atlanta** .... G+
WellStar Cobb Hospital, **Austell** .... G+ E
WellStar Douglas Hospital, **Douglasville** .... S+
WellStar Kennestone Hospital, **Marietta** .... G+ E+
WellStar North Fulton Hospital, **Roswell** .... G+ G+ E+
WellStar Spalding Regional Hospital, **Griffin** .... G+ E

HAWAII

Adventist Health Castle Medical Center, **Kailua** .... G+
Kaiser Foundation Hospital-Moanalua Medical Center, **Honolulu** .... G+ G+ S+
Kuakini Medical Center, **Honolulu** .... S
Maui Memorial Medical Center, **Wailuku** .... G+ HR G+ HR
Pali Momi Medical Center, **Aiea** .... G+ E+
Straub Medical Center, **Honolulu** .... G+ HR
The Queen's Medical Center at Punchbowl, **Honolulu** ...... S G+ E+
The Queen's Medical Center West Oahu, **Ewa Beach** .... G+ E+
Wahiawa General Hospital, **Wahiawa** ....
Wilcox Medical Center, **Lihue** .... G+ E

IDAHO

Eastern Idaho Regional Medical Center, **Idaho Falls** .... G+ E+ G+
Kootenai Health, **Coeur d'Alene** .... G
St. Luke's Boise and Meridian Medical Centers, **Boise** ...... G+

ILLINOIS

Advocate BroMenn Medical Center, **Normal** .... G+ E
Advocate Christ Medical Center, **Oak Lawn** .... G+ E G
Advocate Condell Medical Center, **Libertyville** .... G+ E
Advocate Good Samaritan Hospital, **Downers Grove** .... G+ HR S
Advocate Good Shepherd Hospital, **Barrington** .... G+ E+
Advocate Illinois Masonic Medical Center, **Chicago** .... G+ E+
Advocate Lutheran General Hospital, **Park Ridge** .... G+ E
Advocate Sherman Hospital, **Elgin** .... S+ HR G+ HR
Advocate South Suburban Hospital, **Hazel Crest** .... G+ E
Advocate Trinity Hospital, **Chicago** .... G+ E
Amita Alexian Brothers Medical Center, **Elk Grove Village** .... G+ E
Amita Health Adventist Medical Center La Grange, **La Grange** .... S+ E+
Amita St. Alexius Medical Center, **Hoffman Estates** .... G+ E
Carle Foundation Hospital, **Urbana** .... S G+ E+
Centegra Hospital – Huntley, **Huntley** .... S+ E
Centegra Hospital – McHenry, **McHenry** .... G+ E
Centegra Hospital – Woodstock, **Woodstock** .... G+
Decatur Memorial Hospital, **Decatur** .... G+ E
Edward Hospital, **Naperville** .... G+ E
Elmhurst Hospital, **Elmhurst** .... HR
FHN Memorial Hospital, **Freeport** .... G+
Herrin Hospital, **Herrin** .... G G+ HR
Holy Cross Hospital, **Chicago** .... G+ HR
HSHS St. Elizabeth's Hospital, **Belleville** .... S+ HR
HSHS St. John's Hospital, **Springfield** .... G+ HR G+ E+
Little Company of Mary Hospital and Health Care Centers,
   Evergreen Park .... S+ E G
Loyola University Medical Center, **Maywood** .... G+ E
MacNeal Hospital, **Berwyn** .... G+ HR
Memorial Hospital of Carbondale, **Carbondale** .... G G HR G+ HR G+
Memorial Medical Center, **Springfield** .... G+ G+ E+
Mercy Hospital & Medical Center, **Chicago** .... G+
Mercyhealth Hospital-Rockton Avenue, **Rockford** .... G+ HR
MetroSouth Medical Center, **Blue Island** .... G+ E
Mount Sinai Hospital, **Chicago** .... G HR S
Northwest Community Hospital, **Arlington Heights** .... G+ E
Northwestern Medicine Central DuPage Hospital, **Winfield** .... S+ HR G+ E+
Northwestern Medicine Delnor Hospital, **Geneva** .... S+ HR S G+ E
Northwestern Medicine Lake Forest Hospital, **Lake Forest** ... G+ HR
Northwestern Memorial Hospital, **Chicago** .... G+ E+
OSF HealthCare Saint Anthony's Health Center, **Alton** ..... S+ E
OSF Saint Anthony Medical Center, **Rockford** .... G+ E+
OSF Saint Francis Medical Center, **Peoria** .... G+ E+
OSF St. Joseph Medical Center, **Bloomington** .... G+ HR
Palos Community Hospital, **Palos Heights** ....
Presence Resurrection Medical Center, **Chicago** .... G+ E S
Presence Saint Francis Hospital, **Evanston** .... G+ E
Presence Saint Joseph Hospital – Elgin, **Elgin** .... G
Presence Saint Joseph Hospital Chicago, **Chicago** .... G+ HR
Presence Saints Mary and Elizabeth Medical Center, **Chicago** .... S+ HR
Riverside Medical Center, **Kankakee** .... G+ E
Rush Copley Medical Center, **Aurora** .... G G+ HR G S
Rush Oak Park Hospital, **Oak Park** .... G+ E
Rush University Medical Center, **Chicago** .... G+ E+
Silver Cross Hospital, **New Lenox** .... G+ HR
SSM Health Good Samaritan, **Mount Vernon** .... S+
SSM Health St. Mary's Hospital, **Centralia** .... S+
Swedish American a Division of UW Health, **Rockford** ...... G+ E
Trinity Medical Center, **Rock Island** .... S+
UChicago Medicine, **Chicago** .... G+ HR
UI Health Hospital & Clinics, **Chicago** .... G+ HR G+ E+
UnityPoint Health-Proctor, **Peoria** .... S+ E
UnityPoint Methodist, **Peoria** .... G G+ S G+
West Suburban Medical Center, **Oak Park** .... S

INDIANA

Baptist Health Floyd, **New Albany** .... G+ E+
Community Hospital – North, **Indianapolis** .... S+ E
Community Hospital East, **Indianapolis** .... S+

(INDIANA CONTINUED)

Hospital	Awards
Community Hospital of Anderson, **Anderson**	G+ HR
Community Hospital South, **Indianapolis**	S+ HR
Community Hospital, Community Healthcare System, **Munster**	S+ HR
Deaconess, **Evansville**	S+ HR
Elkhart General Hospital, **Elkhart**	S HR
Franciscan Health Indianapolis, **Indianapolis**	G+ HR E+
Franciscan Health Lafayette East, **Lafayette**	HR
Franciscan Health Michigan City, **Michigan City**	G+
Indiana University Health Ball Memorial Hospital, **Muncie**	
Indiana University Health Methodist Hospital, **Indianapolis**	S+ G+ E+
IU Health Bloomington Hospital, **Bloomington**	G+
IU Health West Hospital, **Avon**	G+ HR
Lutheran Hospital, **Fort Wayne**	G+ E
Memorial Hospital, **South Bend**	S+ HR
Memorial Hospital and Health Care Center, **Jasper**	S+ E
Methodist Hospitals, Inc., **Gary**	G+ E+
Parkview Health, **Fort Wayne**	G+ E+
Porter Regional Hospital, **Valparaiso**	G+ S
St. Catherine Hospital, Inc., **East Chicago**	G+ HR
St. Mary Medical Center, **Hobart**	G+ HR
St. Vincent Anderson Regional Hospital, **Anderson**	S+
St. Vincent Evansville, **Evansville**	S+ E
Union Hospital, **Terre Haute**	S+ HR

IOWA

Hospital	Awards
Allen Hospital, **Waterloo**	S+ S
Genesis Medical Center, **Davenport**	S+ E G+ S
Iowa Methodist, **Des Moines**	S
Mary Greeley Medical Center, **Ames**	S
Mercy Iowa City, **Iowa City**	G+ HR
Mercy Medical Center – Des Moines, **Des Moines**	G+ E
Mercy Medical Center – Dubuque, **Dubuque**	G+ HR S S
Mercy Medical Center – North Iowa, **Mason City**	S
Mercy Medical Center – Sioux City, **Sioux City**	G+ S+ E+ G G
Methodist Jennie Edmunson, **Council Bluffs**	S S
UnityPoint Health Trinity Regional Medical Center, **Fort Dodge**	S
UnityPoint Health-St. Luke's, **Sioux City**	G G
UnityPoint Health-St. Luke's Hospital, **Cedar Rapids**	G+ S
University of Iowa Hospitals and Clinics, **Iowa City**	G+ E

KANSAS

Hospital	Awards
Hays Med, **Hays**	G+ E+
Hutchinson Regional Medical Center, **Hutchinson**	G+ E+
Lawrence Memorial Hospital, **Lawrence**	G+ G+ E+
Menorah Medical Center, **Overland Park**	G+ E+
Olathe Medical Center, **Olathe**	G+ E
Providence Medical Center, **Kansas City**	S+ HR
Saint Catherine Hospital, **Garden City**	G+ E+
Saint Luke's South Hospital, **Overland Park**	G+ E+
Salina Regional Health Center, **Salina**	G+ E+
Shawnee Mission Medical Center, **Shawnee Mission**	G+ G+ E G+
Stormont-Vail HealthCare, **Topeka**	G+ HR G+ G+ G
The University of Kansas Health System, **Kansas City**	G+ HR G+ E+
The University of Kansas Health System St. Francis Campus, **Topeka**	G+ HR
Via Christi Hospital Pittsburg, **Pittsburg**	S+ E
Via Christi Hospital St. Francis, **Wichita**	G+ E
Wesley Medical Center, **Wichita**	G+ HR

KENTUCKY

Hospital	Awards
Baptist Health LaGrange, **LaGrange**	G+
Baptist Health Lexington, **Lexington**	G+ HR G+ E+
Baptist Health Louisville, **Louisville**	G+ E+
Jewish Hospital, **Louisville**	G+ HR G+
King's Daughters Medical Center, **Ashland**	G+ HR
Lake Cumberland Regional Hospital, **Somerset**	G+ HR
Norton Audubon Hospital, **Louisville**	S+ E G
Norton Brownsboro Hospital, **Louisville**	G+ E G
Norton Hospital, **Louisville**	S+
Norton Women's and Kosair Children's Hospital, **Louisville**	S+
Owensboro Health Regional Hospital, **Owensboro**	S+ HR

Hospital	Awards
Paul B. Hall Regional Medical Center, **Paintsville**	G+
Pikeville Medical Center, **Pikeville**	G+ E
Saint Joseph Hospital, **Lexington**	G+ E
St. Elizabeth Edgewood, **Edgewood**	G HR G+
St. Elizabeth Florence, **Florence**	G G HR G+ HR
St. Elizabeth Ft. Thomas, **Fort Thomas**	G G
Sts. Mary and Elizabeth Hospital, **Louisville**	G+ E+
The Medical Center at Bowling Green, **Bowling Green**	S+ E
TriStar Greenview Regional Hospital, **Bowling Green**	S+
University of Kentucky Hospital, **Lexington**	G G+ E+
University of Louisville Hospital, **Louisville**	G+ E+

LOUISIANA

Hospital	Awards
East Jefferson General Hospital, **Metairie**	G+ HR
Lakeview Regional Medical Center, a campus of Tulane Medical Center, **Covington**	G+
Leonard J. Chabert Medical Center, **Houma**	G+
Ochsner Medical Center – Kenner, **Kenner**	S+ E+
Ochsner Medical Center – New Orleans, **New Orleans**	G+ E
Our Lady of Lourdes Regional Medical Center, **Lafayette**	G+ E+
Our Lady of the Lake Regional Medical Center, **Baton Rouge**	G+
Rapides Regional Medical Center, **Alexandria**	G+ S G+ E
Slidell Memorial Hospital, **Slidell**	G+ HR
St. Francis Medical Center, **Monroe**	S HR
St. Tammany Parish Hospital, **Covington**	S+ G+ E
Touro Infirmary, **New Orleans**	S+ E+
Tulane University Hospital and Clinic, **New Orleans**	G G+ E+
University Health, **Shreveport**	S E+
University Medical Center New Orleans (UMCNO), **New Orleans**	G+ E
West Jefferson Medical Center, **Marrero**	G+ E

MAINE

Hospital	Awards
Central Maine Medical Center, **Lewiston**	G+
Eastern Maine Medical Center, **Bangor**	G+ E+
Maine Medical Center, **Portland**	G
MaineGeneral Medical Center, **Augusta**	S+ E
Mercy Hospital, EMHS member, **Portland**	G+
Pen Bay Medical Center, **Rockport**	G+ HR
St. Mary's Regional Medical Center, **Lewiston**	G+
The Aroostook Medical Center (TAMC), **Presque Isle**	S+
York Hospital, **York**	G

MARYLAND

Hospital	Awards
Adventist HealthCare Shady Grove Medical Center, **Rockville**	G+ E+ S+
Anne Arundel Medical Center, **Annapolis**	G+ E G+
Calvert Memorial Hospital, **Prince Frederick**	G+
Carroll Hospital Center, **Westminster**	S+ E
Doctor's Community Hospital, **Lanham**	G+ E
Greater Baltimore Medical Center, **Baltimore**	G+ HR
Holy Cross Germantown Hospital, **Germantown**	G+ HR
Holy Cross Hospital, **Silver Spring**	G+ E+ S
Howard County General Hospital, **Columbia**	G+ E
Johns Hopkins Bayview Medical Center, **Baltimore**	G+ E+
MedStar Franklin Square Medical Center, **Baltimore**	G+ E+ G
MedStar Good Samaritan Hospital, **Baltimore**	G+
MedStar Montgomery Medical Center, **Olney**	G+
MedStar Southern Maryland Hospital Center, **Clinton**	G+ E
MedStar Union Memorial Hospital, **Baltimore**	G+ E S+ S
Meritus Medical Center, **Hagerstown**	S
Northwest Hospital, **Randallstown**	G+ E+
Peninsula Regional Medical Center, **Salisbury**	G+ HR
Saint Agnes Hospital, **Baltimore**	G+ E+
Sinai Hospital of Baltimore, **Baltimore**	G+ E+ S
Suburban Hospital Johns Hopkins Medicine, **Bethesda**	G+ E
The Johns Hopkins Hospital, **Baltimore**	G+ S+ * G+ HR
Union Hospital of Cecil County, **Elkton**	G+ E
University of Maryland Baltimore Washington Medical Center, **Glen Burnie**	S+ E G
University of Maryland Charles Regional Medical Center, **La Plata**	G+ E
University of Maryland Harford Memorial Hospital, **Havre De Grace**	G+ E
University of Maryland Medical Center, **Baltimore**	G+ HR S

American Heart Association.

*These hospitals received Get With The Guidelines-Resuscitation awards for two or more patient populations.

University of Maryland Prince George's Hospital Center, **Cheverly** .... G+ E S
University of Maryland Shore Medical Center at Easton, **Easton** .... G+ HR
University of Maryland St. Joseph Medical Center, **Towson** .... S+ E+ G+ S
University of Maryland Upper Chesapeake Medical Center, **Bel Air** .... G+ E
Washington Adventist Hospital, **Takoma Park** .... G+ E S
Western Maryland Health System, **Cumberland** .... G+ E S S

MASSACHUSETTS

Addison Gilbert Hospital, **Gloucester** .... G+
Baystate Franklin Medical Center, **Greenfield** .... G+ HR
Baystate Medical Center, **Springfield** .... G+ E+
Baystate Noble Hospital, **Westfield** .... S+
Berkshire Medical Center, **Pittsfield** .... G G+ HR G G+ E
Beth Israel Deaconess Hospital – Milton, **Milton** .... S+ HR
Beth Israel Deaconess Hospital – Needham, **Needham** .... S+
Beth Israel Deaconess Hospital – Plymouth, **Plymouth** .... G+ HR
Beth Israel Deaconess Medical Center, **Boston** .... G+ HR S+ G+ E
Beverly Hospital, **Beverly** .... G+ HR
Boston Children's Hospital, **Boston** .... S ★ S+
Boston Medical Center, **Boston** .... G+ HR
Brigham and Women's Faulkner Hospital, **Boston** .... G S
Brigham and Women's Hospital, **Boston** .... S+ E+
Carney Hospital, **Dorchester Center** .... G+
Cooley Dickinson Hospital, **Northampton** .... G+ HR
Emerson Hospital, **Concord** .... G+
Falmouth Hospital, member Cape Cod Healthcare, **Falmouth** .... G+
Good Samaritan Medical Center, **Brockton** .... S HR S+
Holyoke Medical Center, **Holyoke** .... G+ E+
Lahey Hospital & Medical Center, Burlington, **Burlington** .... G+ G+ E
Lawrence Memorial Hospital, **Medford** .... S+
Lowell General Hospital-Main Campus, **Lowell** .... S+ E
Lowell General Hospital-Saints Campus, **Lowell** .... G+ E+
Massachusetts General Hospital, **Boston** .... G+
Melrose-Wakefield Hospital, **Melrose** .... G+
Mercy Medical Center, **Springfield** .... G+ HR
MetroWest Medical Center-Framingham Union Hospital, **Framingham** .. G+ G+ HR S+
MetroWest Medical Center-Leonard Morse Hospital, **Natick** .... G+
Milford Regional Medical Center, **Milford** .... G+
Mount Auburn Hospital, **Cambridge** .... G+ E+
Nashoba Valley Medical Center, **Ayer** .... G+
Newton-Wellesley Hospital, **Newton** .... S G+ HR G+ E+
North Shore Medical Center-Salem Hospital, **Salem** .... G+
North Shore Medical Center-Union Hospital, **Lynn** .... G+
Norwood Hospital, A Steward Family Hospital, **Norwood** .... G+ HR
Saint Anne's Hospital, **Fall River** .... G+
Saint Vincent Hospital, **Worcester** .... G+ E+
Signature Healthcare Brockton Hospital, **Brockton** .... S+ HR E+
South Shore Hospital, **South Weymouth** .... G
Southcoast Health Charlton Memorial Hospital, **Fall River** .... G+ HR
Southcoast Health St. Luke's Hospital, **New Bedford** .... S+ E+
Steward St. Elizabeth's Medical Center, **Brighton** .... G+ HR S+ E+
Sturdy Memorial Hospital, **Attleboro** .... G+ HR G
Tufts Medical Center, **Boston** .... S G+ E+
UMass Memorial Medical Center, **Worcester** .... G G+ E+
UMass Memorial-Marlborough Hospital, **Worcester** .... S+

MICHIGAN

Ascension St. John Hospital, **Detroit** .... S+ E
Beaumont Hospital, Grosse Pointe, **Grosse Pointe** .... G+
Beaumont Hospital, Troy, **Troy** .... G HR
Borgess Medical Center, **Kalamazoo** .... G+ HR
Bronson Methodist Hospital, **Kalamazoo** .... G+ E+
Covenant HealthCare, **Saginaw** .... G+ E
DMC Detroit Receiving Hospital, **Detroit** .... G+ E
Genesys Regional Medical Center, **Grand Blanc** .... G+ E
Henry Ford Hospital and Health Network, **Detroit** .... G+ HR
Henry Ford West Bloomfield Hospital, **West Bloomfield** .... S+ E
Hurley Medical Center, **Flint** .... G+ E
Lakeland Healthcare, **Saint Joseph** .... G+ E
McLaren – Flint, **Flint** .... S+ E
McLaren Greater Lansing, **Lansing** .... S+ E

McLaren Macomb, **Mount Clemens** .... S+ E
McLaren Northern Michigan, **Petoskey** .... G+ E+
Mercy Health Saint Mary's, **Grand Rapids** .... G+ HR G+ E+
Metro Health-University of Michigan Health, **Wyoming** .... G+ HR
Munson Medical Center, **Traverse City** .... S+ E
ProMedica Monroe Regional Hospital, **Monroe** .... S+ E
Sparrow Hospital, **Lansing** .... G+ E
Spectrum Health Grand Rapids, **Grand Rapids** .... S+ E+
St. Joseph Mercy Ann Arbor, **Ypsilanti** .... G+ E+
St. Joseph Mercy Livingston Hospital, **Ann Arbor** .... G+
St. Joseph Mercy Oakland, **Pontiac** .... G+ E+
St. Mary's of Michigan, **Saginaw** .... S+ E
University of Michigan Health System, **Ann Arbor** .... S+ G+ E+

MINNESOTA

CentraCare St. Cloud Hospital, **Saint Cloud** .... G+ G+ ★ G+ E+ G
Essentia Health East. St. Mary's Medical Center, **Duluth** .... G+ HR G+ E+
Essentia Health-St. Joseph's Medical Center, **Brainerd** .... S+
Fairview Lakes Hospital, **Wyoming** .... S+
Fairview Northland Hospital, **Princeton** .... S+
Fairview Range Hospital, **Hibbing** .... G+ HR
Fairview Southdale Hospital, **Edina** .... G+ G+ E+
Hennepin County Medical Center, **Minneapolis** .... G+ E+
Mayo Clinic Hospital, Saint Marys Campus, **Rochester** .... G+ E+
Mercy Hospital, **Coon Rapids** .... G+
North Memorial Health Hospital, **Robbinsdale** .... G+ E
Olmsted Medical Center, **Rochester** .... S+
Park Nicollet Methodist Hospital, **Saint Louis Park** .... G+ G+ E S+
Regions Hospital, **Saint Paul** .... G+ E
St. Luke's, **Duluth** .... G+ E G G
University of Minnesota Heart Care at Fairview Ridges Hospital, **Burnsville** ...... G+
University of Minnesota Medical Center, **Minneapolis** .... G+ HR

MISSISSIPPI

Baptist Memorial Hospital – DeSoto, **Southaven** .... G+ E
Baptist Memorial Hospital – North Mississippi, **Oxford** .... S+
Forrest General Hospital, **Hattiesburg** .... G+ HR
Gilmore Memorial Hospital, **Amory** .... S
Memorial Hospital at Gulfport, **Gulfport** .... S+ E+
Merit Health Wesley, **Hattiesburg** .... G+ HR G+
Methodist Olive Branch Hospital, **Olive Branch** .... S+
MS Baptist Medical Center, **Jackson** .... G+ HR G+ E+
Ocean Springs Hospital (Singing River Health System), **Ocean Springs** .... G+ E
OCH Regional Medical Center, **Starkville** .... G+ HR
River Oaks Hospital, **Jackson** .... G+ HR
Singing River Hospital (Singing River Health System), **Pascagoula** .... G+ E
St. Dominic Memorial Hospital, **Jackson** .... G+ E
University of Mississippi Health Care, **Jackson** .... G+ E

MISSOURI

Barnes-Jewish Hospital, **St. Louis** .... S+ HR G+ E+ G
Barnes-Jewish St. Peters Hospital, **Saint Peters** .... G+
Belton Regional Medical Center, **Belton** .... G+ E
Boone Hospital, **Columbia** .... G+ E+ S S
Capital Region Medical Center, **Jefferson City** .... S+ E
Centerpoint Medical Center, **Independence** .... G+ HR G+ E
Cox Medical Center Branson, **Branson** .... G+ E
Cox Monett Hospital, **Monett** .... S+
CoxHealth, **Springfield** .... G+ E+
Lake Regional Hospital, **Osage Beach** .... G+ E
Liberty Hospital, **Liberty** .... G+ HR S S
Mercy Hospital Jefferson, **Crystal City** .... S+ HR
Mercy Hospital Joplin, **Joplin** .... S
Mercy Hospital Springfield, **Springfield** .... G+ E
Mercy Hospital St. Louis, **St. Louis** .... G+ E
Mosaic Life Care, **Saint Joseph** .... G+ E
Phelps County Regional Medical Center, **Rolla** .... G+ E
Poplar Bluff Regional Medical Center, **Poplar Bluff** .... S+
Progress West Hospital, **O'Fallon** .... G+ E
Research Medical Center, **Kansas City** .... G+ HR G+ E+
Saint Luke's East Hospital, **Lees Summit** .... G+ E

American Heart Association.

(MISSOURI CONTINUED)

Saint Luke's Hospital of Kansas City, **Kansas City** ... G+ HR G+ E+ G
Saint Luke's North Hospital, **Kansas City** ... G+ E G
Southeast Health, **Cape Girardeau** ... S+ HR S
SSM Health DePaul Hospital, **Bridgeton** ... G+ E+
SSM Health Saint Louis University Hospital, **St. Louis** ... G+ E+
SSM Health St. Clare Hospital, **Fenton** ... G+ E+
SSM Health St. Joseph Hospital – St. Charles, **Saint Charles** ... G+ HR
SSM Health St. Mary's Hospital, **St. Louis** ... G+ E+
SSM St. Joseph Hospital Lake St. Louis, **Lake St Louis** ... G+ HR
St. Anthony's Medical Center, **St. Louis** ... G+ HR G+ E+
St. Luke's Des Peres Hospital, **St. Louis** ...
St. Luke's Hospital, **Chesterfield** ... S+ HR
St. Mary's Medical Center, **Blue Springs** ... S+ G+ E+
University of Missouri Health Care, **Columbia** ... G+ HR

MONTANA

Benefis Health System, **Great Falls** ... G+ HR S+
Billings Clinic, **Billings** ... G
Bozeman Health Deaconess Hospital, **Bozeman** ... S+ S
Kalispell Regional Medical Center, **Kalispell** ... S+ HR G+ S+ S
Providence St. Patrick Hospital, **Missoula** ... G S G+ E S S

NEBRASKA

CHI Health Good Samaritan Hospital, **Kearney** ... G+ HR
CHI Health St. Elizabeth, **Lincoln** ... G+ G+ E
Faith Regional Health Services, **Norfolk** ... S+ E+
Great Plains Health, **North Platte** ... G+ E+ S S
Nebraska Medicine, **Omaha** ... G+ E+
Nebraska Medicine – Bellevue, **Bellevue** ... G+ HR
Nebraska Methodist Hospital, **Omaha** ... S+ HR
Regional West Medical Center, **Scottsbluff** ... S+ E+

NEVADA

Centennial Hills Hospital Medical Center, **Las Vegas** ... G+ E S
Desert Springs Hospital Medical Center, **Las Vegas** ... G+ E
Dignity Health St. Rose Dominican Hospital-Rose de Lima Campus,
  Henderson ... S G+
Dignity Health St. Rose Dominican Hospital-San Martin Campus,
  Las Vegas ... S+ HR S
Dignity Health St. Rose Dominican Hospital-Siena Campus,
  Henderson ... G+ HR G+
Henderson Hospital, **Henderson** ... S+
MountainView Hospital, **Las Vegas** ... G HR
Northern Nevada Medical Center, **Sparks** ... G+ E S S
Renown Regional Medical Center, **Reno** ... G G+ E
Saint Mary's Regional Medical Center, **Reno** ... S+ HR G+ E+
Southern Hills Hospital, **Las Vegas** ... G+
Spring Valley Hospital Medical Center, **Las Vegas** ... G+ E G+
Summerlin Hospital Medical Center, **Las Vegas** ... G+ HR S
Sunrise Hospital & Medical Center, **Las Vegas** ... G+ E+
University Medical Center of Southern Nevada, **Las Vegas** ... S S+ E
Valley Hospital Medical Center, **Las Vegas** ... G+ E+ S

NEW HAMPSHIRE

Catholic Medical Center, **Manchester** ... G+ E
Concord Hospital, **Concord** ... G+ HR
Dartmouth-Hitchcock Medical Center, **Lebanon** ... G G+ S G+ E+
Elliot Health System, **Manchester** ... S
Exeter Hospital, **Exeter** ... S
Parkland Medical Center, **Derry** ... S+ HR
Portsmouth Regional Hospital, **Portsmouth** ... G+ E
Southern New Hampshire Medical Center, **Nashua** ... G+
St. Joseph Hospital, **Nashua** ... S+ G+ E
Wentworth-Douglass Hospital, **Dover** ... S+

NEW JERSEY

Capital Health Medical Center – Hopewell, **Pennington** ... G+ E+
Capital Health Regional Medical Center, **Trenton** ... G+ E+
CarePoint Health – Bayonne Medical Center, **Bayonne** ... G+ G
CarePoint Health – Christ Hospital, **Jersey City** ... G+ HR G+ S+

CarePoint Health – Hoboken University Medical Center, **Hoboken** ... G+
CentraState Medical Center, **Freehold** ... S+ HR G+ E
Chilton Medical Center, **Pompton Plains** ... G+ E+
Cooper University Health Care, **Camden** ... S+ E
Deborah Heart and Lung Center, **Browns Mills** ... HR
Hackensack Meridian Health Bayshore Medical Center, **Holmdel** ... G+ E
Hackensack Meridian Health Hackensack University Medical Center,
  Hackensack ... G+ E+
Hackensack Meridian Health Jersey Shore University Medical Center,
  Neptune ... G+ G+ E
Hackensack Meridian Health JFK Medical Center, **Edison** ... G+ E
Hackensack Meridian Health Mountainside Medical Center, **Montclair** ... G+
Hackensack Meridian Health Ocean Medical Center, **Brick** ... G+ G+ E+
Hackensack Meridian Health Palisades Medical Center,
  North Bergen ... G+ HR G+ E
Hackensack Meridian Health Raritan Bay Medical Center,
  Perth Amboy and Old Bridge ... S+ HR
Hackensack Meridian Health Riverview Medical Center, **Red Bank** ... G+ G+ E+
Hackensack Meridian Health Southern Ocean Medical Center,
  Manahawkin ... G+ HR
Hackettstown Medical Center, **Hackettstown** ... S+ E+
Holy Name Medical Center, **Teaneck** ... S G+
Inspira Medical Center Elmer, **Elmer** ... G
Inspira Medical Center Vineland, **Vineland** ... G+
Inspira Medical Center Woodbury, **Woodbury** ... G
Jefferson Cherry Hill Hospital, **Cherry Hill** ... G+ E
Jefferson Stratford Hospital, **Stratford** ... G+ E
Jefferson Washington Township Hospital, **Turnersville** ... G+ E+
Jersey City Medical Center-Barnabas Health, **Jersey City** ... G+ HR
Monmouth Medical Center, **Long Branch** ... G+ E
Morristown Medical Center, **Morristown** ... G+ E
Newark Beth Israel Medical Center, **Newark** ... G
Newton Medical Center, **Newton** ... G+ E+
Our Lady of Lourdes Medical Center, **Camden** ... G+ HR
Overlook Medical Center, **Summit** ... G+ E
Penn Medicine Princeton Medical Center, **Plainsboro** ... S+
Robert Wood Johnson University Hospital, **New Brunswick** ... G+ E
Robert Wood Johnson University Hospital Hamilton, **Hamilton** ... G+ G+ HR
Robert Wood Johnson University Hospital Somerset, **Somerville** ... G+ E
Saint Clare's Denville Hospital, **Denville** ... G+
Saint Clare's Hospital, **Denville and Dover** ... G+ E
Saint Peter's University Hospital, **New Brunswick** ... G+ HR
St. Francis Medical Center, **Trenton** ... G+
St. Joseph's University Medical Center, **Paterson** ... S G+ E G+
St. Joseph's Wayne Hospital, **Wayne** ... S+ HR
St. Luke's Warren Hospital, **Phillipsburg** ... G+
The Valley Hospital, **Ridgewood** ... G G+ E
Trinitas Regional Medical Center, **Elizabeth** ... S
University Hospital, **Newark** ... G+ HR G+ E

NEW MEXICO

Lovelace Medical Center, **Albuquerque** ... S+ HR G+ HR
Presbyterian Hospital, **Albuquerque** ... S+ E+ G+ G
University of New Mexico Hospitals, **Albuquerque** ... G+ HR G+ E+ G

NEW YORK

Albany Med, **Albany** ... G+ HR S+ * G+
Albany Memorial Hospital, **Albany** ... G+
Arnot Ogden Medical Center, **Elmira** ... G+ E+
Auburn Community Hospital, **Auburn** ... G+
Bassett Medical Center, **Cooperstown** ... G G+ E
BronxCare Health System, **Bronx** ... G G+ HR G+ E G G
Brookdale University Hospital Medical Center, **Brooklyn** ... G+ E+
Brookhaven Memorial Hospital Medical Center, **Patchogue** ... G+ E+
Catholic Health-Kenmore Mercy Hospital, **Buffalo** ... G+
Catholic Health-Mercy Hospital of Buffalo, **Buffalo** ... G+
Catholic Health-Mount St. Mary's Hospital, **Lewiston** ... G+
Catholic Health-Sisters of Charity Hospital, Sisters of Charity St. Joseph
  Campus, **Buffalo** ... S+
Catskill Regional Medical Center, **Harris** ... G+
Cohen Children's Medical Center, **New Hyde Park** ... G+

American Heart Association.

Columbia Memorial Hospital, **Hudson** ...... G+

Crouse Hospital, **Syracuse** ...... G+ G+ E+ G

Ellis Hospital, **Schenectady** ...... G+ E+

Erie County Medical Center, **Buffalo** ...... G+ HR G+

F.F. Thompson Hospital, **Canandaigua** ...... G+ HR

Faxton St. Luke's Healthcare, an affiliation of Mohawk Valley Health System,
Utica ...... E

Flushing Hospital Medical Center, **Flushing** ...... G+ HR

Gates Vascular Institute / Buffalo General Medical Center, **Buffalo** ...... G+ E+

Geneva General Hospital, **Geneva** ...... G+

Glen Cove Hospital, **Glen Cove** ...... G+ E+

Good Samaritan Hospital Medical Center, **West Islip** ...... G+

Good Samaritan Hospital, a Member of WMC Health Network, **Suffern** ...... G+ E

Guthrie Corning Hospital, **Corning** ...... G+ E

HealthAlliance: Broadway Campus a Member of the WMC Health Network,
Kingston ...... G+ HR

Highland Hospital, **Rochester** ...... G+ G+

Huntington Hospital, **Huntington** ...... G+ E

Jamaica Hospital Medical Center, **Richmond Hill** ...... S+ G+ E S

John T. Mather Memorial Hospital, **Port Jefferson** ...... G+ E

Kingsbrook Jewish Medical Center, **Brooklyn** ...... G+ HR

Lenox Hill Hospital, **New York** ...... G+ E+

LIJ Medical Center at Forest Hills, **Forest Hills** ...... G+ E

LIJ Valley Stream, **Valley Stream** ...... G+ E

Long Island Jewish Medical Center, **New Hyde Park** ...... G+ E+

Maimonides Medical Center, **Brooklyn** ...... G+ E+

Mercy Medical Center, **Rockville Centre** ...... G+ HR

MidHudson Regional Hospital a Member of the WMC Health Network,
Poughkeepsie ...... G+

Millard Fillmore Suburban Hospital, **Williamsville** ...... S+

Montefiore Medical Center, **Bronx** ...... S

Montefiore Mount Vernon Hospital, **Mount Vernon** ...... G+

Montefiore New Rochelle Hospital, **New Rochelle** ...... S+ HR

Mount Sinai Beth Israel, **New York** ...... G+ HR G+ E+ G

Mount Sinai Brooklyn, **Brooklyn** ...... S+

Mount Sinai Queens, **Astoria** ...... G+ E

Mount Sinai Saint Luke's Hospital, **New York** ...... S+

Mount Sinai St. Luke's & Mount Sinai West, **New York** ...... G+ E

Nassau University Medical Center, **East Meadow** ...... G+ HR G+ E

New York Community Hospital, **Brooklyn** ...... G+ HR

New-York Presbyterian/Hudson Valley Hospital, **Cortlandt Manor** ...... G+ E

Newark–Wayne Community Hospital, **Newark** ...... G+ E

NewYork-Presbyterian Brooklyn Methodist Hospital, **Brooklyn** ...... G+ E+ G

NewYork-Presbyterian Queens, **Flushing** ...... G+ E+ G

NewYork-Presbyterian/Columbia University Medical Center, **New York** ...... G+ E+

NewYork-Presbyterian/Lawrence Hospital, **Bronxville** ...... G+ G+ HR

NewYork-Presbyterian/Lower Manhattan Hospital, **New York** ...... G+ E+

NewYork-Presbyterian/The Allen Hospital, **New York** ...... G+ E+

NewYork-Presbyterian/Weill Cornell Medical Center, **New York** ...... G+ E+

Niagara Falls Memorial Medical Center, **Niagara Falls** ...... G+

North Shore University Hospital, **Manhasset** ...... G+ E+

Northern Dutchess Hospital, **Rhinebeck** ...... S+

Northern Westchester Hospital, **Mount Kisco** ...... G+

Nyack Hospital, **Nyack** ...... G+ E

NYC Health + Hospitals/Bellevue, **New York** ...... G+ HR G G+ E+ G S

NYC Health + Hospitals/Coney Island, **Brooklyn** ...... G+ E+

NYC Health + Hospitals/Elmhurst, **Elmhurst** ...... G+ E+

NYC Health + Hospitals/Harlem, **New York** ...... G+

NYC Health + Hospitals/Jacobi, **Bronx** ...... G+ E+

NYC Health + Hospitals/Kings County, **Brooklyn** ...... G+ S G+ E

NYC Health + Hospitals/Lincoln, **Bronx** ...... S+ G+ E+

NYC Health + Hospitals/Metropolitan, **New York** ...... G+ HR

NYC Health + Hospitals/North Central Bronx, **Bronx** ...... G+ HR

NYC Health + Hospitals/Woodhull, **Brooklyn** ...... G+ S+

NYU Langone Hospital – Brooklyn, **Brooklyn** ...... G+ E+

NYU Langone Tisch Hospital, **New York** ...... G+ G+ E+ G

NYU Winthrop Hospital, **Mineola** ...... S+ G+ E+

Olean General Hospital, Member: Upper Allegheny Health System, **Olean** ...... S+

Orange Regional Medical Center, **Middletown** ...... G+ E

Our Lady of Lourdes Memorial Hospital, **Binghamton** ...... G+

Peconic Bay Medical Center, **Riverhead** ...... G+ E+

Phelps Hospital, **Sleepy Hollow** ...... G+ E+

Plainview Hospital, **Plainview** ...... G+ E

Putnam Hospital Center, **Carmel** ...... G+

Richmond University Medical Center, **Staten Island** ...... G+ E+

Rochester General Hospital, **Rochester** ...... G+ E+

Rome Memorial Hospital, **Rome** ...... S

Saint Joseph's Medical Center, **Yonkers** ...... G+

Samaritan Hospital, **Troy** ...... S+ E

Saratoga Hospital, **Saratoga Springs** ...... S+

SBH Health System, **Bronx** ...... G+ E

South Nassau Communities Hospital, **Oceanside** ...... G+ HR G+ E

Southampton Hospital, **Southampton** ...... G+ E

Southside Hospital, **Bay Shore** ...... G+ E+ G

St. Catherine of Siena Medical Center, **Smithtown** ...... G+ E

St. Charles Hospital, **Port Jefferson** ...... G+

St. Francis Hospital, The Heart Center, **Roslyn** ...... G+ HR G+ E

St. John's Episcopal Hospital, **Far Rockaway** ...... G+ E+

St. John's Riverside Hospital, **Yonkers** ...... G+

St. Joseph Hospital, **Bethpage** ...... G+ E+

St. Luke's Cornwall Hospital, **Newburgh** ...... G+ E+

St. Peter's Hospital, **Albany** ...... G+ G+ E S+

Staten Island University Hospital, **Staten Island** ...... G+ E+

Stony Brook University Hospital, **Stony Brook** ...... S+ G S G+ E

Syosset Hospital, **Syosset** ...... G+ E+

The Brooklyn Hospital Center, **Brooklyn** ...... G+ HR G+ E

The Mount Sinai Hospital, **New York** ...... S+ HR E S

UHS Wilson Medical Center, **Johnson City** ...... G+ HR

United Memorial Medical Center, **Batavia** ...... S+

Unity Hospital, **Rochester** ...... G+ E

University Hospital of Brooklyn-SUNY Downstate Medical Center, **Brooklyn** ...... G+

Upstate University Hospital, **Syracuse** ...... G+ G+ E+

UR Medicine Strong Memorial Hospital, **Rochester** ...... G+ HR G+ G+ E+ G

Vassar Brothers Medical Center, **Poughkeepsie** ...... G+ HR

Westchester Medical Center, **Valhalla** ...... G+

White Plains Hospital, **White Plains** ...... G+ E S

Wyckoff Heights Medical Center, **Brooklyn** ...... G+ E+

NORTH CAROLINA

Angel Medical Center, **Franklin** ...... G+ E+

Cape Fear Valley Medical Center, **Fayetteville** ...... G+ G+ G S+ G+ E G+

CarolinaEast Medical Center, **New Bern** ...... S

Carolinas HealthCare System Blue Ridge – Morganton, **Morganton** ...... S+ E

Carolinas HealthCare System Cleveland, **Shelby** ...... G+ E

Carolinas HealthCare System Kings Mountain, **Kings Mountain** ...... G+

Carolinas HealthCare System NorthEast, **Concord** ...... G+ E+ G+ G

Carolinas HealthCare System Pineville, **Charlotte** ...... G+ E+ G+ G

Carolinas HealthCare System Stanly, **Albemarle** ...... G+ E

Carolinas HealthCare System Union, **Monroe** ...... G+ E

Carolinas HealthCare System University, **Charlotte** ...... G+ HR

Carolinas Medical Center, **Charlotte** ...... G+ E+ G+ G

Carolinas Medical Center – Mercy, **Charlotte** ...... S

CaroMont Regional Medical Center, **Gastonia** ...... G+ HR G+ E

Carteret Health Care Medical Center, **Morehead City** ...... G+ HR G+ G+

Columbus Regional Healthcare, **Whiteville** ...... G+ HR

Cone Health, **Greensboro** ...... G+ G+ E+ S+

Cone Health-Alamance Regional, **Burlington** ...... S

Duke Raleigh Hospital, **Raleigh** ...... G+ E

Duke Regional Hospital, **Durham** ...... G+ E

Duke University Hospital, **Durham** ...... G+ HR G+ E+

Durham VA HealthCare System, **Durham** ...... S+

FirstHealth of the Carolinas Moore Regional Hospital, **Pinehurst** ...... G+ E+

Frye Regional Medical Center, **Hickory** ...... G+ HR G+ HR G+ S

High Point Regional UNC Health Care, **High Point** ...... S+ E+

Hugh Chatham Memorial Hospital, **Elkin** ...... G+ E+

Iredell Memorial Hospital, **Statesville** ...... G+

Mission Hospital McDowell, **Marion** ...... S+ HR

Mission Hospitals, Inc., **Asheville** ...... G+ E+

Nash UNC Health Care, **Rocky Mount** ...... G+ HR G G

New Hanover Regional Medical Center, **Wilmington** ...... G+ E+ G+ G

Novant Health Brunswick Medical Center, **Bolivia** ...... G+

 American Heart Association.

© 2018 American Heart Association

(NORTH CAROLINA CONTINUED)

Novant Health Forsyth Medical Center, **Winston-Salem**............ G+ HR G+ G+
Novant Health Huntersville Medical Center, **Huntersville**............ S+ HR G+ G
Novant Health Matthews Medical Center, **Matthews**............ HR G+ E+
Novant Health Presbyterian Medical Center, **Charlotte**............ G+ HR G+ E+ G
Novant Health Rowan Medical Center, **Salisbury**............ G+ HR G+ HR S
Novant Health Thomasville Medical Center, **Thomasville**............ G+
Onslow Memorial Hospital, **Jacksonville**............ S S+
Pardee UNC Health Care, **Hendersonville**............ S
UNC Hospitals, **Chapel Hill**............ G+ E+ G+ G
UNC Lenoir Health Care, **Kinston**............ S+
UNC REX Healthcare, **Raleigh**............ G+ E G
Vidant Medical Center, **Greenville**............ G+ HR S S+ HR G G
Wake Forest Baptist Medical Center, **Winston-Salem**............ S+ G+ E+
WakeMed Cary Hospital, **Cary**............ S+ E
WakeMed Health & Hospitals-Raleigh Campus, **Raleigh**............ S HR G+ E+
Wayne UNC Health Care, **Goldsboro**............ S+ G+ HR

NORTH DAKOTA

Altru Health System, **Grand Forks**............ G+ E+ S
CHI St. Alexius Health Bismarck, **Bismarck**............ G+ E S
Essentia Health, **Fargo**............ G+ HR
Sanford Bismarck Medical Center, **Bismarck**............ G+ E G S
Sanford Medical Center Fargo, **Fargo**............ S+ E+ G S
Trinity Health, **Minot**............ G+ E+ S

OHIO

Adena Health System, **Chillicothe**............ S+ E
Alliance Community Hospital, **Alliance**............ S
Ashtabula County Medical Center, **Ashtabula**............ G+
Atrium Medical Center, **Franklin**............ G+ E G
Aultman Hospital, **Canton**............ G+ HR G+ HR G+
Cincinnati Children's, **Cincinnati**............ S
Cleveland Clinic, **Cleveland**............ G+ S+ *
Cleveland Clinic Akron General, **Akron**............ G+ E+
Euclid Hospital, **Euclid**............ S+ E
Fairfield Medical Center, **Lancaster**............ G+ E
Fairview Hospital, **Cleveland**............ G+ E+
Fisher Titus Medical Center, **Norwalk**............ S+ E
Genesis Healthcare System, **Zanesville**............ S G+ G+ E
Good Samaritan Hospital, **Dayton**............ G+ E+
Hillcrest Hospital, **Mayfield Heights**............ G+ E+
Kettering Medical Center, **Dayton**............ G+ E+
Licking Memorial Hospital, **Newark**............ G G
Louis Stokes Cleveland VA Medical Center, **Cleveland**............ S+ HR
Marymount Hospital, **Garfield Heights**............ G+ E+
Medina Hospital, **Medina**............ G+ HR
Mercy Health Clermont Hospital, **Batavia**............ S+
Mercy Health-Anderson Hospital, **Cincinnati**............
Mercy Health-Fairfield Hospital, **Fairfield**............ G
Mercy Health-St. Elizabeth Youngstown Hospital, **Youngstown**............ G+ HR G+ E+
Mercy Medical Center, **Canton**............ G+ HR G+
Miami Valley Hospital, **Dayton**............ G+ E+
Mount Carmel Health System, **Columbus**............ G+ E
Mount Carmel St. Ann's, **Westerville**............ G+ E
OhioHealth Marion General Hospital, **Marion**............ S G+ HR
OhioHealth Riverside Methodist Hospital, **Columbus**............ G+ E
ProMedica Flower Hospital, **Sylvania**............ G+ E
ProMedica Toledo Hospital, **Toledo**............ G+ E+
Southwest General Health Center, **Middleburg Heights**............ G+ S+ E+ G+ G
St. Luke's Hospital, **Maumee**............ S+ E
Summa Health Akron City Hospital, **Akron**............ G+ E+
Sycamore Medical Center, **Miamisburg**............ G+
The Jewish Hospital Mercy Health, **Cincinnati**............ S+ E
The MetroHealth System, **Cleveland**............ G+ G+ HR G+
The Ohio State University Wexner Medical Center, **Columbus**............ S G+ E
The University of Toledo Medical Center, **Toledo**............ G+ G+ E
UH Regional Hospitals, Bedford Medical Center and
   Richmond Medical Center, **Richmond Heights**............ G+
Union Hospital, **Dover**............ G+ HR
University Hospitals Cleveland Medical Center, **Cleveland**............ G+ E+

University Hospitals Elyria Medical Center, **Elyria**............ G+ E
University Hospitals Geauga Medical Center, **Chardon**............ G+ E+
University Hospitals Parma Medical Center, **Parma**............ S+ E
University Hospitals St. John Medical Center, **Cleveland**............ S+ E
University of Cincinnati Medical Center, **Cincinnati**............ G+ HR G+ G+
West Chester Hospital, **West Chester**............ G+ S
West Hospital, **Cincinnati**............ HR G+
Western Reserve Hospital, **Cuyahoga Falls**............ G+ HR G+

OKLAHOMA

Hillcrest Medical Center, **Tulsa**............ G+ E+
INTEGRIS Baptist Medical Center, **Oklahoma City**............ G+ E+
INTEGRIS Southwest Medical Center, **Oklahoma City**............ G+ E
McAlester Regional Health Center, **McAlester**............ S+ E
Mercy Hospital Oklahoma City Comprehensive Stroke Center,
   Oklahoma City............ G+ E+
Norman Regional Health System, **Norman**............ S+ E+ S+ S
Saint Francis Hospital, **Tulsa**............ G+ E+
St. Anthony Hospital, **Oklahoma City**............ S+ HR
St. John Medical Center, **Tulsa**............ G+ E+
Stillwater Medical Center, **Stillwater**............ S+ E

OREGON

Asante Rogue Regional Medical Center, **Medford**............ G+
Good Samaritan Regional Medical Center, **Corvallis**............ G+ HR
Kaiser Foundation Hospital Westside, **Hillsboro**............ G+
Kaiser Sunnyside Medical Center, **Clackamas**............ G+ HR
Legacy Emanuel Medical Center, **Portland**............ G+ E
Legacy Good Samaritan Medical Center, **Portland**............ G+ E
Legacy Meridian Park Medical Center, **Tualatin**............ G+ E
Legacy Mount Hood Medical Center, **Gresham**............ G+ E
Oregon Health & Science University, **Portland**............ G+ HR G+ G+
PeaceHealth Sacred Heart Medical Center RiverBend, **Springfield**............ G+ E+
Providence Hood River Memorial Hospital, **Hood River**............ S+
Providence Medford Medical Center, **Medford**............ G+ E+ G
Providence Newberg Medical Center, **Newberg**............ S+ E G
Providence Portland Medical Center, **Portland**............ G+ E+ S+
Providence Seaside Hospital, **Seaside**............ S+
Providence St. Vincent Medical Center, **Portland**............ G+ E+ G
Providence Willamette Falls Medical Center, **Oregon City**............ G+ E+
Samaritan Albany General Hospital, **Albany**............ S+ HR
Samaritan Lebanon Community Hospital, **Lebanon**............ S+ HR
Samaritan Pacific Communities Hospital, **Newport**............ S+
Sky Lakes Medical Center, **Klamath Falls**............ G+ HR
St. Charles Medical Center – Bend, **Bend**............ G S+ E
Tuality Healthcare, **Hillsboro**............ G+ HR

PENNSYLVANIA

Abington Health-Abington Memorial Hospital, **Abington**............ G+ G+ E+ G+
Allegheny General Hospital, **Pittsburgh**............ G G+ HR G+ E+
Allegheny Valley Hospital, **Natrona Hts**............ S+ HR
Aria Health, **Philadelphia**............ G+ E+ G+
Bryn Mawr Hospital, **Bryn Mawr**............ G+ HR S+
Butler Memorial Hospital, **Butler**............ G+ HR
Carlisle Regional Medical Center, **Carlisle**............ G+ E
Chambersburg Hospital, **Chambersburg**............ HR G+ HR
Chester County Hospital, **West Chester**............ E S
Chestnut Hill Hospital, **Philadelphia**............ G+ E
Conemaugh Valley Memorial Hospital, **Johnstown**............ G G+ E
Crozer-Chester Medical Center, **Upland**............ G+ E
Delaware County Memorial Hospital, **Drexel Hill**............ G
Doylestown Hospital, **Doylestown**............ G+ HR G+ G+ E+ G+
Einstein Medical Center – Philadelphia, **Philadelphia**............ G+ E+ G+
Einstein Medical Center Montgomery, **East Norriton**............ G+ E
Evangelical Community Hospital, **Lewisburg**............ G+ HR
Excela Health Latrobe, **Latrobe**............ S+ HR
Excela Health Westmoreland, **Greensburg**............ S+
Forbes Hospital, **Monroeville**............ S+ HR G+ E
Geisinger Community Medical Center, **Scranton**............ G+ E+ G
Geisinger Holy Spirit, **Camp Hill**............ G G+ G+ HR G+

© 2018 American Heart Association

American Heart Association.

*These hospitals received Get With The Guidelines-
Resuscitation awards for two or more patient populations.

Geisinger Medical Center, **Danville** .... G+ E+ G+
Geisinger Wyoming Valley, **Wilkes Barre** .... G+ E G
Grand View Health, **Sellersville** .... G+ HR S+ G+
Hahnemann University Hospital, **Philadelphia** .... G+ G+ E+
Hanover Hospital, **Hanover** .... G+ HR
Heritage Valley Beaver, **Beaver** .... G+ E+
Heritage Valley Sewickley, **Sewickley** .... S+
Holy Redeemer Hospital, **Meadowbrook** .... G+ G
Jeanes Hospital-Temple University Health System, **Philadelphia** .... G+
Jefferson Hospital, **Clairton** .... G+ HR G+
Lancaster General Hospital, **Lancaster** .... G+ E
Lancaster Regional Medical Center, **Lancaster** ..... G+ HR
Lankenau Medical Center, **Wynnewood** .... G+ G
Lansdale Hospital, **Lansdale** .... G+ E
Lehigh Valley Health Network Cedar Crest, **Allentown** ...... G+ E
Lehigh Valley Health Network Muhlenberg, **Bethlehem** ...... G+
Lehigh Valley Hospital – Hazleton, **Hazleton** .... HR G+
Lower Bucks Hospital, **Bristol** .... S+
Mercy Fitzgerald Hospital, **Darby** .... G G+
Mercy Philadelphia Hospital, **Philadelphia** .... G G+
Monongahela Valley Hospital, **Monongahela** .... S G+ G+ E S
Mount Nittany Medical Center, **State College** .... G+ E
Nazareth Hospital, **Philadelphia** .... HR G+ HR
Paoli Hospital, **Paoli** .... G+ E
Penn Highlands DuBois, **DuBois** .... G+ E
Penn Presbyterian Medical Center, **Philadelphia** ... S+ G+ E+ S+
Penn State Hershey Medical Center, **Hershey** .... G+ HR G+ E+
Pennsylvania Hospital, **Philadelphia** .... G+ E+
Phoenixville Hospital, **Phoenixville** .... G+
Pinnacle Health System-West Shore Hospital, **Mechanicsburg** ...... G+
Pocono Medical Center, **East Stroudsburg** .... G+ HR
Pottstown Memorial Medical Center, **Pottstown** .... G+ E+
Reading Hospital, **West Reading** .... G+ HR G+ E G
Regional Hospital of Scranton, **Scranton** .... G+ HR
Riddle Hospital, **Media** .... G+ HR
Robert Packer Hospital, **Sayre** .... S+
Roxborough Memorial Hospital, **Philadelphia** ...... G+ HR
Sacred Heart Hospital, **Allentown** .... G+ HR
Saint Vincent Health System, **Erie** .... G+ HR
Schuylkill Medical Center East Norwegian Street, **Pottsville** ...... G+ HR
Sharon Regional Hospital, **Sharon** .... S+ E
St. Clair Hospital, **Pittsburgh** .... G+ E+
St. Joseph Regional Health Network, **Reading** ...... G+ HR G+
St. Luke's Hospital Quakertown Campus, **Quakertown** ...... G+
St. Luke's Hospital-Anderson Campus, **Easton** ...... G+ HR
St. Luke's Hospital-Miners Campus, **Coaldale** .... G+ HR
St. Luke's University Hospital, **Bethlehem** .... G+ E+
St. Mary Medical Center, **Langhorne** .... G G+ E+ G
Suburban Hospital, **Norristown** .... G+ G+ E+
Temple University Hospital, **Philadelphia** .... S G+ E+
The Children's Hospital of Philadelphia, **Philadelphia** ...... G+ *
The Good Samaritan Health System, **Lebanon** ...... G+ HR G+
The Hospital of the University of Pennsylvania, **Philadelphia** ...... G+ HR G+ E
Thomas Jefferson University Hospital, **Philadelphia** ...... G+ E+
Uniontown Hospital, **Uniontown** .... S S+ G+ E
UPMC Altoona, **Altoona** .... G+ E
UPMC East, **Monroeville** .... G+
UPMC Hamot, **Erie** .... G+ HR G+ E+
UPMC McKeesport, **McKeesport** .... G+ E
UPMC Mercy Pittsburgh, **Pittsburgh** .... G+ E+
UPMC Northwest, **Seneca** .... G+ E
UPMC Passavant, **Pittsburgh** .... G+ E
UPMC Pinnacle Harrisburg, **Harrisburg** .... G+ HR G+ E
UPMC Presbyterian, **Pittsburgh** .... G+ E+
UPMC Shadyside, **Pittsburgh** .... G+
UPMC St. Margaret, **Pittsburgh** .... G+ E
Washington Health System, **Washington** .... G+ E
Wellspan Ephrata Community Hospital, **Stevens** ... G+ G+ HR
WellSpan Gettysburg Hospital, **Gettysburg** .... G+ S+ E+
WellSpan Health-York Hospital, **York** .... G+ G G+ E

PUERTO RICO

Hospital HIMA San Pablo Bayamon, **Bayamon** ...... G+ HR
Hospital HIMA-San Pablo – Caguas, **Caguas** .... G+ HR G+ HR

RHODE ISLAND

Kent Hospital, **Warwick** .... G+ HR
Landmark Medical Center, **Woonsocket** .... S+
Newport Hospital, **Newport** .... S+
Our Lady of Fatima Hospital, **North Providence** .... G+ E+
Rhode Island Hospital, **Providence** .... G+ E+
South County Hospital, **Wakefield** .... G+
The Miriam Hospital, **Providence** .... G+ E

SOUTH CAROLINA

Aiken Regional Medical Center, **Aiken** .... S+ HR
AnMed Health, **Anderson** .... S G+ HR
Beaufort Memorial Hospital, **Beaufort** .... G+ E G S
Bon Secours Saint Francis Health System, **Greenville** ...... G+ HR G+ HR
Bon Secours St. Francis Hospital, **Charleston** ...... G+ E
Coastal Carolina Hospital, **Hardeeville** .... G HR
Conway Medical Center, **Conway** .... G+ E
East Cooper Medical Center, **Mount Pleasant** ...... S+
Grand Strand Medical Center, **Myrtle Beach** .... G+ E
Greenville Memorial Hospital, **Greenville** .... G+ E+
Greer Memorial Hospital, **Greer** .... G+ HR
Hilton Head Hospital, **Hilton Head** .... G+ E
Lexington Medical Center, **West Columbia** .... S+ S G E G
Mary Black Health System, **Spartanburg** .... G+ E+
McLeod Regional Medical Center, **Florence** .... G+ E+
MUSC Health, **Charleston** .... G+ E+
Palmetto Health Baptist Parkridge, **Columbia** ...... S+
Palmetto Health Richland, **Columbia** .... G+ S ★ G+ E+ S+
Piedmont Medical Center, **Rock Hill** .... G G G+ E
Regional Medical Center of Orangeburg & Calhoun Counties, **Orangeburg** ...... G+ HR G G+ E
Roper St. Francis Hospital, **Charleston** .... G+ E+
Self Regional Healthcare, **Greenwood** .... G+ HR S+
Spartanburg Regional Healthcare System, **Spartanburg** ...... S+ E
Springs Memorial Hospital, **Lancaster** .... S+ E+
Summerville Medical Center, **Summerville** .... G+ E
Tidelands Georgetown Memorial Hospital, **Georgetown** ...... G+ E+
Tidelands Waccamaw Community Hospital, **Murrells Inlet** ...... G+ E+
Trident Medical Center, **Charleston** .... G+ G+ HR

SOUTH DAKOTA

Avera Heart Hospital of South Dakota, **Sioux Falls** ...... S S
Avera St. Luke's Hospital, **Aberdeen** .... S+ E
Rapid City Regional Hospital, **Rapid City** .... G+ HR
Sanford USD Medical Center, **Sioux Falls** .... G G G

TENNESSEE

Erlanger Health System, **Chattanooga** .... G+ E+
Fort Sanders Regional Medical Center, **Knoxville** .. G+ E+
Jackson-Madison County General Hospital, **Jackson** ...... S+ E
LeConte Medical Center, **Sevierville** .... S+ E
Methodist Healthcare University Hospital, **Memphis** ...... G+ E+
North Knoxville Medical Center, **Powell** .... G+ E+
NorthCrest Medical Center, **Springfield** .... G+
Parkridge Medical Center, **Chattanooga** .... S+ E
Parkwest Medical Center, **Knoxville** .... S+ HR
Physicians Regional Medical Center, **Knoxville** ..... S+ E+
Saint Francis Hospital – Memphis, **Memphis** .... G+ E+
Saint Thomas Hospital, **Nashville** .... S+ E
Saint Thomas Midtown Hospital, **Nashville** .... S+ E+
Saint Thomas Rutherford Hospital, **Murfreesboro** . S+ E+
St. Francis Hospital – Bartlett, **Bartlett** .... G+ E+
Sumner Regional Medical Center, **Gallatin** .... G+ E+
The University of Tennessee Medical Center, **Knoxville** ...... G+ E+
TriStar Centennial Medical Center, **Brentwood** ..... G+ E+

American Heart Association.

(TENNESSEE CONTINUED)

TriStar Southern Hills Medical Center, **Nashville** .... (G+) (E)
TriStar Summit Medical Center, **Hermitage** .... (G+) (E+)
Vanderbilt University Medical Center, **Nashville** .... (G+) (E+)

TEXAS

Baptist Health System, **San Antonio** .... (G+) (E)
Baylor All Saints Medical Center, **Fort Worth** .... (S) (HR)
Baylor Scott & White Hillcrest Medical Center, **Waco** .... (G+) (G+) (HR)
Baylor Scott & White Lake Pointe, **Rowlett** .... (G+) (G+) (HR)
Baylor Scott & White Medical Center – Irving, **Irving** .... (S+) (HR)
Baylor Scott & White Medical Center – Round Rock, **Round Rock** ..... (G+) (G+) (E+) (G+) (S)
Baylor Scott & White Medical Center – Temple, **Temple** .... (G+) (E+) (G+)
Baylor Scott & White Medical Center Grapevine, **Grapevine** .... (G+) (E)
Baylor Scott & White Medical Center Lakeway, **Lakeway** .... (G+) (E+)
Baylor Scott & White Medical Center – College Station, **College Station** .... (S+) (HR)
Baylor Scott & White Medical Center – McKinney, **McKinney** ....
Baylor University Medical Center at Dallas, **Dallas** .... (G+) (E+)
Bayshore Medical Center, **Pasadena** .... (G+)
Ben Taub Hospital, **Houston** .... (G+) (E+) (G+) (G)
BSA, **Amarillo** .... (S+) (HR)
Cedar Park Regional Medical Center, **Cedar Park** .... (S+) (HR)
Central Texas Medical Center, **San Marcos** .... (G+) (E)
CHI St. Joseph Health Regional, **Bryan** .... (S+) (HR)
CHI St. Luke's Health Memorial Lufkin, **Lufkin** .... (S+) (E)
CHI St. Luke's Health-Baylor St. Luke's Medical Center, **Houston** .... (G+) (E+)
CHI St. Luke's Health-The Woodlands Hospital, **The Woodlands** .... (G+) (E+) (S)
CHRISTUS Hospital-St. Elizabeth & St. Mary, **Beaumont** .... (G+) (E+)
CHRISTUS Santa Rosa Health, **San Antonio** .... (G+) (HR) (G+)
CHRISTUS Spohn Hospital Corpus Christi – Shoreline, **Corpus Christi** .... (G+) (HR)
CHRISTUS St. Michael Health System, **Texarkana** .... (G+) (E)
Citizens Medical Center, **Victoria** .... (G+) (HR) (S) (G)
Clear Lake Regional Medical Center, **Webster** .... (G+) (E+) (S)
Connally Memorial Medical Center, **Floresville** .... (S+)
Conroe Regional Medical Center, **Conroe** .... (G+) (E) (S+)
Corpus Christi Medical Center, **Corpus Christi** .... (G+) (E) (S)
Covenant Medical Center, **Lubbock** .... (S+) (HR)
Cuero Regional Hospital, **Cuero** .... (S)
Cypress Fairbanks Medical Center, **Houston** .... (G+) (HR)
Del Sol Medical Center, **El Paso** .... (G+) (E+)
Dell Seton Medical Center at The University of Texas, **Austin** .... (G+) (E+)
DeTar Healthcare System, **Victoria** .... (G+) (HR)
Doctors Hospital at Renaissance, **Edinburg** .... (G+) (HR) (G+) (E+)
Good Shepherd Medical Center, **Longview** .... (G+) (E+)
Good Shepherd Medical Center – Marshall, **Marshall** .... (G+) (E)
HCA-West Houston Medical Center, **Houston** .... (G+) (E) (G)
Hendrick Medical Center, **Abilene** .... (G+) (E+)
Houston Methodist Hospital, **Houston** .... (G+) (E+)
Houston Methodist San Jacinto Hospital, **Baytown** .... (G+) (G+) (E+)
Houston Methodist St. John Hospital, **Nassau Bay** .... (G+) (E+)
Houston Methodist Sugar Land Hospital, **Sugar Land** .... (G+) (E+)
Houston Methodist The Woodlands Hospital, **The Woodlands** .... (S+)
Houston Methodist West Hospital, **Houston** .... (G+) (E+)
Houston Methodist Willowbrook Hospital, **Houston** .... (G+) (E+)
Houston Northwest Medical Center, **Houston** .... (G+) (E+)
Huntsville Memorial Hospital, **Huntsville** .... (G+) (HR)
JPS Health Network, **Fort Worth** .... (S+) (E)
Kingwood Medical Center, **Kingwood** .... (G+) (E+)
Knapp Medical Center, **Weslaco** .... (G+) (E)
Las Palmas Medical Center, **El Paso** .... (G+)
Medical Center Hospital, **Odessa** .... (G+) (HR)
Medical City Dallas Hospital, **Dallas** .... (G+) (S+) *
Memorial Hermann Greater Heights Hospital, **Houston** .... (G+) (E+)
Memorial Hermann Katy Hospital, **Katy** .... (G+) (E+)
Memorial Hermann Memorial City Medical Center, **Houston** .... (G+) (E+)
Memorial Hermann Northeast Hospital, **Humble** .... (S+) (HR)
Memorial Hermann Pearland Hospital, **Pearland** .... (G+) (HR)
Memorial Hermann Southeast Hospital, **Houston** .... (G+) (HR)
Memorial Hermann Southwest Hospital, **Houston** .... (G+) (E+)
Memorial Hermann The Woodlands, **The Woodlands** .... (G+) (E+)
Memorial Hermann-Texas Medical Center, **Houston** .... (G+) (E+)

Methodist Charlton Medical Center, **Dallas** .... (S+) (E) (G+) (S)
Methodist Dallas Medical Center, **Dallas** .... (G+) (E+)
Methodist Hospital, **San Antonio** .... (G+) (E)
Methodist Mansfield Medical Center, **Mansfield** .... (G+) (E) (S)
Methodist Richardson Medical Center, **Richardson** .... (G+) (S+)
Methodist Stone Oak Hospital, **San Antonio** .... (G+) (E+)
Metroplex Hospital, **Killeen** .... (G+) (HR) (G+)
Metropolitan Methodist Hospital, **San Antonio** .... (G+) (HR)
Midland Memorial Hospital, **Midland** .... (S)
North Cypress Medical Center, **Cypress** .... (G+) (HR) (G) (S)
Northeast Methodist Hospital, **San Antonio** .... (S+) (HR)
OakBend Medical Center, **Richmond** .... (G+) (HR)
OakBend Medical Center Williams Way Campus, **Richmond** .... (G+)
Parkland Health & Hospital System, **Dallas** .... (G+) (G+) (E) (G) (G)
Providence Health Center, **Waco** .... (G+) (HR)
Rio Grande Regional Hospital, **McAllen** .... (S+) (HR)
Seton Medical Center Austin, **Austin** .... (G+) (E+) (G+)
Seton Medical Center Hays, **Kyle** .... (G+) (E) (G)
Seton Medical Center Williamson, **Round Rock** .... (G+) (E+)
Shannon Medical Center, **San Angelo** .... (G+) (G+) (G) (G)
Southwest General Hospital, **San Antonio** .... (G+)
St. David's Georgetown Hospital, **Georgetown** .... (G+) (HR) **(G)**
St. David's Medical Center, **Austin** .... (G+) (E+) (G) (S)
St. David's North Austin Medical Center, **Austin** .... (G+) (G+) (S)
St. David's Round Rock Medical Center, **Round Rock** .... (G+) (E) (G+) (S)
St. David's South Austin Medical Center, **Austin** .... (G+) (HR) (G+) (G)
St. Joseph Medical Center, **Houston** .... (G+) (E+)
Texas Health Arlington Memorial Hospital, **Arlington** .... (G+) (E+)
Texas Health Denton, **Denton** .... (G+)
Texas Health Fort Worth, **Fort Worth** .... (S+) (E+) (S+)
Texas Health Heart and Vascular Hospital, **Arlington** .... (G+)
Texas Health Hurst Euless Bedford, **Bedford** .... (G)
Texas Health Presbyterian Hospital Dallas, **Dallas** .... (G+) (E) (G+)
Texas Health Presbyterian Hospital Plano, **Plano** .... (G+)
Texoma Medical Center, **Denison** .... (S+) (E+)
The Heart Hospital Baylor Plano, **Plano** .... (HR)
The Hospitals of Providence East Campus, **El Paso** .... (G+)
The Hospitals of Providence Memorial Campus, **El Paso** .... (G+)
The Hospitals of Providence Sierra Campus, **El Paso** .... (G+) (G+)
The Hospitals of Providence Transmountain Campus, **El Paso** .... (S+)
The University of Texas Medical Branch-Galveston Campus, **Galveston** .... (G) (S) (G+) (E+)
Titus Regional Medical Center, **MT Pleasant** .... (G+) (E)
United Regional Healthcare System, **Wichita Falls** .... (S+) (E)
University Health System, **San Antonio** .... (G+) (E)
University Medical Center, **Lubbock** .... (G+) (HR)
University Medical Center of El Paso, **El Paso** .... (G+) (HR)
UT Health Tyler, **Tyler** .... (G+) (HR)
UT Southwestern Medical Center, **Dallas** .... (G+) (E+)
Valley Baptist Medical Center – Brownsville, **Brownsville** .... (G+) (E+)
Valley Baptist Medical Center – Harlingen, **Harlingen** .... (G+) (E+)
Valley Regional Medical Center, **Brownsville** .... (G+) (E+)
Wadley Regional Medical Center, **Texarkana** .... (G+) (E+)

UTAH

Davis Hospital and Medical Center, **Layton** .... (G+) (E+)
Dixie Regional Medical Center, **Saint George** .... (G+) (E+)
Intermountain Medical Center, **Murray** .... (G+) (E+)
Jordan Valley Medical Center/JVMC-West Valley Campus/Mountain Point Medical Center, a Campus of JVMC, **West Jordan** .... (S) (G+) (E+)
Lakeview Hospital, **Bountiful** .... (G+) (HR)
McKay-Dee Hospital, **Ogden** .... (G+) (E+)
Mountain View Hospital – Payson Utah, **Payson** .... (G+)
Ogden Regional Medical Center, **Ogden** .... (G+)
St. Mark's Hospital, **Salt Lake City** .... (G+) (E+)
Timpanogos Regional Hospital, **Orem** .... (G+)
University Of Utah Health, **Salt Lake City** .... (S+) (HR) (G+) (E+)
Utah Valley Hospital, **Provo** .... (G+) (HR)

VERMONT

The University of Vermont Medical Center, **Burlington** .... (S+) (G+) (E)

American Heart Association.

*These hospitals received Get With The Guidelines-Resuscitation awards for two or more patient populations.

VIRGINIA

Augusta Health, **Fishersville** .... G+ HR
Bon Secours DePaul Medical Center, **Norfolk** .... G+ E+ S
Bon Secours Mary Immaculate Hospital, **Newport News** .... S+
Bon Secours Maryview Medical Center, **Portsmouth** .... G+ E+ G+
Bon Secours Memorial Regional Medical Center,
    Mechanicsville .... G S G+ HR S
Bon Secours Rappahannock General Hospital, **Kilmarnock** .... G+ E
Bon Secours Richmond Community Hospital, **Richmond** .... S
Bon Secours St. Francis Medical Center, **Midlothian** .... S+ HR S+
Bon Secours St. Mary's Hospital, **Richmond** .... G+ G+ E
Carilion Roanoke Memorial Hospital, **Roanoke** .... G+ HR
Centra Lynchburg General Hospital, **Lynchburg** .... G+ HR G+ E+ G+
Chesapeake Regional Medical Center, **Chesapeake** .... S+ E+ G
Inova Alexandria Hospital, **Alexandria** .... G+ E+
Inova Fair Oaks Hospital, **Fairfax** .... G+ HR
Inova Fairfax Hospital, **Falls Church** .... G+ E+
Inova Loudoun Hospital, **Leesburg** .... G+ E+
Inova Mount Vernon Hospital, **Alexandria** .... G+ E+
John Randolph Medical Center, **Hopewell** .... G+ E+
Martha Jefferson Hospital, **Charlottesville** .... S+ E
Mary Washington Hospital, **Fredericksburg** .... S+ E
Novant Health UVA Health System Culpeper Medical Center, **Culpeper** .... G+
Novant Health UVA Health System Haymarket Medical Center, **Haymarket** ...... S+
Novant Health UVA Health System Prince William Medical Center,
    Manassas .... G+ G+ HR
Reston Hospital Center, **Reston** .... G+ E
Riverside Regional Medical Center, **Newport News** .... G+ E+
Sentara Leigh Hospital, **Norfolk** .... S+ E
Sentara Louise Obici Memorial Hospital, **Suffolk** .... S+ E
Sentara Norfolk General Hospital/Sentara Heart Hospital, **Norfolk** ... S+ E+
Sentara Northern Virginia Medical Center, **Woodbridge** .... S+ E
Sentara Princess Anne Hospital, **Virginia Beach** .... S+ E+
Sentara Virginia Beach General Hospital, **Virginia Beach** .... S+ E+
Southampton Memorial Hospital, **Franklin** .... S+ HR
StoneSprings Hospital Center, **Dulles** .... G+
The University of Virginia Health System, **Charlottesville** ...... G+ HR G+ E+ G
Twin County Regional Healthcare, **Galax** .... G+ HR
VCU Community Memorial Hospital, **South Hill** .... G+ E+
Virginia Commonwealth University Medical Center, **Richmond** ..... G+ E+
Winchester Medical Center, **Winchester** .... G

WASHINGTON

Cascade Valley Hospital, **Arlington** .... S+
CHI Franciscan St Joseph Medical Center, **Tacoma** .... G+ E
Confluence Health-Central Washington Hospital, **Wenatchee** ... G+ E+ G
EvergreenHealth, **Kirkland** .... G+ E
EvergreenHealth Monroe, **Monroe** .... S+
Harborview Medical Center, **Seattle** .... G+ E+ S
Harrison Medical Center, **Bremerton** .... G+ E
Highline Medical Center, **Burien** .... G+
Jefferson Healthcare, **Port Townsend** .... G+
Legacy Salmon Creek Medical Center, **Vancouver** .... S+ E+
MultiCare Auburn Medical Center, **Auburn** .... S G+
MultiCare Deaconess Hospital, **Spokane** .... G+ E+
MultiCare Good Samaritan Hospital, **Puyallup** .... G S G+ E+
MultiCare Tacoma General/Allenmore Hospital, **Tacoma** .... S
MultiCare Valley Hospital, **Spokane Valley** .... S
Northwest Hospital & Medical Center, **Seattle** .... G+ E+
Overlake Medical Center, **Bellevue** .... G+ E+
PeaceHealth Southwest Medical Center, Stroke & Telestroke Program,
    Vancouver .... S+ E
PeaceHealth St. John Medical Center, **Longview** .... S+
PeaceHealth St. Joseph Medical Center, **Bellingham** .... G+ E+
Providence Centralia Hospital, **Centralia** .... S G S+ E
Providence Regional Medical Center Everett, **Everett** .... G+ E+
Providence Sacred Heart Medical Center & Children's Hospital, **Spokane** ... G+ E+
Providence St. Mary Medical Center, **Walla Walla** .... S+ HR
Providence St. Peter Hospital, **Olympia** .... G S+ S+ E

Saint Anthony Hospital, **Gig Harbor** .... S+ HR
Skagit Valley Hospital, **Mount Vernon** .... G+ E
Swedish Edmonds, **Edmonds** .... G+ E+
Swedish Medical Center-Cherry Hill Campus, **Seattle** .... G+ E+
Swedish Medical Center, Issaquah and Redmond Ambulatory
    Care Center, **Issaquah** .... G+ HR
Trios Health, **Kennewick** .... G+ HR S
UW Medicine | Valley Medical Center, **Renton** .... G+ E+
Virginia Mason Medical Center, **Seattle** .... G+ E S
Virginia Mason Memorial Hospital, **Yakima** .... G G+ E+

WEST VIRGINIA

Cabell Huntington Hospital, **Huntington** .... S+ G+ E
Camden Clark Medical Center, **Parkersburg** .... G
Davis Medical Center, **Elkins** .... S+
Mon Health Medical Center, **Morgantown** .... G+
Ohio Valley Medical Center, Inc., **Wheeling** .... S+
St. Mary's Medical Center, **Huntington** .... G+ G+ G+ HR
United Hospital Center, **Bridgeport** .... S+ HR G+ G+ E+
West Virginia University Hospital, Inc., **Morgantown** ...... G+ HR G+ E+
Wheeling Hospital, **Wheeling** .... G+

WISCONSIN

Ascension-All Saints, **Racine** .... G+ G+ E
Aspirus Wausau Hospital, **Wausau** .... S
Aurora BayCare Medical Center, **Green Bay** .... G G+ S G+ E+
Aurora Lakeland Medical Center, **Elkhorn** .... G+ HR G+ E+
Aurora Medical Center – Grafton, **Grafton** .... G+ G+ E
Aurora Medical Center – Kenosha, **Kenosha** .... G+ HR G+
Aurora Medical Center – Oshkosh, **Oshkosh** .... G+ E+
Aurora Medical Center Manitowoc County, **Two Rivers** .... S+
Aurora Medical Center Summit, **Oconomowoc** .... G+ G+ E
Aurora Medical Center Washington County, **Hartford** .... G+
Aurora Memorial Hospital Burlington, **Burlington** .... G+ HR G+
Aurora Sheboygan Memorial Medical Center, **Sheboygan** ..... S G+ E+
Aurora Sinai Medical Center, **Milwaukee** .... G+ HR G+
Aurora St. Luke's Medical Center, **Milwaukee** .... G+ HR G+ E+
Aurora St. Luke's South Shore, **Cudahy** .... G+ HR G+ HR
Aurora West Allis Medical Center, **West Allis** .... G+ G+ E+
Bellin Memorial Hospital, **Green Bay** .... G+ HR
Beloit Memorial Hospital, **Beloit** .... G+ E
Columbia-St. Mary's Hospital, **Milwaukee** .... G+ E
Columbia-St. Mary's Hospital – Ozaukee, **Mequon** .... G+ E
Froedtert Hospital, **Milwaukee** .... G+ S+ E+
Gundersen Lutheran Medical Center, **La Crosse** .... G+ E+
Marshfield Medical Center, **Marshfield** .... G+ E+
Mayo Clinic Health System in Eau Claire, **Eau Claire** .... G+
Mayo Clinic Health System LaCrosse, **La Crosse** .... G+ E
Mercy Hospital and Trauma Center, **Janesville** .... G+ G+ E
Mercy Medical Center – Oshkosh, **Oshkosh** .... S+
Oconomowoc Memorial Hospital, **Oconomowoc** .... G+ HR
SSM Health St. Clare Hospital, **Baraboo** .... HR
SSM Health St. Mary's Hospital – Madison, **Madison** .... G+ E+ G+
St. Agnes Hospital, **Fond Du Lac** .... S+ G+ E
St. Elizabeth Hospital, **Appleton** .... S+ E
St. Mary's Hospital Medical Center, **Green Bay** .... G+ E
St. Mary's Janesville Hospital, **Janesville** .... S+
St. Nicholas Hospital, **Sheboygan** .... S+
Theda Clark Medical Center, **Neenah** .... G+ E
United Hospital System-St. Catherine's Medical Center Campus,
    Pleasant Prairie .... S+ E
UnityPoint Health – Meriter, **Madison** .... G G+
UW Health, **Madison** .... G+ E+ G
Waukesha Memorial Hospital, **Waukesha** .... G+ E
Wheaton Franciscan Healthcare – Elmbrook, **Brookfield** .... G+ HR
Wheaton Franciscan Healthcare – St. Joseph, **Milwaukee** ..... G+ E+

WYOMING

Cheyenne Regional Medical Center, **Cheyenne** .... S+ G+
Wyoming Medical Center, **Casper** .... S G+ E+

American
Heart
Association.

Diets That Deliver

U.S. News looks at how well 40 eating plans live up to the hype

As frustrated dieters know, losing weight is hard, and most diets don't work. This is why U.S. News produces its Best Diets rankings, based on the views of a panel of nationally recognized experts (Page 85) who considered the effectiveness of some of the best-known eating plans, whether the aim is to lose weight, improve heart health, or manage diabetes.

Our panelists reviewed the research, added their own fact-finding, and rated the diets from 1 to 5 (the top score) in a number of areas: short-term weight loss (the likelihood of losing significant weight during the

first 12 months); long-term weight loss (the likelihood of maintaining significant weight loss for two years or more); diabetes prevention and management; heart health (effectiveness at preventing cardiovascular disease and reducing risk for heart patients); ease of compliance; nutritional completeness (how well a plan meets federal dietary guidelines); and safety (whether, for example, it omits key nutrients).

Which plan can help you achieve your goals? Check out the results in these pages. For more on the plans, visit **usnews.com/bestdiets.**

How the Plans Compare Overall

Forty diets were rated from 1 to 5 on multiple measures. Rank is based on a score compiled from panelists' average scores for each measure. The results:

Rank	Diet	Overall score	Short-term weight loss	Long-term weight loss	For diabetes	For heart health	Nutrition	Safety	Easy to follow
1	DASH	4.1	3.0	3.3	3.5	4.4	4.8	4.8	3.4
1	Mediterranean	4.1	2.9	3.1	3.7	4.2	4.8	4.8	3.6
3	Flexitarian	4.0	3.4	3.2	3.4	3.8	4.5	4.7	3.5
4	Weight Watchers	3.9	4.0	3.5	3.4	3.2	4.5	4.5	3.5
5	MIND	3.8	2.7	2.8	3.3	3.8	4.5	4.4	3.3
5	TLC	3.8	3.0	2.7	3.0	4.0	4.6	4.6	2.8
5	Volumetrics	3.8	3.8	3.3	3.4	3.3	4.4	4.5	3.0
8	Mayo Clinic	3.7	3.2	3.0	3.4	3.4	4.5	4.4	3.0
9	Ornish	3.6	3.4	3.0	3.2	4.2	4.1	4.2	2.0
10	Fertility	3.5	2.5	2.3	3.0	3.0	4.2	4.2	3.2
10	Vegetarian	3.5	3.1	3.0	3.1	3.6	4.0	4.1	2.6
12	Jenny Craig	3.4	3.7	3.0	3.3	2.9	3.8	3.8	3.0
12	Traditional Asian	3.4	2.8	2.9	2.7	3.1	4.2	4.3	2.4
14	Anti-Inflammatory	3.3	2.5	2.4	2.9	3.3	3.7	4.0	2.6
15	Flat Belly	3.2	3.1	2.4	2.6	3.0	3.8	3.8	2.7
15	Nutritarian	3.2	3.2	2.6	3.1	3.4	3.6	3.8	1.7
15	Spark Solution	3.2	3.1	2.5	2.5	2.5	3.9	4.1	2.4
18	Engine 2	3.1	3.6	2.9	3.2	3.7	3.2	3.5	1.6
19	Biggest Loser	3.0	3.8	2.3	3.0	2.9	3.6	3.3	2.2
19	Nutrisystem	3.0	3.7	2.5	2.8	2.5	3.1	3.4	2.5
19	Vegan	3.0	3.6	3.2	3.4	3.8	2.6	3.2	1.5
22	Eco-Atkins	2.9	3.4	2.5	2.7	3.1	3.1	3.2	1.6
22	Glycemic-Index	2.9	2.6	2.1	2.6	2.3	3.7	3.8	2.0
22	South Beach	2.9	3.4	2.4	2.6	2.5	3.3	3.4	2.6
22	Zone	2.9	3.2	2.4	2.5	2.8	3.4	3.5	2.1
26	Abs	2.8	2.7	1.9	2.3	2.5	3.3	3.5	2.6
26	Macrobiotic	2.8	2.9	2.6	2.8	3.1	2.9	3.2	1.7
26	SlimFast	2.8	3.8	2.6	2.7	2.4	2.8	3.1	2.6
29	HMR	2.7	4.0	2.2	2.7	2.5	2.8	3.0	2.4
29	Medifast	2.7	3.8	2.1	2.7	2.7	2.7	2.9	2.2
31	Acid Alkaline	2.4	2.3	1.9	2.1	2.2	2.5	3.0	2.0
32	Paleo	2.3	2.8	2.2	2.5	2.0	2.2	2.6	1.8
32	Raw Food	2.3	3.6	2.8	2.7	2.7	2.1	2.2	1.1
32	Supercharged Hormone	2.3	2.8	2.0	2.1	2.1	2.5	2.6	1.9
35	Fast	2.2	3.0	2.0	2.0	2.1	2.4	2.3	2.0
36	Atkins	2.1	3.7	2.2	2.4	1.8	1.6	2.2	1.8
37	Body Reset	2.0	2.6	1.3	1.6	1.6	2.0	2.6	1.6
37	Whole30	2.0	2.8	1.7	1.9	1.8	2.0	2.5	1.4
39	Dukan	1.9	3.1	1.9	2.0	1.5	1.6	2.1	1.5
39	Ketogenic	1.9	3.5	2.0	2.3	2.0	1.4	1.7	1.4

Best
Weight-Loss Diets

Diets are ranked by the average of the scores experts assigned them for producing short- and long-term results.

Rank	Diet	Avg. score
1	Weight Watchers	3.7
2	Volumetrics	3.5
3	Jenny Craig	3.4
3	Vegan	3.4
5	Flexitarian	3.3
6	DASH	3.2
6	Engine 2	3.2
6	Ornish	3.2
6	Raw Food	3.2
6	SlimFast	3.2

Best
Diets for the Heart

With these plans, you can take aim at cholesterol, blood pressure or triglycerides, as well as weight.

Rank	Diet	Avg. score
1	DASH	4.4
2	Mediterranean	4.2
2	Ornish	4.2
4	TLC	4.0
5	Flexitarian	3.8
5	MIND	3.8
5	Vegan	3.8
8	Engine 2	3.7
9	Vegetarian	3.6
10	Mayo Clinic	3.4
10	Nutritarian	3.4

Best
Diabetes Diets

These plans scored highest for both managing and preventing the condition.

Rank	Diet	Avg. score
1	Mediterranean	3.7
2	DASH	3.5
3	Flexitarian	3.4
3	Mayo Clinic	3.4
3	Vegan	3.4
3	Volumetrics	3.4
3	Weight Watchers	3.4
8	Jenny Craig	3.3
8	MIND	3.3
10	Engine 2	3.2
10	Ornish	3.2

Best
Plant-Based Diets

These diets emphasize minimally processed foods from plants and are good bets for weight loss.

Rank	Diet	Avg. score
1	Mediterranean	4.1
2	Flexitarian	4.0
3	Ornish	3.6
4	Vegetarian	3.5
5	Traditional Asian	3.4
6	Anti-Inflammatory	3.3
7	Nutritarian	3.2
8	Engine 2	3.1
9	Vegan	3.0
10	Eco-Atkins	2.9

Best
Commercial Diets

Nutritional value, ease of use and safety are counted, as well as weight-loss effectiveness.

Rank	Diet	Avg. score
1	Weight Watchers	3.9
2	Jenny Craig	3.4
3	Flat Belly	3.2
3	Nutritarian	3.2
5	Biggest Loser	3.0
5	Nutrisystem	3.0
7	South Beach	2.9
7	Zone	2.9
9	SlimFast	2.8
10	HMR	2.7
10	Medifast	2.7

Easiest-to-Follow
Diets

The ranking is based on ease of use and a diet's ability to deliver weight loss and good nutrition.

Rank	Diet	Avg. score
1	Mediterranean	3.6
2	Flexitarian	3.5
2	Weight Watchers	3.5
4	DASH	3.4
5	MIND	3.3
6	Fertility	3.2
7	Jenny Craig	3.0
7	Mayo Clinic	3.0
7	Volumetrics	3.0
10	TLC	2.8

The Expert Panel

Twenty-five panelists reviewed detailed assessments of the U.S. News list of 40 diets and rated them on a number of key measures, described on Page 84.

Kathie Beals
Associate professor, clinical, division of nutrition, University of Utah

Amy Campbell
Nutrition and wellness consultant and writer

Lawrence Cheskin
Director, Johns Hopkins Weight Management Center

Michael Dansinger
Founding director of the Diabetes Reversal Program at Tufts Medical Center

Meredith Dillon
Registered dietitian specializing in pediatric Type 1 and Type 2 diabetes at Children's National Medical Center

Marion Franz
Nutrition and health consultant, Nutrition Concepts by Franz, Inc.

Teresa Fung
Professor of nutrition, Simmons College

Hollie Gelberg
Clinical/research dietitian at the Department of Veterans Affairs Greater Los Angeles Healthcare System

Andrea Giancoli
Nutrition communications consultant

Michael Greger
Physician, author and internationally recognized speaker on nutrition, food safety and public health issues

Stephan Guyenet
Neurobiologist and writer who specializes in the role of the brain in eating behavior and body fatness

David Katz
Director, Yale-Griffin Prevention Research Center

Penny Kris-Etherton
Distinguished professor of nutrition, Pennsylvania State University

James Levine
Obesity expert and endocrinologist at Mayo Clinic

JoAnn Manson
Professor of women's health, Harvard Medical School

Yasmin Mossavar-Rahmani
Associate professor of clinical epidemiology and population health, Albert Einstein College of Medicine

Elisabetta Politi
Nutrition director, Duke Diet and Fitness Center

Rebecca Reeves
Adjunct assistant professor, University of Texas School of Public Health

Eric Rimm
Professor of epidemiology and nutrition and director of the Program in Cardiovascular Epidemiology at the Harvard T.H. Chan School of Public Health

Susan Roberts
Professor of nutrition, Tufts University and founder of the iDiet weight-loss program

Lisa Sasson
Clinical associate professor of nutrition, food studies and public health, New York University

Laurence Sperling
Founder and director of the Heart Disease Prevention Center at Emory University

Anne Thorndike
Assistant professor of medicine at Harvard Medical School and an associate physician at Massachusetts General Hospital

Jill Weisenberger
Author, health and wellness coach, and internationally recognized expert in nutrition and diabetes

Adrienne Youdim
Associate clinical professor of medicine, UCLA David Geffen School of Medicine, Cedars Sinai Medical Center

AMERICA'S
Healthiest Communities

What makes this Virginia enclave stand out from all the rest?

by **Gaby Galvin** *and* **Steve Sternberg**

FALLS CHURCH, VA. — For decades, the educated and affluent have flocked to northern Virginia, which boasts excellent schools, high-quality health care and easy access to the nation's capital.

But of all the communities in the area – indeed, the country – one tops the rest when it comes to measuring the crucial factors that combine to shape the health and well-being of its residents.

That community, Falls Church, holds the No. 1 spot in the inaugural U.S. News rankings of the Healthiest Communities in America. The project, created with the Aetna Foundation, scores nearly 3,000 counties across several dozen metrics that extend well beyond those typically associated with health like obesity rate and access to doctors, parks,

and fresh produce. U.S. News also gathered and weighed data on the many social factors that are increasingly recognized as major determinants of physical and mental well-being (story, Page 38), including income and employment, housing and public safety, educational achievement and exposure to crime. The goals: to examine how location and circumstances affect the overall health of Americans and to educate health leaders, policymakers and the public. "Our behavior is shaped by the world around us," says Steven Woolf, director

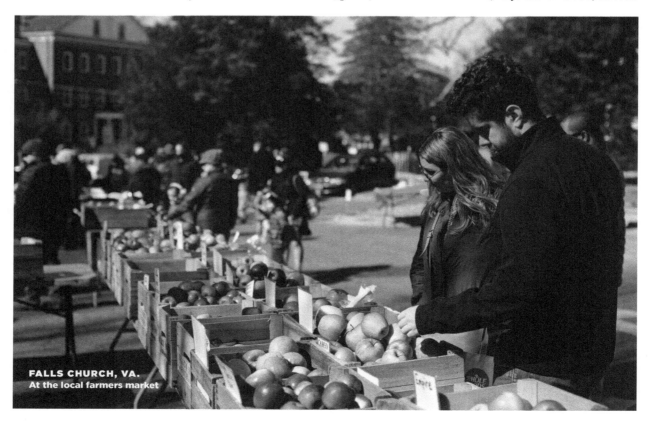

FALLS CHURCH, VA.
At the local farmers market

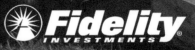

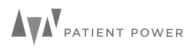
40 Star Performers

Besides creating an overall ranking of America's Healthiest Communities, U.S. News measured them in peer groups based on how rural or urban they are and their economic strength. Below, see how the top 10 in each group stack up on a sampling of key metrics. For full details on the project, visit usnews.com/healthiestcommunities.

Peer group rank	Community	Overall score (out of 100)	Years of life expectancy	Heart disease prevalence[1]	Obesity prevalence (adults)	Walkability index (20=best)	Adults who don't get exercise[2]	Population within 0.5 mile of a park	Preventable hospital admissions[3]	Population with no health insurance	High school graduation rate	Adults with advanced degree[4]	Unemployment rate	Poverty rate	Median household income
URBAN, HIGH PERFORMING
1	Falls Church city, Va.	100.00	81.81	20.56%	26.90%	16.15	20.70%	88.65%	2,547.0	3.60%	97.50%	81.80%	2.7%	2.72%	$120,522
2	Douglas County, Colo.	98.37	83.72	18.98%	16.60%	9.00	9.90%	57.40%	2,672.0	5.03%	90.00%	64.71%	2.7%	3.96%	$102,964
3	Broomfield County, Colo.	93.87	80.02	18.86%	17.50%	10.42	11.80%	87.75%	2,375.0	6.84%	83.41%	60.32%	2.9%	6.52%	$81,898
4	Los Alamos County, N.M.	93.65	83.49	15.09%	19.50%	5.39	12.30%	91.14%	2,283.0	5.79%	87.00%	71.86%	4.2%	6.12%	$101,934
5	Dukes County, Mass.	92.41	82.05	20.60%	21.10%	8.58	16.40%	28.63%	3,449.0	8.11%	NA	49.06%	5.0%	11.66%	$64,222
6	Fairfax city, Va.	91.59	83.73	20.30%	21.50%	14.77	15.70%	91.48%	2,919.0	11.30%	NA	60.35%	3.0%	6.99%	$105,297
7	Hamilton County, Ind.	91.59	81.78	25.47%	25.40%	7.81	16.30%	12.09%	3,013.0	6.65%	95.70%	62.45%	3.2%	4.71%	$86,222
8	Loudoun County, Va.	90.41	83.19	21.83%	21.30%	7.99	18.20%	34.16%	3,837.0	7.97%	93.00%	64.34%	3.2%	4.02%	$123,453
9	Ozaukee County, Wis.	90.29	82.13	22.33%	26.20%	7.21	17.60%	48.62%	2,847.0	4.13%	95.69%	54.74%	3.5%	5.18%	$76,433
10	Delaware County, Ohio	89.57	81.43	25.53%	27.50%	7.07	17.60%	27.53%	3,441.0	4.40%	94.71%	58.55%	3.5%	4.54%	$91,955
URBAN, UP-AND-COMING
1	Island County, Wash.	71.84	81.93	17.39%	27.20%	8.70	17.70%	27.36%	2,438.0	8.76%	83.09%	42.90%	6.0%	9.64%	$58,815
2	Bennington County, Vt.	71.62	79.49	23.26%	24.10%	6.53	18.80%	37.08%	3,974.0	5.29%	84.50%	41.38%	3.8%	13.50%	$49,573
3	Montgomery County, Va.	71.18	79.38	22.70%	24.40%	8.92	20.70%	41.62%	3,298.0	7.83%	85.00%	53.09%	4.0%	24.84%	$46,663
4	Latah County, Idaho	70.27	81.01	15.36%	24.50%	6.65	15.80%	41.78%	2,856.0	8.90%	86.20%	53.54%	3.3%	21.64%	$42,439
5	Transylvania County, N.C.	69.67	80.33	20.77%	24.70%	5.99	20.50%	54.18%	2,452.0	18.18%	85.00%	38.04%	4.9%	12.62%	$45,114
6	Leelanau County, Mich.	68.58	83.10	22.59%	25.50%	5.00	21.70%	14.87%	2,969.0	8.92%	66.70%	49.65%	4.7%	10.40%	$56,189
7	Sibley County, Minn.	68.25	80.88	17.51%	33.00%	5.08	25.00%	37.11%	5,610.0	5.88%	90.83%	27.63%	4.3%	10.69%	$56,990
8	Kennebec County, Maine	68.24	78.53	21.47%	30.80%	6.55	19.60%	7.06%	3,048.0	8.83%	86.64%	34.99%	3.6%	13.84%	$46,917
9	Marquette County, Mich.	68.11	79.31	24.55%	28.70%	6.45	19.60%	11.95%	2,737.0	10.60%	87.10%	37.78%	5.6%	16.98%	$45,409
10	Kitsap County, Wash.	68.01	79.66	17.08%	29.30%	9.73	17.40%	42.17%	2,434.0	8.77%	82.22%	41.23%	5.8%	10.64%	$62,941
RURAL, HIGH PERFORMING
1	Routt County, Colo.	90.56	82.73	15.35%	14.00%	6.61	12.10%	30.71%	2,617.0	11.22%	92.15%	58.13%	2.7%	10.17%	$64,963
2	Ouray County, Colo.	90.46	83.00	10.81%	17.90%	6.23	12.30%	35.01%	2,935.0	14.19%	84.38%	57.44%	3.8%	7.77%	$61,624
3	Sublette County, Wyo.	89.21	80.48	17.56%	23.20%	6.45	16.20%	24.09%	2,737.0	15.05%	93.08%	31.14%	6.4%	8.06%	$81,772
4	Grand County, Colo.	87.80	82.73	14.09%	16.90%	6.89	12.00%	20.76%	2,299.0	19.83%	91.57%	46.16%	2.7%	10.76%	$63,628
5	Teton County, Wyo.	87.09	83.46	17.35%	12.50%	6.85	10.90%	32.96%	2,439.0	16.85%	97.50%	59.28%	3.4%	7.38%	$75,325
6	Winneshiek County, Iowa	86.26	82.62	20.26%	25.00%	6.32	16.90%	43.53%	2,274.0	5.08%	96.35%	40.42%	3.6%	8.15%	$54,429
7	Chaffee County, Colo.	86.01	81.22	16.15%	20.50%	7.72	14.90%	73.41%	1,963.0	14.37%	77.00%	41.30%	2.7%	8.72%	$51,092
8	Morgan County, Utah	85.97	81.47	22.18%	21.50%	6.04	14.30%	45.60%	2,032.0	10.31%	92.00%	44.83%	3.0%	5.42%	$74,314
9	Pitkin County, Colo.	84.57	86.52	24.24%	14.50%	7.04	8.60%	56.50%	2,384.0	14.25%	94.16%	66.03%	3.4%	9.85%	$71,196
10	Mono County, Calif.	83.24	82.96	14.31%	22.30%	10.15	15.70%	2.83%	2,620.0	23.75%	NA	40.34%	5.3%	4.87%	$56,944
RURAL, UP-AND-COMING
1	Jefferson County, Wash.	74.81	81.26	15.77%	23.70%	9.83	14.20%	26.47%	967.0	10.14%	76.40%	43.76%	7.3%	12.01%	$49,279
2	Lincoln County, Wash.	71.90	80.03	18.74%	31.10%	6.52	21.20%	46.03%	2,960.0	10.57%	83.60%	31.40%	5.7%	15.27%	$46,069
3	Dolores County, Colo.	67.72	79.50	14.66%	19.60%	4.57	16.10%	16.28%	2,406.0	11.01%	90.00%	29.72%	4.0%	21.49%	$31,875
4	Emery County, Utah	67.05	77.99	21.23%	25.20%	5.46	21.60%	18.93%	3,122.0	13.04%	92.00%	24.87%	6.3%	11.16%	$49,787
5	Keweenaw County, Mich.	65.02	80.20	26.24%	30.30%	2.82	19.80%	4.27%	3,798.0	9.68%	77.13%	36.14%	8.4%	15.35%	$37,813
6	Tillamook County, Oregon	64.93	79.00	18.81%	28.30%	8.53	16.40%	24.02%	2,857.0	12.58%	84.30%	27.20%	5.0%	17.43%	$42,581
7	Wallowa County, Oregon	64.90	80.42	19.31%	23.70%	6.34	15.80%	11.09%	2,844.0	10.93%	82.98%	34.43%	6.7%	15.29%	$40,581
8	Big Stone County, Minn.	64.85	79.89	26.37%	28.20%	6.36	17.90%	25.00%	5,770.0	5.99%	94.92%	28.53%	4.9%	14.39%	$47,794
9	Garfield County, Wash.	64.70	80.56	20.94%	33.10%	6.17	25.40%	25.07%	2,568.0	10.72%	88.84%	40.02%	6.0%	11.45%	$45,855
10	Lexington city, Va.	64.58	80.26	21.70%	26.70%	9.88	20.40%	18.73%	3,108.0	6.54%	NA	47.22%	6.3%	20.24%	$34,017

NA = Not available. Data are from various years. [1]Percentage of Medicare beneficiaries with heart disease (2007-2015). [2]Percentage of adults who did not get leisure-time physical activity in past month (2013). [3]Among Medicare beneficiaries per 100,000 population (2015). [4]Age 25 and up with at least an associate degree (2015). [5]Share voting in 2016 presidential election. [6]Per 100,000 population (2014).

Home-ownership rate	Voter participation rate[5]	Violent crime rate[6]
58.7%	84.5%	92.83
79.4%	87.4%	114.32
68.4%	86.8%	61.44
74.2%	80.5%	261.26
79.9%	87.9%	235.59
70.0%	75.8%	127.57
78.3%	76.5%	44.25
77.1%	84.4%	88.47
76.7%	80.2%	51.55
81.5%	77.2%	89.13
67.8%	68.2%	131.94
71.9%	56.1%	151.93
54.2%	56.6%	117.42
54.0%	60.7%	119.62
76.7%	65.3%	168.43
84.9%	83.2%	41.62
78.7%	70.5%	34.91
70.3%	68.9%	150.14
68.6%	60.0%	158.04
67.2%	60.6%	322.92
69.1%	76.4%	207.85
71.7%	84.8%	49.57
73.5%	58.0%	97.18
72.7%	75.7%	257.89
60.5%	74.4%	319.33
77.0%	67.6%	23.69
75.5%	72.4%	75.77
83.2%	78.7%	41.47
65.2%	78.5%	138.64
59.5%	54.4%	353.38
75.0%	79.2%	187.99
79.0%	71.2%	84.68
77.1%	84.9%	64.02
82.6%	58.8%	30.07
88.7%	78.8%	154.20
72.4%	67.3%	70.73
67.4%	75.1%	23.66
79.0%	67.4%	56.78
68.2%	71.6%	204.32
57.5%	39.1%	37.66

emeritus of the Virginia Commonwealth University Center on Society and Health. "People's ability to change behavior is driven by conditions in which they live."

Indeed, research reveals that how long – and how well – you live is tied to your community, your neighborhood, and sometimes even your block, says David Fleming, vice president of global health programs at the nonprofit global health organization PATH.

The U.S. News analysis makes use of the National Committee on Vital and Health Statistics' pioneering Measurement Framework for Community Health and Well-Being, developed by an expert committee appointed to advise the U.S. Department of Health and Human Services. Guided by that framework, the project scores and ranks communities on 80 indicators across 10 categories: community vitality, equity, economy, education, environment, food and nutrition, population health, housing, public safety and infrastructure. Complete data and details on the methodology can be found at usnews. com/healthiestcommunities.

Additionally, rankings in four peer groups, defined by their population density and the strength of their economic performance – urban high performing, urban up-and-coming, rural high performing and rural up-and-coming – were created to enable better comparisons of similar communities. The top 10 performers in each peer group are featured in the table at left. A team of population health experts from the University of Missouri Center for Applied Research and Engagement Systems – a research group skilled in community health assessment – helped develop the project's methodology and carried out the analysis.

A strong economy, first-rate school system and safe neighborhoods helped Falls Church earn top honors in the overall ranking. Only around 1 in 10 of its residents smoke – half the state and national average – and residents generally have lower rates of chronic diseases, data show. On average, they live to about age 82, a decade longer than residents of Baltimore, a city just 50 miles north in Maryland. In addition, Falls Church sits at No. 1 among the smaller category of high-performing urban counties like it.

In Falls Church, health is built into much of daily life, with the city often partnering with local businesses, community groups and the school system

to promote wellness initiatives. Its handful of public schools focus on students' mental health, mindfulness, healthy eating and physical fitness, with an early morning exercise class hosted at the middle school and an annual "Stress Less Week" at George Mason High School featuring therapy dogs and yoga classes. School lunches are often made with locally sourced ingredients, including lettuce grown hydroponically at the high school.

Beyond the school system, healthy food is accessible through a large new grocery store and weekly farmers market. Residents benefit from accessible primary care doctors and widespread health insurance coverage, likely due in part to the city's above-average share of workers employed by the federal government. Falls Church leadership also

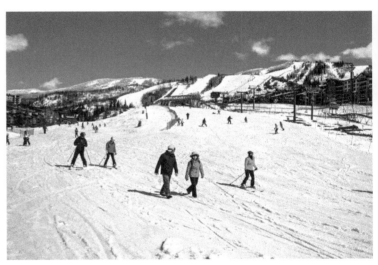

ROUTT COUNTY, COLORADO. Skiers and snowboarders hit the slopes at Steamboat Springs.

prioritizes environmentally friendly initiatives, with plans for a new bike share and an emphasis on things like safer, cleaner sidewalks.

"We're trying to create a more walkable, bikeable, vibrant downtown," Mayor David Tarter says. It doesn't hurt that Falls Church is among the wealthiest and most highly educated U.S. communities. Around a quarter of its households earn $200,000 or more annually, according to U.S. Census Bureau estimates, and the poverty rate is around 3 percent. About 80 percent of adults 25 or older hold at least an associate degree, more than double the rate in Virginia and the rest of the U.S.

Its strong score in the community vitality category, which measures rates of homeownership and voter participation, for example, also helped propel it to the top of the standings. Residents are politically engaged, and there's a high concentra-

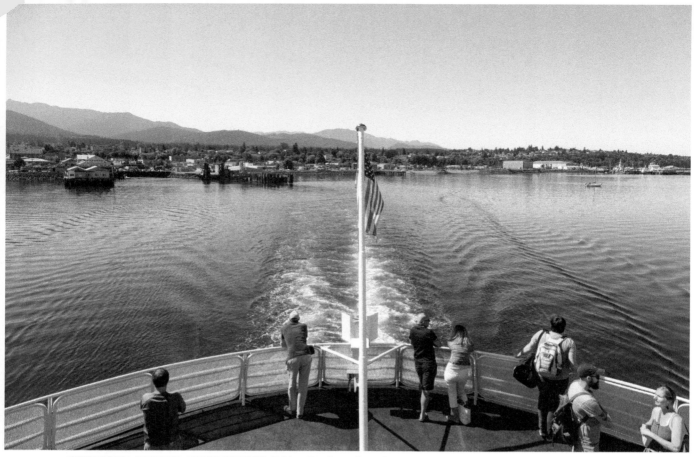

JEFFERSON COUNTY, WASHINGTON. Taking the ferry from Port Townsend to nearby Vancouver Island

tion of registered nonprofits in the region.

Falls Church has seen a flurry of development in recent years, increasing residents' access to services. But while the new development has boosted the local economy and helped the city fund services for a growing population, it has also fueled concerns of displacement among some small-business owners. "The new buildings, which are beautiful and nice" and offer needed amenities, are much more expensive, says resident Sally Cole, executive director of the Falls Church Chamber of Commerce. "As more and more development happens, it's going to be harder for the independent businesses to stay."

One redevelopment project forced Esmat Niazy, who lives nearby in Vienna, Virginia, to move his family's Afghan restaurant after more than 30 years in the same location. Uncertainty over whether he'd have to relocate "has been a strain on my wallet," but he says customers like his new space just minutes away.

Another challenge: As new residents are drawn by the city's schools and sense of community, its growth has tested it in areas of equity and housing affordability – issues that plague other top-ranked communities. Nearly a third of its households spend more than 30 percent of their incomes on monthly housing costs. And income inequality and racial gaps in educational attainment exist in the increasingly diverse community, which is about 70 percent non-Hispanic white.

To help moderate- and low-income residents stay, the city implemented a voluntary program in which developers can set aside 6 percent of all new apartments for households meeting certain income thresholds. Participating developers are considered for exemptions from some building height and use requirements.

"This is a very high-income area, and the poverty rate is low, but it's not nonexistent," says Nancy Vincent, who leads the city's Housing and Human Services department. "There's a group of low-income folks, and quite a few low-income seniors in the city. These folks are an important part of the community and culture of the city, and it would be a huge loss for them not to live here."

To highlight racial inequality and discrimination, as well as strengthen business ties in the community, Cole's chamber has partnered with the region's Arab American Business Council to host events where members network and learn about challenges facing minority business owners. Marwan Ahmad, who heads the business council, says city leadership has been "very open and very inviting to us as businesses and individuals." He hopes neighboring Fairfax County and Virginia as a whole "will follow suit, because this is a good example of how we can work together."

Knowing how all these social factors interact to create a healthier community – or a sicker one – is an important first step toward targeting resources where they'll do the most good, Fleming says. "Rather than thinking about what we should be doing about diabetes, smoking, poverty and education," he says, "we should be thinking what we could be doing in communities across all these domains."

The need for better understanding and action is clear. Disparities in health and well-being across the U.S. are staggering, says Ali Mokdad, a professor of health metrics sciences at the University of Washington's Institute for Health Metrics and Evaluation. People living in Florida's Union County, for example, have a life expectancy of 68, while people in Summit County, Colorado, No. 26 in the overall ranking, can expect an average lifespan of 87 years. ●

Achieving
the Distinction
that Matters

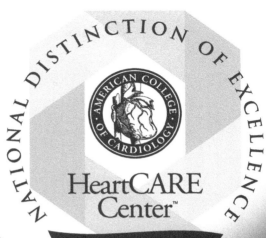

NATIONAL DISTINCTION OF EXCELLENCE

AMERICAN COLLEGE · OF CARDIOLOGY

HeartCARE Center™

2018

Photo: CHRISTUS Trinity Mother Frances Health System

The first HeartCARE Center awardee: CHRISTUS Trinity Mother Frances Louis and Peaches Owen Heart Hospital - Tyler

THE AMERICAN COLLEGE OF CARDIOLOGY CELEBRATES AND CONGRATULATES THESE OUTSTANDING CARDIOVASCULAR TEAMS AS OUR INAUGURAL HEARTCARE CENTER AWARDEES:

CHRISTUS TRINITY MOTHER FRANCES LOUIS AND PEACHES OWEN HEART HOSPITAL — TYLER

REGIONAL HOSPITAL OF SCRANTON – COMMONWEALTH HEALTH

CHESTER COUNTY HOSPITAL – PENN MEDICINE

LAWRENCE GENERAL HOSPITAL

MANY OTHER FACILITIES WILL SOON JOIN THEIR RANKS AND EARN THE ULTIMATE RECOGNITION FOR THEIR HARD WORK AND DEDICATION TO PATIENTS.

Achieving the HeartCARE Center distinction confirms your standing as a provider of world-class cardiovascular care.

CV programs that demonstrate a commitment to comprehensive process improvement, disease and procedure-specific accreditation, professional excellence and community engagement are solid contenders for this prestigious recognition. In little less than two months since the inception of this national distinction of excellence, four facilities have been named HeartCARE Centers.

Seek the recognition that makes a difference from the organization that has set the standard for world-class cardiovascular science and patient care guidelines for nearly 70 years. It tells peers, patients and the community that your commitment to quality patient care and successful outcomes stands head and shoulders above the rest.

ACC.org/HeartCARECenter

Pharmacist Picks

The experts share their top
over-the-counter choices

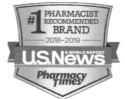

#1 PHARMACIST RECOMMENDED BRAND 2018-2019
U.S.News & WORLD REPORT
Pharmacy Times

ike many people, when you're suffering from a migraine, allergies or some other ailment, you probably make a beeline to a nearby pharmacy looking for a remedy that will offer prompt relief. But trying to figure out your best option among the crowded drugstore shelves can be a challenge. For some people, the which-should-I-pick decision comes down to price. For others, it may be a simple matter of brand loyalty ("My family always used ..."). For still others, it's whichever medication gets the most compelling pitch in advertisements or commercials. Often, it's been a decision people have had to make randomly, without any real guidance.

But help has arrived in the form of pharmacists, whose mission includes educating patients on how and when to take a prescribed medicine, advising them on possible side effects, and warning about potential drug interactions.

For more than 20 years, the industry trade publication Pharmacy Times has surveyed thousands of pharmacists nationwide to pinpoint their top recommendations for a range of over-the-counter products. The results, published each year in its OTC Guide, are then shared widely among pharmacists throughout the nation to help them guide consumers' buying decisions. And now this inside intel is available to you, too.

U.S. News and Pharmacy Times have combed through the survey responses to show how different brands stack up in more than 150 over-the-counter product categories. The tables that follow here reveal the top brand-name picks for a number of popular product types, including decongestants, sunscreen, infant formulas, migraine relievers and remedies for upset stomachs. Percentages have been rounded.

Though you should always read package labels for ingredients, directions and warnings, don't hesitate to consult with your pharmacist as you navigate the drugstore aisles. For the full results in all 150-plus categories, visit usnews.com/tophealthproducts.

ACID REDUCERS

Product	% Pharmacists recommending
Prilosec OTC	40%
Zantac	26%
Pepcid	16%
Nexium 24HR	14%
Prevacid 24HR	1%
Zegerid OTC	1%

ACNE PRODUCTS

Product	% Pharmacists recommending
Differin Gel	27%
Neutrogena	22%
Clearasil	21%
PanOxyl	13%
Clean & Clear Persa-Gel 10	5%
OXY	5%

ADHESIVE BANDAGES

Product	% Pharmacists recommending
BAND-AID	74%
Nexcare	17%
Curad	9%

ANTIBIOTICS/ ANTISEPTICS (TOPICAL)

Product	% Pharmacists recommending
NEOSPORIN	75%
Polysporin	12%
HIBICLENS	6%
Bacitraycin Plus	3%
Betadine	3%

ANTIHISTAMINES (ORAL)

Product	% Pharmacists recommending
Claritin	39%
Zyrtec	38%
Allegra Allergy	9%
Benadryl	8%
Chlor-Trimeton	4%

ARTHRITIS TREATMENT (ORAL)

Product	% Pharmacists recommending
Aleve	33%
Tylenol Arthritis Pain	30%
Advil	23%
Motrin	14%

ARTIFICIAL TEARS

Product	% Pharmacists recommending
Systane	36%
Refresh	33%
Tears Naturale	10%
GenTeal	6%
Hypo Tears	3%
Visine	3%

ATHLETE'S FOOT/ ANTIFUNGAL PRODUCTS

Product	% Pharmacists recommending
Lamisil	45%
Lotrimin	41%
Tinactin	8%
Zeasorb	4%
Micatin	1%

BLOOD PRESSURE MONITORS

Product	% Pharmacists recommending
Omron	85%
LifeSource	11%
HoMedics	4%

BURN TREATMENTS

Product	% Pharmacists recommending
NEOSPORIN	32%
Dermoplast	16%
Lanacane Spray	12%
ALOCANE	11%
Curad Silver Solution	8%
A+D Ointment	7%

CHOLESTEROL MANAGEMENT

Product	% Pharmacists recommending
Nature Made Fish Oil	37%
Metamucil	22%
Nature's Bounty Fish Oil	14%
Slo-Niacin	11%
Schiff MegaRed	8%
Nature Made CholestOff	5%

COLD REMEDIES

Product	% Pharmacists recommending
Cepacol	37%
Halls Defense	17%
Zicam	17%
Cold-EEZE	16%
Sucrets	4%

CONTACT LENS SOLUTIONS

Product	% Pharmacists recommending
OPTI-FREE	50%
Biotrue	14%
renu multi-purpose solution	14%
Boston ADVANCE	7%
Clear Care Cleaning & Disinfecting Solution	7%
COMPLETE Multi-Purpose Solution EASY RUB Formula	5%

COUGH SUPPRESSANTS

Product	% Pharmacists recommending
Delsym	50%
Mucinex DM	28%
Robitussin	20%
NyQuil	2%
Zarbee's Naturals	1%

DANDRUFF SHAMPOO

Product	% Pharmacists recommending
Head & Shoulders	31%
Nizoral	27%
Selsun Blue	27%
T/Gel	13%
Denorex	2%

DECONGESTANTS (ORAL)

Product	% Pharmacists recommending
Sudafed (pseudoephedrine)	49%
Mucinex D	10%
Advil Cold & Sinus	9%
Claritin-D	9%
Sudafed PE (phenylephrine)	9%
Zyrtec-D	8%
Allegra-D	6%

DIAPER RASH PRODUCTS

Product	% Pharmacists recommending
Desitin Diaper Rash	30%
A+D Diaper Rash Ointment	28%
Boudreaux's Butt Paste	12%
Triple Paste	7%
Calmoseptine	6%
Balmex	5%

DIGITAL THERMOMETERS

Product	% Pharmacists recommending
Braun ThermoScan	30%
Omron	25%
Vicks	22%
3M Nexcare	16%
Exergen Temporal Artery Thermometer	7%

FIBER SUPPLEMENTS

Product	% Pharmacists recommending
Metamucil	48%
Benefiber	27%
FiberCon	10%
Citrucel	9%
Konsyl	3%

FLU TREATMENT PRODUCTS

Product	% Pharmacists recommending
DayQuil Cold & Flu	21%
Tylenol Cold + Flu Severe	20%
NyQuil Cold & Flu	17%
Theraflu	17%
Coricidin HBP Cold & Flu	13%
Alka-Seltzer Plus Cold + Flu	9%

HAND SANITIZERS

Product	% Pharmacists recommending
Purell	83%
Germ-X	17%

INFANT FORMULAS

Product	% Pharmacists recommending
Enfamil	48%
Similac	37%
Gerber Good Start	8%
Earth's Best	4%
Similac Soy Isomil	3%

MIGRAINE RELIEVERS

Product	% Pharmacists recommending
Excedrin Migraine	74%
Aleve	13%
Advil Migraine	10%
Tylenol	3%

MULTIVITAMINS

Product	% Pharmacists recommending
Centrum	51%
One A Day	22%
Nature Made	14%
Nature's Bounty	7%
vitafusion MultiVites	2%

PRENATAL VITAMINS

Product	% Pharmacists recommending
One A Day Prenatal	44%
Nature Made Multi Prenatal	22%
Centrum Specialist Prenatal	11%
Nature's Bounty Prenatal	8%
vitafusion PreNatal	8%
21st Century Prenatal	3%

SLEEP AIDS

Product	% Pharmacists recommending
Unisom	53%
Vicks ZzzQuil	14%
Sominex	9%
Nature Made Sleep	7%
Nytol	4%
Simply Sleep	4%

SUNSCREEN

Product	% Pharmacists recommending
Neutrogena	32%
Coppertone	28%
Banana Boat	14%
Bullfrog	7%
CeraVe	6%

TOOTHPASTE

Product	% Pharmacists recommending
Crest	36%
Colgate	29%
Sensodyne	26%
Aquafresh	4%
Arm & Hammer	3%

UPSET STOMACH REMEDIES

Product	% Pharmacists recommending
Pepto-Bismol	61%
Emetrol	21%
Alka-Seltzer	12%
Kaopectate	6%

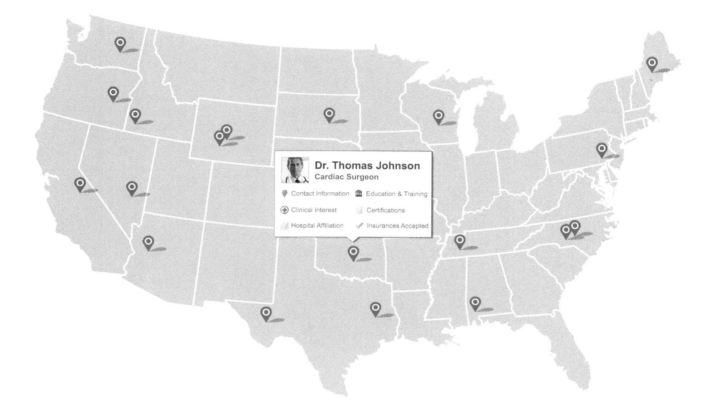

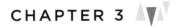

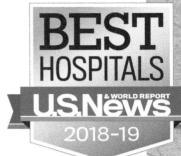

Best Hospitals

Operating at No. 1
Mayo Clinic

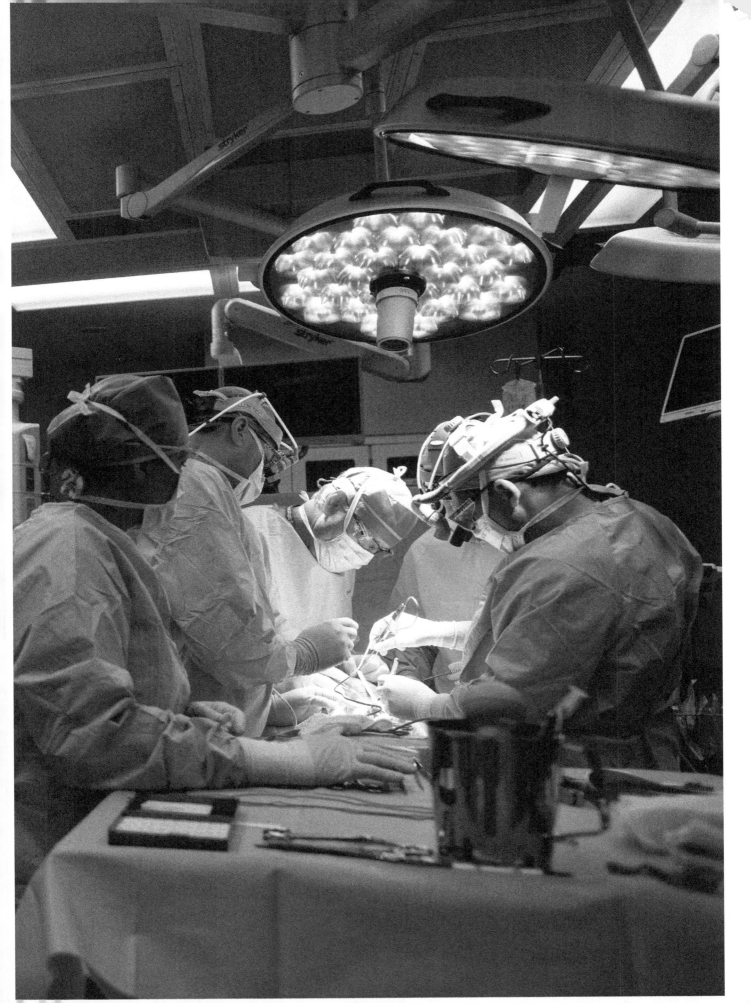

The Honor Roll

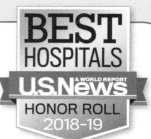

The 20 medical centers below excel in treating patients with complex diagnoses and those with relatively routine needs. Each hospital is nationally ranked in nine or more of the 16 Best Hospitals specialties and is rated "high performing" in most or all of nine common procedures and conditions (full ratings at usnews.com/best-hospitals). Honor Roll standing is based on points. A hospital that was ranked No. 1 in all 16 specialties and rated high performing in all nine procedures and conditions would have received 448 points. The 20 highest scorers qualified for the Honor Roll.

1 Mayo Clinic
Rochester, Minn., 414 points

2 Cleveland Clinic
385 points

3 Johns Hopkins Hospital
Baltimore, 355 points

4 Massachusetts General Hospital
Boston, 354 points

5 U. of Michigan Hospitals-Michigan Medicine
Ann Arbor, 324 points

6 UCSF Medical Center
San Francisco, 296 points

7 UCLA Medical Center
Los Angeles, 267 points

8 Cedars-Sinai Medical Center
Los Angeles, 252 points

9 Stanford Health Care-Stanford Hospital
Stanford, Calif., 250 points

10 New York-Presbyterian Hospital-Columbia and Cornell
New York, 242 points

11* Barnes-Jewish Hospital
St. Louis, 241 points

11* Mayo Clinic-Phoenix
241 points

13 Northwestern Memorial Hospital
Chicago, 228 points

14 Hospitals of the University of Pennsylvania-Penn Presbyterian
Philadelphia, 225 points

15* NYU Langone Hospitals
New York, 208 points

15* UPMC Presbyterian Shadyside
Pittsburgh, 208 points

17 Vanderbilt University Medical Center
Nashville, Tenn., 198 points

18 Mount Sinai Hospital
New York, 192 points

19 Duke University Hospital
Durham, N.C., 178 points

20 Brigham and Women's Hospital
Boston, 177 points

*Denotes a tie

A Guide to the Rankings

How we identified 158 outstanding hospitals in 16 specialties

by **Ben Harder** and **Avery Comarow**

The mission of the Best Hospitals annual rankings, now in their 29th year, remains the same as always: to help guide patients who need an especially high level of care to the right place. These are patients whose surgery or condition is complex or difficult. Or whose advanced age, physical infirmity or existing medical condition puts them at heightened risk.

Such people account for a small fraction of hospital patients, but they add up to millions of individuals, and most hospitals may not be able to meet their needs. A hospital ranked by U.S. News in cardiology and heart surgery, say, is likely to have the experience and expertise to operate safely on a patient 85 or 90 years old with a leaky heart valve. The typical community hospital cannot supply the special techniques and precautions needed, and should instead send such a patient to a hospital that can. Many community hospitals do that. But not all.

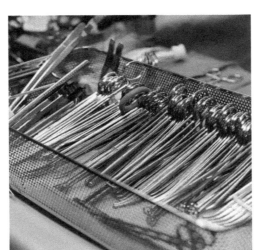

The following pages offer hospital rankings in 16 specialties, from cancer to urology. Of 4,656 hospitals evaluated this year, only 158 performed well enough to be ranked in any specialty. Based on input from experts and medical studies, we have refined the methodology over time to improve the rankings' usefulness to consumers.

In 12 of 16 specialties, hard data from the federal government and other sources were the main factors determining whether a hospital was ranked. Some kinds of data, such as death rates, are intimately related to quality. Numbers of patients and the balance of nurses to patients are examples of data that are also important, although the quality connection may seem less evident. To capture medical experts' opinions, we also factored in results from annual surveys of specialist physicians who were asked to name hospitals they consider tops in their specialty for difficult cases.

Hospitals in the other four specialties (ophthalmology, psychiatry, rehabilitation and rheumatology) were ranked solely on the basis of the annual physician surveys. That's because so few patients die in these specialties that mortality rates, which carry heavy weight in the 12 other specialties, mean little.

To be considered for ranking in the 12 data-driven specialties, a hospital had to meet any of four criteria: It had to be a teaching hospital, or be affiliated with a medical school, or have at least 200 beds, or have at least 100 beds and offer at least four out of eight advanced medical technologies. This year 2,264 hospitals met that test.

The hospitals next had to meet a volume requirement in each specialty – a minimum number of Medicare inpatients from 2014 to 2016 who received certain procedures and treatment for specific conditions. The minimum number of patients for cardiology and heart surgery, for example, was 1,391, of which 500 had to be surgical. A hospital that fell short was still eligible if it was nominated in the specialty by at least 1 percent of the physicians responding to the 2016, 2017 and 2018 surveys.

At the end of the process, 1,897 hospitals remained candidates for ranking in at least one specialty. Each received a U.S. News score of 0 to 100 based on four elements: patient survival; patient safety; care-related factors such as nursing, volume, technology, and special accreditations and recognitions; and expert opinion. The 50 top performers in each of the 12 specialties were ranked. Scores and data for the rest, as well as more detail on the methodology, are available at usnews.com/best-hospitals. The four elements and their weights in brief:

Survival score (37.5 percent). Success at keeping patients alive was judged by the proportion of Medicare inpatients with certain conditions who died within 30 days of admission in 2014, 2015 and 2016. That rate was adjusted to account for

Canon–a bright future in healthcare.

Healthcare IT

Offering leading-edge diagnostic support systems and network solutions utilizing ICT.

Diagnostic Imaging Systems

Meeting clinical needs with high resolution imaging from CT, MRI, X-ray and Ultrasound systems.

Canon

Introducing Canon Medical Systems

Technology that's made for life.
Canon—having welcomed Toshiba Medical Systems Corporation,
a company renowned in the field of medical imaging,
into the Canon Group—celebrates today on January 4th, 2018,
the birth of Canon Medical Systems Corporation.
Made for Partnerships. Made for Patients. Made for You.
Based on our "Made for Life," philosophy, we aim to support the wellbeing,
safety and security of humankind globally.

Canon Medical Systems will contribute to even further developments in healthcare
through three pillars of advanced technology: Diagnostic Imaging Systems,
Healthcare IT and In-vitro Diagnostic Systems.

In-vitro Diagnostic Systems

Supporting examination
workflows with high resolution
and rapid analysis of blood
and other specimens
taken from patients.

Images are for reference purposes only.

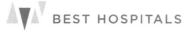

the severity of patients' illnesses, the complexity of their care, and risk-elevating factors such as advanced age, obesity, high blood pressure and poverty (as reflected in whether they received Medicaid). Industry-standard software was used to adjust each patient's risk in calculating survival odds. To avoid penalizing institutions that receive the sickest patients, we excluded from our analysis all patients who were transferred into a hospital from another hospital. In the tables that follow, a score of 10 indicates the best chance of survival (and 1 the worst) relative to other hospitals.

Patient safety score (5 percent). Every hospital harms patients unnecessarily. This score reflects efforts to prevent the four kinds of harm listed in the box below.

Other care-related indicators (30 percent). Trauma center status, arthritis center certification, and availability of intensive care specialists are examples.

Expert opinion (27.5 percent). This part of a hospital's total score was drawn from the last three years of annual physician surveys. Specialists were asked to name up to five hospitals, setting aside location and cost, that they consider best in their area of expertise for patients with the most difficult medical problems. In the 2018 survey alone, responses were tallied from some 21,000 physicians.

USNEWS.COM/BESTHOSPITALS

Visit usnews.com regularly while researching your health care choices, as U.S. News often adds content aimed at helping patients and families make the best possible decisions about their medical care. We also update the Best Hospitals, Best Children's Hospitals, and Best Regional Hospitals data on the website when new data become available.

The figures shown under "% of specialists recommending hospital" in the ranking tables are the average percentages of specialists in 2016, 2017 and 2018 who recommended a hospital. In many cases, hospitals with low scores on the physician surveys but strong clinical numbers outrank centers with stronger reputations.

In the four survey-based specialties, a hospital had to be cited by at least 5 percent of responding physicians in the latest three years of U.S. News surveys to be ranked. That created lists of 11 hospitals in psychiatry, 12 in ophthalmology, and 13 each in rehabilitation and rheumatology.

If you've consulted past editions of Best Hospitals, you're bound to notice some hospitals that have risen or fallen in the rankings. Don't make too much of modest year-to-year movements. It takes multiple years of progressive change to know if a hospital is truly improving or worsening.

No hospital, no matter how excellent, is best for every patient. You'll want to add your own fact-gathering to ours and consult with your doctor or other health professional. ●

A Glossary of Terms

FACT accreditation level: hospital meets Foundation for the Accreditation of Cellular Therapy standards as of March 1, 2018, for harvesting and transplanting stem cells from a patient's own bone marrow and tissue (level 1) and from a donor (level 2) to treat cancer.

Intensivists: at least one critical-care specialist manages patients in intensive care units.

NAEC epilepsy center: designated by the National Association of Epilepsy Centers as of March 1, 2018, as a regional or national referral facility (level 4) for staffing, technology and training in epilepsy care.

NCI cancer center: designated by the National Cancer Institute as of March 1, 2018, as a clinical or comprehensive cancer hospital.

NIA Alzheimer's center: designated by the National Institute on

Aging as of March 7, 2018, as an Alzheimer's Disease Center, indicating high quality of research and clinical care.

Number of patients: estimated number of Medicare inpatients in 2014, 2015 and 2016 who received certain high-level care as defined by U.S. News. Based on an adjustment to the number of such patients with traditional Medicare insurance. In geriatrics, only patients ages 75 and older are included.

A Nurse Magnet hospital: recognized by the American Nurses Credentialing Center as of January 2, 2018, for nursing excellence.

Nurse staffing score: relative balance of nonsupervisory registered nurses (inpatient and outpatient) to average daily number of all patients. Inpatient staffing receives greater weight. Agency and temporary nurses are not counted.

Patient safety score: indicates ability to protect patients from four types of preventable harm: death from preventable postsurgical complications, major postsurgical bleeding and bruising, postsurgical respiratory failure, and injury during surgery.

Patient services score: number of services offered out of the number considered important to quality (such as genetic testing in cancer and an Alzheimer's center in geriatrics).

% of specialists recommending hospital: percentage of physicians responding to U.S. News surveys in 2016, 2017 and 2018 who named the hospital as among the best in their specialty for especially challenging cases and procedures, setting aside location and cost.

Rank: based on U.S. News score except in ophthalmology, psychiatry, rehabilitation and rheumatology, where specialist recommendations determine rank.

Survival score: reflects patient survival rate in the specialty within 30 days of admission.

Technology score: reflects availability of technologies considered important to a high quality of care, such as PET/CT scanner in pulmonology and diagnostic radio-isotope services in urology.

Transparency score: indicates whether hospital publicly reports heart outcomes through the American College of Cardiology and the Society of Thoracic Surgeons.

Trauma center: indicates Level 1 or 2 trauma center certification. Such a center can care properly for the most severe injuries.

U.S. News score: summary of quality of hospital inpatient care. In most specialties, survival is worth 37.5 percent, operational quality data such as nurse staffing and patient volume 30 percent, specialists' recommendations 27.5 percent, and patient safety 5 percent.

CEDARS-SINAI®

HONORED

TO BE AMONG THE TOP 10 HOSPITALS IN THE NATION.

Cedars-Sinai is proud to be ranked in the top 10 of
U.S. News & World Report's Best Hospitals
Honor Roll, and to be among the very best in multiple
specialties. Thank you for trusting us to deliver
the expert care you and your family deserve, when
you need it most.

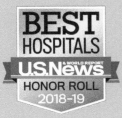

RANKED #8 IN THE NATIONAL HONOR ROLL

RANKED #3 IN THE NATION FOR CARDIOLOGY & HEART SURGERY
RANKED #3 IN THE NATION FOR GASTROENTEROLOGY & GI SURGERY
RANKED #9 IN THE NATION FOR ORTHOPAEDICS

ALSO RANKED AMONG THE NATION'S BEST IN:
CANCER
DIABETES & ENDOCRINOLOGY
EAR, NOSE & THROAT
GERIATRICS
GYNECOLOGY
NEPHROLOGY
NEUROLOGY & NEUROSURGERY
PULMONOLOGY
UROLOGY

©2018 Cedars-Sinai

CANCER

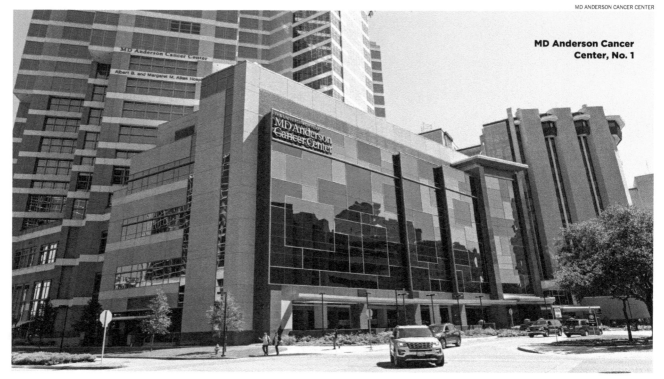

MD Anderson Cancer Center, No. 1

Rank	Hospital	U.S. News score	Survival score (10=best)	Patient safety score (9=best)	Number of patients	Nurse staffing score (higher is better)	A Nurse Magnet hospital	NCI cancer center	FACT accreditation level (2=best)	Patient services score (8=best)	% of specialists recommending hospital
1	University of Texas MD Anderson Cancer Center, Houston	100.0	10	5	7,855	2.0	Yes	Yes	2	8	53.3%
2	Memorial Sloan-Kettering Cancer Center, New York	97.4	10	5	6,241	2.1	Yes	Yes	2	8	50.6%
3	Mayo Clinic, Rochester, Minn.	95.3	10	5	4,019	2.8	Yes	Yes	2	8	22.3%
4	Dana-Farber/Brigham and Women's Cancer Center, Boston	83.0	10	5	3,161	2.3	Yes	Yes	2	8	26.6%
5	Cleveland Clinic	80.9	10	6	2,554	2.1	Yes	Yes	2	8	8.7%
6	Johns Hopkins Hospital, Baltimore	80.3	10	4	1,855	2.1	Yes	Yes	2	8	17.6%
7	Seattle Cancer Care Alliance/U. of Washington Medical Ctr.	78.5	10	5	1,580	2.0	Yes	Yes	2	8	8.1%
8	H. Lee Moffitt Cancer Center and Research Institute, Tampa	76.6	10	4	3,264	1.2	Yes	Yes	2	7	7.0%
8	UCSF Medical Center, San Francisco	76.6	10	6	2,089	2.1	Yes	Yes	2	8	5.4%
10	Hosps. of the U. of Pennsylvania-Penn Presby., Philadelphia	75.8	10	6	3,037	2.4	Yes	Yes	2	8	6.8%
11	Mayo Clinic-Phoenix	74.1	10	6	1,761	2.9	Yes	Yes	2	8	2.7%
12	Massachusetts General Hospital, Boston	72.6	9	5	2,866	2.4	Yes	Yes	2	8	9.9%
12	Northwestern Memorial Hospital, Chicago	72.6	10	5	1,723	1.8	Yes	Yes	2	8	2.2%
14	Stanford Health Care-Stanford Hospital, Stanford, Calif.	72.4	10	5	2,126	2.5	Yes	Yes	2	8	5.9%
15	Siteman Cancer Center, St. Louis	72.3	10	5	3,402	2.2	Yes	Yes	2	8	4.0%
15	U. of Michigan Hospitals-Michigan Medicine, Ann Arbor	72.3	10	7	2,128	2.7	Yes	Yes	2	8	3.7%
17	USC Norris Cancer Hosp.-Keck Med. Ctr. of USC, Los Angeles	71.7	10	6	1,345	2.4	No	Yes	2	8	1.0%
18	University of Iowa Hospitals and Clinics, Iowa City	70.2	10	5	1,356	1.8	Yes	Yes	2	8	1.4%
19	Wake Forest Baptist Medical Center, Winston-Salem, N.C.	70.0	10	5	2,652	1.6	Yes	Yes	2	8	1.5%
20	Ohio State University James Cancer Hospital, Columbus	69.9	10	5	3,206	2.1	Yes	Yes	2	8	4.8%
21	City of Hope Helford Clinical Research Hosp., Duarte, Calif.	69.4	10	5	2,152	2.4	No	Yes	2	8	5.0%
21	UCLA Medical Center, Los Angeles	69.4	10	5	2,053	3.0	Yes	Yes	2	8	5.0%
23	UPMC Presbyterian Shadyside, Pittsburgh	68.9	10	5	3,820	1.9	Yes	Yes	2	8	4.1%
24	MUSC Health-University Medical Center, Charleston, S.C.	68.7	10	5	1,082	2.3	Yes	Yes	2	8	0.4%

(CONTINUED ON PAGE 106)

Terms are explained on Page 102.

▶ **More** @ usnews.com/besthospitals

WE SPEED
LIFE-CHANGING DISCOVERIES
TO LIFE

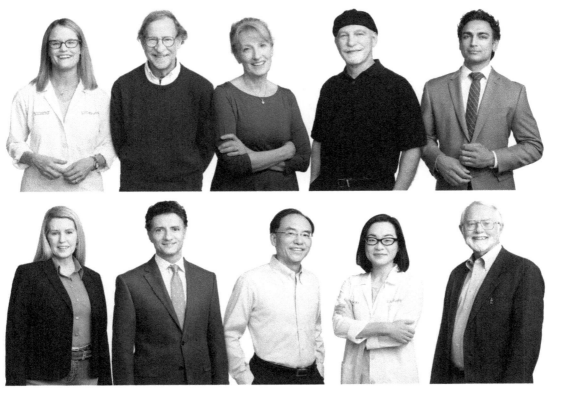

It's not enough to promise future cures. We have to find them today. This is the passion that drives us. We are City of Hope doctors and researchers, advancing science that saves lives. Our work has led to the development of four of the most widely used cancer-fighting drugs. We've pioneered CAR T cell therapy and are turning your immune system into cancer's worst enemy. We're making precision medicine a reality by using your genes to determine the best treatment for your cancer. At City of Hope, our patients depend on us for extraordinary answers. That's why we work like there's no tomorrow. Find out more at **CityofHope.org**

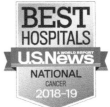

BEST HOSPITALS
U.S.News & WORLD REPORT
NATIONAL CANCER 2018–19

the **MIRACLE** of **SCIENCE** with **SOUL**™ City of Hope®

CANCER (CONTINUED)

Rank	Hospital	U.S. News score	Survival score (10=best)	Patient safety score (9=best)	Number of patients	Nurse staffing score (higher is better)	A Nurse Magnet hospital	NCI cancer center	FACT accreditation level (2=best)	Patient services score (8=best)	% of specialists recommending hospital
25	New York-Presbyterian Hospital-Columbia and Cornell, N.Y.	68.5	10	4	4,424	2.9	No	Yes	2	8	3.5%
26	Jefferson Health-Thomas Jefferson U. Hospitals, Philadelphia	68.4	10	5	2,082	2.2	Yes	Yes	2	8	2.1%
26	University of Colorado Hospital, Aurora	68.4	10	5	1,803	1.9	Yes	Yes	2	8	1.5%
28	OHSU Hospital, Portland, Ore.	67.9	10	5	1,648	2.0	Yes	Yes	2	8	1.2%
28	University Hospitals Seidman Cancer Center, Cleveland	67.9	10	5	1,538	2.6	Yes	Yes	2	8	1.1%
30	Mayo Clinic Jacksonville, Fla.	67.8	10	6	961	2.1	Yes	Yes	2	8	2.8%
30	Roswell Park Comprehensive Cancer Center, Buffalo	67.8	10	5	1,257	1.9	No	Yes	2	8	2.1%
32	University of Maryland Medical Center, Baltimore	67.7	10	3	1,073	2.9	Yes	Yes	2	8	0.5%
33	University of Chicago Medical Center	67.2	10	7	1,818	2.4	No	Yes	2	8	3.8%
33	University of Minnesota Medical Center, Minneapolis	67.2	10	5	1,680	2.0	No	Yes	2	8	0.4%
35	Duke University Hospital, Durham, N.C.	67.1	9	6	2,047	2.1	Yes	Yes	2	8	5.4%
36	University of California, Davis Medical Center, Sacramento	66.8	10	5	1,509	2.8	Yes	Yes	2	8	0.4%
36	University of North Carolina Hospitals, Chapel Hill	66.8	10	5	1,538	1.8	Yes	Yes	2	8	2.4%
38	U. of Kentucky Albert B. Chandler Hospital, Lexington	66.1	10	5	1,015	1.9	Yes	Yes	2	8	1.2%
39	Vanderbilt University Medical Center, Nashville, Tenn.	65.8	9	6	1,844	2.5	Yes	Yes	2	8	2.9%
40	University of Virginia Medical Center, Charlottesville	65.6	10	5	962	2.1	Yes	Yes	2	8	0.8%
41	Cedars-Sinai Medical Center, Los Angeles	65.5	10	5	2,650	2.6	Yes	No	2	8	1.5%
42	University of Kansas Hospital, Kansas City	65.3	10	5	1,501	2.1	Yes	Yes	2	8	0.8%
43	University of Wisconsin Hospitals, Madison	65.1	10	5	1,349	2.1	Yes	Yes	2	8	0.7%
44	NYU Langone Hospitals, New York, N.Y.	64.4	10	5	1,699	2.3	Yes	Yes	1	8	1.4%
45	UC San Diego Health - Moores Cancer Center	64.0	10	5	1,315	2.0	Yes	Yes	2	8	1.6%
46	Indiana University Health Medical Center, Indianapolis	63.3	10	5	1,564	2.0	Yes	Yes	2	8	0.5%
47	Mount Sinai Hospital, New York	62.3	9	6	1,933	1.9	Yes	Yes	2	8	0.8%
48	Huntsman Cancer Institute at the U. of Utah, Salt Lake City	62.2	10	5	1,153	1.8	No	Yes	2	8	0.7%
49	Beth Israel Deaconess Medical Center, Boston	62.1	10	5	1,405	1.6	No	Yes	2	8	0.5%
49	Rush University Medical Center, Chicago	62.1	10	5	1,505	2.2	Yes	No	2	8	1.2%

Terms are explained on Page 102.

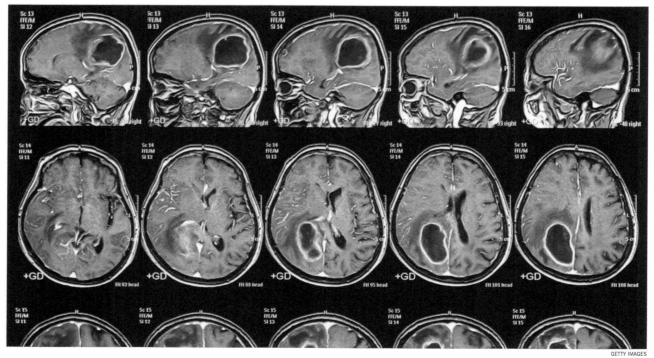

GETTY IMAGES

⏵ More @ usnews.com/besthospitals

CARDIOLOGY & HEART SURGERY

SMIDT HEART INSTITUTE

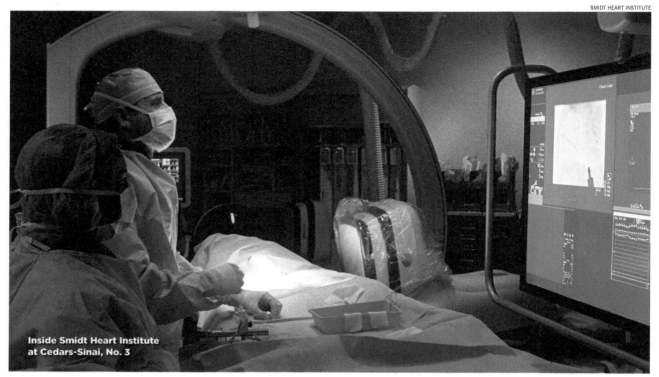

Inside Smidt Heart Institute at Cedars-Sinai, No. 3

Rank	Hospital	U.S. News score	Survival score (10=best)	Patient safety score (9=best)	Trans-parency score (3=best)	Number of patients	Nurse staffing score (higher is better)	A Nurse Magnet hospital	Technology score (6=best)	Patient services score (7=best)	Intensivists	% of specialists recom-mending hospital
1	Cleveland Clinic	100.0	10	6	3	14,270	2.1	Yes	6	7	Yes	42.7%
2	Mayo Clinic, Rochester, Minn.	99.6	10	5	3	13,557	2.8	Yes	6	7	Yes	38.6%
3	Smidt Heart Institute at Cedars-Sinai, Los Angeles	84.3	10	5	3	12,171	2.6	Yes	6	7	Yes	8.1%
4	New York-Presbyterian Hospital-Columbia and Cornell, N.Y.	83.3	10	4	3	16,804	2.9	No	6	7	Yes	14.7%
5	Massachusetts General Hospital, Boston	79.8	10	5	3	8,992	2.4	Yes	6	7	Yes	17.9%
6	Hosps. of the U. of Pennsylvania-Penn Presby., Philadelphia	78.0	10	6	3	11,078	2.4	Yes	6	7	Yes	8.6%
7	Northwestern Memorial Hospital, Chicago	76.9	10	5	3	4,919	1.8	Yes	6	7	Yes	5.5%
8	Brigham and Women's Hospital, Boston	76.7	10	5	3	6,562	2.3	No	6	7	Yes	15.3%
8	U. of Michigan Hospitals-Michigan Medicine, Ann Arbor	76.7	10	7	3	6,268	2.7	Yes	6	7	Yes	4.5%
10	Mount Sinai Hospital, New York	75.8	10	6	3	9,425	1.9	Yes	6	7	Yes	4.2%
11	Johns Hopkins Hospital, Baltimore	74.3	10	4	3	4,300	2.1	Yes	6	7	Yes	13.8%
12	Barnes-Jewish Hospital, St. Louis	73.0	10	5	3	8,049	2.2	Yes	6	7	Yes	3.2%
13	Stanford Health Care-Stanford Hospital, Stanford, Calif.	72.4	10	5	3	4,709	2.5	Yes	6	7	Yes	6.4%
14	Houston Methodist Hospital	72.3	10	5	3	8,328	2.0	Yes	6	7	Yes	4.9%
15	Duke University Hospital, Durham, N.C.	72.2	9	6	3	6,605	2.1	Yes	6	7	Yes	11.6%
16	UCLA Medical Center, Los Angeles	71.3	10	5	3	5,499	3.0	Yes	6	7	Yes	4.0%
17	Vanderbilt University Medical Center, Nashville, Tenn.	70.9	10	6	3	6,397	2.5	Yes	6	7	Yes	3.1%
18	University of Alabama at Birmingham Hospital	69.7	10	6	3	6,065	1.8	Yes	6	7	Yes	1.4%
19	Minneapolis Heart Institute at Abbott Northwestern Hospital	67.7	10	5	3	12,253	2.4	Yes	6	7	Yes	0.9%
20	Morristown Medical Center, Morristown, N.J.	67.6	10	5	3	8,335	2.1	Yes	5	7	Yes	0.5%
21	Baylor Scott and White The Heart Hospital Plano, Texas	67.5	10	6	3	4,992	2.0	Yes	5	7	Yes	1.6%
22	Texas Heart Inst. at Baylor St. Luke's Medical Ctr., Houston	67.2	10	5	3	7,012	1.6	Yes	5	6	Yes	8.0%
23	Scripps La Jolla Hospitals, La Jolla, Calif.	67.0	10	6	3	5,464	3.1	Yes	5	7	Yes	1.1%
24	Ohio State University Wexner Medical Center, Columbus	66.9	10	5	3	7,344	2.1	Yes	6	7	Yes	1.3%

(CONTINUED ON PAGE 114)

Terms are explained on Page 102.

▶ **More** @ usnews.com/besthospitals

MORRISTOWN MEDICAL CENTER
#1 HOSPITAL IN NJ

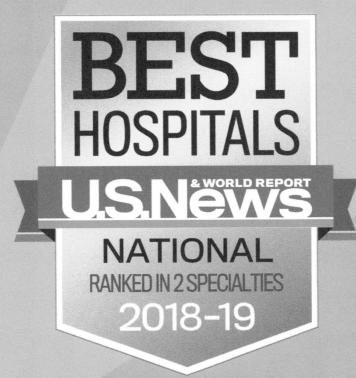

BEST HOSPITALS
U.S.News **& WORLD REPORT**
NATIONAL
RANKED IN 2 SPECIALTIES
2018-19

With nationally recognized leadership
in Cardiology & Heart Surgery and
Gastroenterology & GI Surgery

 Atlantic Health System
Morristown Medical Center

To learn more visit **atlantichealth.org**/usnews

Congratulations
to the Recipients of the
ACTION Registry®
2018 Performance
Achievement Award

Rewarding Excellence. Driving Success.

The ACTION Registry® (now the Chest Pain – MI Registry™) Performance Achievement
Award recognizes a hospital's success in implementing a higher standard of care for
heart attack patients by meeting aggressive performance measures as outlined by the
American College of Cardiology (ACC) and the American Heart Association (AHA) clinical
guidelines and recommendations.
The Registry helps hospitals:

- Improve patient outcomes using relevant data to drive decision making

- Apply the ACC/AHA clinical guidelines

- Improve the quality of care for heart attack patients through hospital-wide
  evaluation of performance standards

The ACTION Registry (now the Chest Pain – MI Registry) is the nation's largest and most
authoritative quality improvement registry with 1.5 million patient records and more than
10 years of proven success driving positive health outcomes for patients.

View hospitals participating in the registry
at *CardioSmart.org/ChestPainMI.*

**AMERICAN
COLLEGE *of*
CARDIOLOGY**

Chest Pain – MI Registry™
Formerly the ACTION Registry®

Providence Alaska Medical Center
Anchorage, AK

Adventist Health Bakersfield
Bakersfield, CA

California Pacific Medical Center
San Francisco, CA

Doctors Medical Center of Modesto
Modesto, CA

El Camino Hospital
Mountain View, CA

John Muir Medical Center – Concord Campus
Concord, CA

John Muir Medical Center – Walnut Creek Campus
Walnut Creek, CA

Palomar Medical Center
Escondido, CA

St. Josephs Medical Center of Stockton
Stockton, CA

Littleton Adventist Hospital
Littleton, CO

Medical Center of Aurora
Aurora, CO

Medical Center of the Rockies
Loveland, CO

Mercy Regional Medical Center
Durango, CO

North Colorado Medical Center
Greeley, CO

Parker Adventist Hospital
Parker, CO

Parkview Medical Center
Pueblo, CO

Penrose Hospital
Colorado Springs, CO

Porter Adventist Hospital
Denver, CO

Sky Ridge Medical Center
Lone Tree, CO

St. Anthony Hospital
Lakewood, CO

St. Francis Medical Center
Colorado Springs, CO

UCH – Memorial Hospital
Colorado Springs, CO

Saint Francis Hospital & Medical Center
Hartford, CT

Baptist Hospital, Inc.
Pensacola, FL

Mount Sinai Medical Center
Miami Beach, FL

West Florida Hospital
Pensacola, FL

Dekalb Medical Center
Decatur, GA

Gwinnett Hospital System
Lawrenceville, GA

Piedmont Fayette Hospital
Fayetteville, GA

Redmond Regional Medical Center
Rome, GA

St. Joseph's Hospital
Savannah, GA

Saint Alphonsus Regional Medical Center
Boise, ID

Adventist Hinsdale Hospital
Hinsdale, IL

Adventist La Grange Memorial Hospital
LaGrange, IL

Advocate Sherman Hospital
Downers Grove, IL

Carle Foundation Hospital
Urbana, IL

Loyola University Medical Center
Maywood, IL

Memorial Hospital Carbondale
Carbondale, IL

OSF HealthCare Saint Francis Medical Center
Peoria, IL

OSF Saint Anthony Medical Center
Rockford, IL

OSF Saint Joseph Medical Center
Bloomington, IL

Prairie Heart Institute at St. John's Hospital
Springfield, IL

Riverside Medical Center
Kankakee, IL

RUSH – Copley Medical Center
Aurora, IL

Columbus Regional Hospital
Columbus, IN

Community Hospital
Munster, IN

Deaconess Hospital
Evansville, IN

Goshen Hospital
Goshen, IN

Indiana University Health Ball Memorial Hospital
Muncie, IN

Indiana University Health Methodist Hospital
Indianapolis, IN

Indiana University Health Saxony Hospital
Fishers, IN

Riverview Health
Noblesville, IN

St. Vincent Evansville
Evansville, IN

The Heart Hospital at Deaconess Gateway, LLC
Newburgh, IN

Mercy Iowa City
Iowa City, IA

Mercy Medical Center
Sioux City, IA

Mercy Medical Center – Des Moines
Des Moines, IA

Saint Lukes Hospital
Cedar Rapids, IA

UnityPoint Health, St Luke's Sioux City
Sioux City, IA

Menorah Medical Center
Overland Park, KS

Olathe Medical Center
Olathe, KS

Stormont – Vail HealthCare
Topeka, KS

The University of Kansas Hospital
Kansas City, KS

University of Kansas Health System St. Francis Campus
Topeka, KS

Baptist Health Paducah
Paducah, KY

Saint Elizabeth Healthcare Edgewood
Edgewood, KY

St. Francis Medical Center
Monroe, LA

Johns Hopkins Bayview Medical Center
Baltimore, MD

Saint Agnes Hospital
Baltimore, MD

UM Baltimore Washington Medical Center
Glen Burnie, MD

University of Maryland Saint Joseph Medical Center
Towson, MD

Washington Adventist Hospital
Takoma Park, MD

Edward W Sparrow Hospital Assoc
Lansing, MI

Metro Health Hospital
Wyoming, MI

CentraCare Heart & Vascular Center
Saint Cloud, MN

Essentia Health – St. Mary's Medical Center
Duluth, MN

Essentia Health – Fargo
Fargo, MN

St. Luke's Hospital
Duluth, MN

Forrest General Hospital
Hattiesburg, MS

Magnolia Regional Health Center
Corinth, MS

North Mississippi Medical Center
Tupelo, MS

Southwest MS Regional Medical Center
McComb, MS

St. Dominic – Jackson Memorial Hospital
Jackson, MS

University of Mississippi Medical Center
Jackson, MS

Barnes Jewish Hospital/ Washington University
Saint Louis, MO

Capital Region Medical Center
Jefferson City, MO

Centerpoint Medical Center
Independence, MO

Mercy Hospital Joplin
Joplin, MO

MERCY Hospital Springfield
Springfield, MO

North Kansas City Hospital
North Kansas City, MO

Research Medical Center
Kansas City, MO

Saint Francis Medical Center
Cape Girardeau, MO

Saint Luke's East Hospital
Lee's Summitt, MO

Saint Luke's Hospital of Kansas City
Kansas City, MO

Saint Luke's North Hospital – Barry Road
Kansas City, MO

Southeast Missouri Hospital
Cape Girardeau, MO

SSM Health St. Mary's Hospital – Madison
St. Louis, MO

Billings Clinic (formerly Deaconess)
Billings, MT

Bozeman Health Deaconess Hospital
Bozeman, MT

Community Medical Center
Missoula, MT

Kalispell Regional Medical Center Inc
Kalispell, MT

Providence St. Patrick Hospital
Missoula, MT

Faith Regional Health Services
Norfolk, NE

Northern Nevada Medical Center
Sparks, NV

Saint Mary's Regional Medical Center
Reno, NV

Bayshore Community Hospital
Holmdel, NJ

Inspira Medical Center – Woodbury
Woodbury, NJ

Jersey Shore University Medical Center
Neptune, NJ

Ocean Medical Center
Brick, NJ

Riverview Medical Center
Red Bank, NJ

Lovelace Medical Center
Albuquerque, NM

Presbyterian Healthcare Services
Albuquerque, NM

Mercy Hospital of Buffalo
Buffalo, NY

CarolinaEast Medical Center
New Bern, NC

Carolinas HealthCare System NorthEast
Charlotte, NC

Carolinas HealthCare System Pineville
Charlotte, NC

Carolinas Medical Center
Charlotte, NC

Duke University Hospital
Durham, NC

Frye Regional Medical Center
Hickory, NC

Mission Hospital, Inc.
Asheville, NC

Moses H. Cone Memorial Hospital
Greensboro, NC

New Hanover Regional Medical Center
Wilmington, NC

North Carolina Baptist Hospital
Winston– Salem, NC

Novant Health Forsyth Medical Center
Winston– Salem, NC

Novant Health Presbyterian Medical Center
Charlotte, NC

Novant Health – Rowan Medical Center
Salisbury, NC

University of North Carolina Hospitals
Chapel Hill, NC

Vidant Medical Center
Greenville, NC

Sanford Medical Center Fargo
Fargo, ND

Aultman Hospital
Canton, OH

Platinum *continued from previous page*

EMH Regional Medical Center
Elyria, OH

Licking Memorial Hospital
Newark, OH

Mercy Medical Center
Canton, OH

Saint Ritas Medical Center
Lima, OH

Southwest General Health Center
Middleburg Heights, OH

The Christ Hospital Health Network
Cincinnati, OH

The MetroHealth System
Cleveland, OH

The Ohio State University Medical Center
Columbus, OH

University Hospitals St. John Medical Center
Westlake, OH

Oregon Health & Science University
Portland, OR

Butler Memorial Hospital
Butler, PA

Doylestown Hospital
Doylestown, PA

Meadville Medical Center
Meadville, PA

Sharon Regional Health System
Sharon, PA

UPMC Pinnacle Harrisburg
Harrisburg, PA

UPMC Pinnacle West Shore Hospital
Harrisburg, PA

AnMed Health
Anderson, SC

Beaufort Memorial Hospital
Beaufort, SC

Bon Secours St. Francis Health System
Greenville, SC

McLeod Regional Medical Center
Florence, SC

Spartanburg Regional Healthcare System
Spartanburg, SC

Trident Medical Center
Charleston, SC

Avera Heart Hospital of South Dakota
Sioux Falls, SD

Rapid City Regional Hospital
Rapid City, SD

Sanford USD Medical Center
Sioux Falls, SD

Baptist Memorial Hospital – Memphis
Memphis, TN

Baptist Memorial Hospital – Desoto
Memphis, TN

Blount Memorial Hospital
Maryville, TN

Bristol Regional Medical Center
Bristol, TN

Chattanooga – Hamilton County Hospital Authority
Chattanooga, TN

Holston Valley Medical Center
Kingsport, TN

Jackson Madison County General Hospital
Jackson, TN

University of Tennessee Medical Center (UHS)
Knoxville, TN

Baylor Scott & White Medical Center – Round Rock
Round Rock, TX

Baylor Scott & White Medical Center – Irving
Irving, TX

Baylor Scott & White Medical Center – Garland
Garland, TX

Baylor Scott & White Health (Temple)
Temple, TX

Ben Taub Hospital
Houston, TX

CHRISTUS Good Shepherd Medical Center
Longview, TX

Christus Spohn Hospital Corpus Christi – Shoreline
Corpus Christi, TX

Memorial Hermann The Woodlands Medical Center
Spring, TX

Methodist Charlton Medical Center
Dallas, TX

Methodist Stone Oak Hospital
San Antonio, TX

Metroplex Hospital
Killeen, TX

Metropolitan Methodist Hospital
San Antonio, TX

Parkland Health & Hospital System
Dallas, TX

Shannon Medical Center
San Angelo, TX

Centra Lynchburg General Hospital
Lynchburg, VA

Inova Alexandria Hospital
Alexandria, VA

Inova Fairfax Hospital/Inova Heart & Vascular Institute
Falls Church, VA

Inova Loudoun Hospital
Leesburg, VA

Sentara Careplex Hospital
Hampton, VA

Sentara Leigh Hospital
Norfolk, VA

Sentara Martha Jefferson Hospital
Charlottesville, VA

Sentara Norfolk General Hospital
Norfolk, VA

Sentara Northern Virginia Medical Center
Woodbridge, VA

Sentara Princess Anne Hospital
Virginia Beach, VA

Sentara Virginia Beach General Hospital
Virginia Beach, VA

Sentara Williamsburg Regional Medical Center
Williamsburg, VA

University of Virginia Medical Center
Charlottesville, VA

Winchester Medical Center Inc.
Winchester, VA

Astria Regional Medical Center & Astria Heart Inst
Yakima, WA

Harrison Medical Center
Bremerton, WA

Providence Sacred Heart Medical Center
Spokane, WA

St. Joseph Medical Center
Tacoma, WA

Saint Mary's Medical Center
Huntington, WV

Wheeling Hospital
Wheeling, WV

Aspirus Wausau Hospital
Wausau, WI

Aurora Grafton
Grafton, WI

Aurora St. Lukes Medical Center
Milwaukee, WI

Holy Family Memorial
Manitowoc, WI

Meriter Hospital
Madison, WI

University of Wisconsin Hospital & Clinics
Madison, WI

Cheyenne Regional Medical Center
Cheyenne, WY

Wyoming Medical Center
Casper, WY

Hospital totalCor
Sao Paulo, Brazil

2018 Gold Performance Achievement Award

ACTION Registry

NCDR

French Hospital Medical Center
San Luis Obispo, CA

NorthBay Medical Center
Fairfield, CA

Tri-City Medical Center
Oceanside, CA

Rose Medical Center
Denver, CO

Christiana Care Health System
Newark, DE

Piedmont Athens Regional
Athens, GA

Edward Hospital
Naperville, IL

Memorial Medical Center
Springfield, IL

Northwestern Medicine Central DuPage Hospital
Winfield, IL

Northwestern Medicine Delnor Hospital
Geneva, IL

Rush University Medical Center
Chicago, IL

Franciscan Health Indianapolis
Indianapolis, IN

Terrebonne General Medical Center
Houma, LA

Frederick Memorial Hospital
Frederick, MD

Holland Hospital
Holland, MI

Westchester County Medical Center
Valhalla, NY

Nash UNC Healthcare
Rocky Mount, NC

Adena Regional Medical Center
Chillicothe, OH

Fairview Hospital
Cleveland, OH

Hillcrest Hospital
Mayfield Hts, OH

Lima Memorial Health System
Lima, OH

Mercy Hospital Anderson
Cincinnati, OH

Hillcrest Medical Center
Tulsa, OK

Legacy Emanuel Medical Center
Portland, OR

Legacy Good Samaritan
Portland, OR

Legacy Meridian Park
Tualatin, OR

Mercy Fitzgerald Hospital
Darby, PA

UPMC Susquehanna
Williamsport, PA

Greenville Memorial Hospital
Greenville, SC

Fort Sanders Regional Medical Center
Knoxville, TN

East Texas Medical Center
Tyler, TX

Methodist Hospital
San Antonio, TX

Northeast Methodist Hospital
San Antonio, TX

Seton Medical Center Austin
Austin, TX

Seton Medical Center Hays
Kyle, TX

Seton Medical Center Williamson
Round Rock, TX

St. David's South Austin Medical Center
Austin, TX

Congratulations to the Recipients of the

ACTION Registry 2018 Performance Achievement Award

2018
Silver Performance Achievement Award

ACTION Registry

NCDR

Crestwood Medical Center
Huntsville, AL

Thomas Hospital
Fairhope, AL

Exempla Good Samaritan Medical Center
Lafayette, CO

Lutheran Medical Center
Wheat Ridge, CO

McKee Medical Center
Loveland, CO

Saint Marys Hospital and Regional Medical Center
Grand Junction, CO

Swedish Medical Center
Englewood, CO

Memorial Health University Medical Center
Savannah, GA

Piedmont Rockdale Hospital
Conyers, GA

Southern Regional Medical Center
Riverdale, GA

Wellstar Cobb Hospital
Austell, GA

Wellstar Douglas Hospital
Douglasville, GA

Wellstar Kennestone Regional Medical Center
Marietta, GA

Centegra Hospital – McHenry
McHenry, IL

Franciscan Health Olympia Fields
Olympia Fields, IL

MacNeal Hospital
Berwyn, IL

Northwestern Lake Forest Hospital
Lake Forest, IL

Presence Saints Mary and Elizabeth Medical Center
Chicago, IL

Franciscan Health Lafayette East
Lafayette, IN

Indiana University Health Bloomington
Bloomington, IN

Indiana University Health West Hospital
Indianapolis, IN

Iowa Methodist Medical Center
Des Moines, IA

Hays Medical Center
Hays, KS

Shawnee Mission Medical Center
Shawnee Mission, KS

St. Luke's South Hospital
Overland Park, KS

Baptist Health Lexington
Lexington, KY

Baptist Health Louisville
Louisville, KY

Pikeville Medical Center
Pikeville, KY

Christus St. Patrick Hospital
Lake Charles, LA

Lafayette General Medical Center
Lafayette, LA

Lafayette General Southwest
Lafayette, LA

Anne Arundel Medical Center
Annapolis, MD

Johns Hopkins Hospital
Baltimore, MD

MedStar Union Memorial Hospital
Baltimore, MD

Sinai Hospital of Baltimore
Baltimore, MD

Suburban Hospital
Bethesda, MD

McLaren Bay Region
Bay City, MI

Delta Regional Medical Center
Greenville, MS

Jeff Anderson Regional Medical Center
Meridian, MS

Merit Health Wesley Medical Center
Hattiesburg, MS

Citizens Memorial Hospital
Bolivar, MO

Heartland Regional Medical Center
St. Joseph, MO

Liberty Hospital
Liberty, MO

Mercy Hospital St. Louis
St. Louis, MO

The Nebraska Medical Center
Omaha, NE

Renown Regional Medical Center
Reno, NV

Chilton Medical Center
Pompton Plains, NJ

Overlook Medical Center
Summit, NJ

Robert Wood Johnson University Hospital Somerset
Somerville, NJ

UR Medicine Strong Memorial Hospital
Rochester, NY

Catawba Valley Medical Center
Hickory, NC

WakeMed Raleigh Campus
Raleigh, NC

Sanford Medical Center Bismarck
Bismarck, ND

Fairfield Medical Center
Lancaster, OH

Firelands Regional Medical Center
Sandusky, OH

Mercy Health Fairfield Hospital
Fairfield, OH

Mercy Health West Hospital
Cincinnati, OH

The University of Toledo Medical Center
Toledo, OH

AllianceHealth Deaconess
Oklahoma City, OK

Hillcrest Hospital South
Tulsa, OK

Norman Regional Health System
Norman, OK

Providence Medford Medical Center
Medford, OR

Providence Portland Medical Center
Portland, OR

Providence Saint Vincent Medical Center
Portland, OR

Chambersburg Hospital
Chambersburg, PA

Hanover Hospital
Hanover, PA

Self Regional Healthcare
Greenwood, SC

Baptist Memorial Hospital North Mississippi
Memphis, TN

NEA Baptist Memorial Hospital
Memphis, TN

Parkwest Medical Center
Knoxville, TN

Baylor Scott & White Hillcrest Medical Center
Waco, TX

Bexar County Hospital District d/b/a University Health System
San Antonio, TX

CHI/St Luke's the Woodlands Hospital
The Woodlands, TX

Memorial Hermann Northeast
Humble, TX

Memorial Hermann Sugar Land
Sugar Land, TX

Methodist Texsan Hospital
San Antonio, TX

Mother Frances Hospital
Tyler, TX

Providence Healthcare Network
Waco, TX

Seton Medical Center Harker Heights
Harker Heights, TX

Texas Health Harris Methodist HEB
Bedford, TX

Texas Health Presbyterian Hospital of Dallas
Dallas, TX

The Heart Hospital Baylor Plano
Plano, TX

St. Marks Hospital/ Northern Utah Healthcare Corp.
Salt Lake City, UT

University of Utah Hospitals and Clinics
Salt Lake City, UT

Augusta Health
Fishersville, VA

Johnston Memorial Hospital
Abingdon, VA

Novant Health UVA Prince William Hospital
Manassas, VA

Rockingham Memorial Hospital
Harrisonburg, VA

Sentara Halifax Regional Hospital
South Boston, VA

VCU – Medical College Of Virginia
Richmond, VA

St. Francis Hospital
Federal Way, WA

Virginia Mason Medical Center
Seattle, WA

Marshfield Medical Center
Marshfield, WI

HCOR – Hospital Do Coracao
Sao Paulo, Brazil

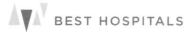

CARDIOLOGY & HEART SURGERY
(CONTINUED)

Rank	Hospital	U.S. News score	Survival score (10=best)	Patient safety score (9=best)	Trans-parency score (3=best)	Number of patients	Nurse staffing score (higher is better)	A Nurse Magnet hospital	Technology score (6=best)	Patient services score (7=best)	Intensivists	% of specialists recom-mending hospital
24	University of Kansas Hospital, Kansas City	66.9	10	5	3	4,205	2.1	Yes	6	7	Yes	0.5%
26	University Hospitals Cleveland Medical Center	66.4	10	5	3	4,413	2.6	Yes	6	7	Yes	1.5%
27	Loyola University Medical Center, Maywood, Ill.	66.1	10	5	3	3,332	2.4	Yes	6	7	Yes	1.1%
28	Memorial Hermann-Texas Medical Center, Houston	66.0	10	5	3	4,351	2.2	Yes	6	7	Yes	1.2%
29	Mayo Clinic-Phoenix	65.7	10	6	2	4,055	2.9	Yes	6	7	Yes	1.6%
30	Beaumont Hospital-Royal Oak, Mich.	65.6	10	6	3	9,864	1.9	Yes	5	7	Yes	0.9%
30	UCSF Medical Center, San Francisco	65.6	10	6	3	2,645	2.1	Yes	6	6	Yes	2.8%
32	Sentara Norfolk Gen. Hosp.-Sentara Heart Hosp., Norfolk, Va.	65.4	10	5	3	6,246	1.6	Yes	6	7	Yes	0.4%
33	NYU Langone Hospitals, New York, N.Y.	65.0	9	5	3	7,659	2.3	Yes	5	7	Yes	3.2%
34	University of California, Davis Medical Center, Sacramento	64.8	10	5	3	4,070	2.8	Yes	5	7	Yes	0.2%
35	Aurora St. Luke's Medical Center, Milwaukee	64.7	10	3	3	9,571	2.2	Yes	6	7	Yes	1.0%
36	Cleveland Clinic Fairview Hospital, Cleveland	64.6	10	6	3	4,045	1.9	Yes	5	7	Yes	0.1%
37	UPMC Presbyterian Shadyside, Pittsburgh	64.5	9	5	3	9,730	1.9	Yes	6	7	Yes	2.5%
38	St. Luke's Hospital of Kansas City, Mo.	64.4	10	5	3	5,211	1.6	Yes	6	7	Yes	0.9%
39	Jefferson Health-Thomas Jefferson U. Hospitals, Philadelphia	63.1	10	5	3	4,514	2.2	Yes	6	7	Yes	1.0%
40	UC San Diego Health - Sulpizio Cardiovascular Center	62.9	10	5	3	3,573	2.0	Yes	6	7	Yes	0.5%
41	OHSU Hospital, Portland, Ore.	62.7	10	5	3	3,857	2.0	Yes	6	7	Yes	0.6%
42	University of Colorado Hospital, Aurora	62.1	10	5	2	4,650	1.9	Yes	6	7	Yes	1.1%
43	Banner University Medical Center Phoenix	62.0	10	5	0	3,597	2.3	Yes	5	7	Yes	0.4%
44	University of Virginia Medical Center, Charlottesville	61.9	10	5	3	3,990	2.1	Yes	6	7	Yes	0.9%
45	Keck Hospital of USC, Los Angeles	61.8	10	6	3	2,295	2.4	No	6	7	Yes	1.4%
46	Indiana University Health Medical Center, Indianapolis	61.5	10	5	3	4,403	2.0	Yes	6	7	Yes	0.5%
46	Mayo Clinic Jacksonville, Fla.	61.5	10	6	2	2,473	2.1	Yes	6	7	Yes	1.2%
48	University of Wisconsin Hospitals, Madison	61.4	10	5	3	3,605	2.1	Yes	6	7	Yes	0.5%
49	MedStar Heart and Vascular Institute, Washington, D.C.	61.2	10	4	3	8,820	2.3	No	6	7	Yes	1.8%
49	St. Cloud Hospital, St. Cloud, Minn.	61.2	9	5	3	9,024	2.2	Yes	5	7	Yes	0.0%

Terms are explained on Page 102.

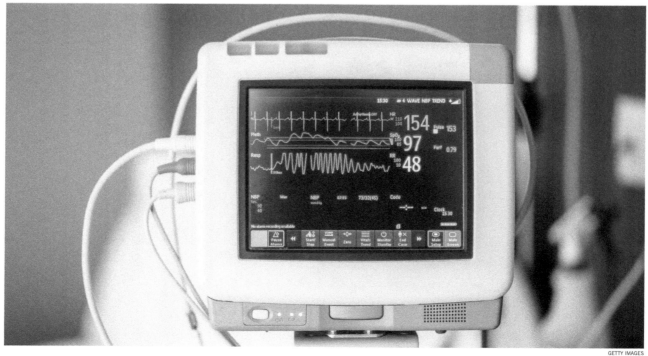

GETTY IMAGES

▶ **More** @ usnews.com/besthospitals

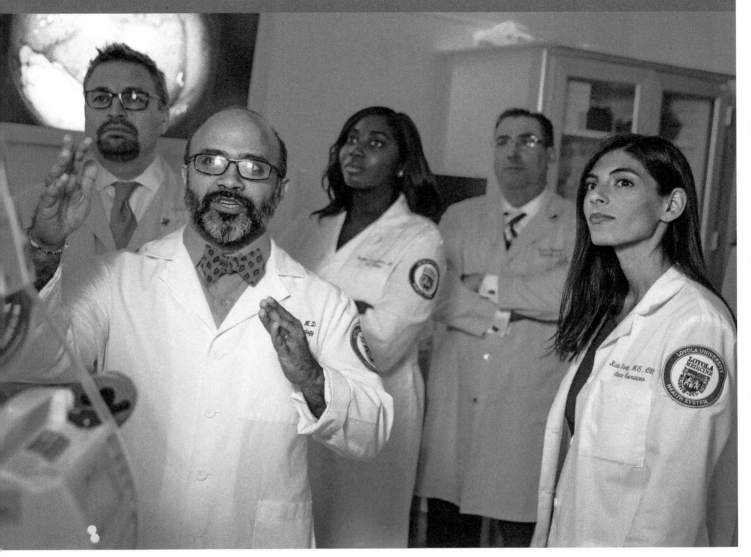
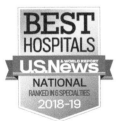
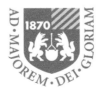
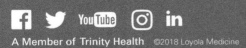

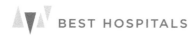

DIABETES & ENDOCRINOLOGY

Rank	Hospital	U.S. News score	Survival score (10=best)	Patient safety score (9=best)	Number of patients	Nurse staffing score (higher is better)	A Nurse Magnet hospital	Technology score (4=best)	Patient services score (8=best)	Intensivists	% of specialists recommending hospital
1	Mayo Clinic, Rochester, Minn.	100.0	10	5	777	2.8	Yes	4	8	Yes	45.4%
2	Johns Hopkins Hospital, Baltimore	86.8	10	4	354	2.1	Yes	4	8	Yes	18.3%
3	Massachusetts General Hospital, Boston	83.1	8	5	515	2.4	Yes	4	8	Yes	28.9%
4	Cleveland Clinic	80.5	8	6	646	2.1	Yes	4	8	Yes	16.2%
5	Hosps. of the U. of Pennsylvania-Penn Presby., Philadelphia	79.1	9	6	578	2.4	Yes	4	8	Yes	8.9%
6	UCSF Medical Center, San Francisco	78.5	10	6	394	2.1	Yes	4	8	Yes	9.0%
6	University of Colorado Hospital, Aurora	78.5	10	5	588	1.9	Yes	4	8	Yes	5.6%
8	New York-Presbyterian Hospital-Columbia and Cornell, N.Y.	78.1	8	4	1,369	2.9	No	4	8	Yes	11.6%
9	UCLA Medical Center, Los Angeles	76.6	9	5	557	3.0	Yes	4	8	Yes	5.7%
10	Barnes-Jewish Hospital, St. Louis	76.3	9	5	608	2.2	Yes	4	8	Yes	7.0%
11	UPMC Presbyterian Shadyside, Pittsburgh	74.4	10	5	695	1.9	Yes	4	8	Yes	3.5%
12	University of Washington Medical Center, Seattle	73.3	10	5	175	2.0	Yes	4	8	Yes	7.3%
13	U. of Michigan Hospitals-Michigan Medicine, Ann Arbor	73.2	9	7	390	2.7	Yes	4	8	Yes	5.5%
14	Beaumont Hospital-Royal Oak, Mich.	72.6	10	6	946	1.9	Yes	4	8	Yes	0.1%
15	Cedars-Sinai Medical Center, Los Angeles	72.5	9	5	886	2.6	Yes	4	8	Yes	2.5%
16	DMC Harper University Hospital, Detroit	72.2	10	5	237	1.7	Yes	4	8	Yes	0.2%
17	Stanford Health Care-Stanford Hospital, Stanford, Calif.	72.1	10	5	439	2.5	Yes	4	8	Yes	3.5%
18	University of Kansas Hospital, Kansas City	71.9	10	5	337	2.1	Yes	4	8	Yes	0.2%
19	Scripps La Jolla Hospitals, La Jolla, Calif.	71.7	10	6	353	3.1	Yes	4	8	Yes	0.5%
20	Providence Portland Medical Center, Portland, Ore.	71.4	10	4	251	1.5	Yes	3	8	Yes	0.0%
21	Ohio State University Wexner Medical Center, Columbus	71.1	10	5	587	2.1	Yes	4	8	Yes	2.6%
21	UT Southwestern Medical Center, Dallas	71.1	10	5	336	2.3	Yes	4	8	Yes	2.9%
23	Abbott Northwestern Hospital, Minneapolis	70.7	10	5	422	2.4	Yes	4	8	Yes	0.0%
24	Tampa General Hospital	70.6	10	3	440	2.1	Yes	4	8	Yes	0.0%
25	VCU Medical Center, Richmond, Va.	70.5	10	5	188	2.4	Yes	4	8	Yes	0.1%
26	MedStar Georgetown University Hospital, Washington, D.C.	70.4	10	5	135	1.1	Yes	4	8	Yes	0.5%
27	Brigham and Women's Hospital, Boston	70.1	9	5	433	2.3	No	4	8	Yes	10.5%
28	University of Alabama at Birmingham Hospital	70.0	10	6	441	1.8	Yes	4	8	Yes	1.0%
28	West Virginia University Hospitals, Morgantown, W.Va.	70.0	10	6	276	2.8	Yes	4	8	Yes	0.4%
30	Indiana University Health Medical Center, Indianapolis	69.5	10	5	386	2.0	Yes	4	8	Yes	0.2%
31	Mayo Clinic-Phoenix	69.1	9	6	362	2.9	Yes	4	8	Yes	1.1%
31	Sentara Norfolk General Hospital, Norfolk, Va.	69.1	10	5	244	1.6	Yes	4	8	Yes	1.2%
33	U. of Kentucky Albert B. Chandler Hospital, Lexington	69.0	10	5	216	1.9	Yes	4	8	Yes	0.1%
34	Yale New Haven Hospital, New Haven, Conn.	68.5	8	4	812	2.0	Yes	4	8	Yes	5.6%
35	Bon Secours St. Francis Hospital, Charleston, S.C.	68.4	10	5	129	1.4	Yes	4	8	Yes	0.0%
36	Mount Sinai Hospital, New York	68.0	8	6	617	1.9	Yes	4	8	Yes	5.1%
37	Orange Coast Memorial Med. Ctr., Fountain Valley, Calif.	67.6	10	5	137	2.2	Yes	4	8	Yes	0.0%
38	University of Maryland Medical Center, Baltimore	67.3	10	3	172	2.9	Yes	4	8	Yes	0.6%
39	Montefiore Medical Center, Bronx, N.Y.	66.9	9	4	1,154	2.3	No	4	8	Intensivists	1.4%
39	OHSU Hospital, Portland, Ore.	66.9	9	5	251	2.0	Yes	4	8	Yes	2.9%
39	UF Health Shands Hospital, Gainesville, Fla.	66.9	10	5	300	1.9	Yes	4	8	Yes	0.5%
42	Houston Methodist Hospital	66.7	9	5	583	2.0	Yes	4	8	Yes	0.3%
42	University Hospitals Cleveland Medical Center	66.7	9	5	394	2.6	Yes	4	8	Yes	0.8%
44	Penn Medicine Chester County Hospital, West Chester, Pa.	66.4	10	5	164	1.8	Yes	4	8	Yes	0.0%
45	Queen's Medical Center, Honolulu	66.3	10	4	382	1.7	Yes	4	8	Yes	0.0%
46	Providence Little Company of Mary Med. Ctr. Torrance, Calif.	66.0	10	5	246	2.8	Yes	4	8	Yes	0.0%
47	NYU Langone Hospitals, New York, N.Y.	65.9	8	5	633	2.3	Yes	4	8	Yes	2.9%
48	University of California, Davis Medical Center, Sacramento	65.8	9	5	318	2.8	Yes	4	8	Yes	0.2%
49	Flagler Hospital, St. Augustine, Fla.	65.4	10	5	213	1.6	Yes	3	7	Yes	0.0%
49	Miami Valley Hospital, Dayton, Ohio	65.4	9	5	387	2.5	Yes	4	8	Yes	0.0%

Terms are explained on Page 102.

More @ usnews.com/besthospitals

EAR, NOSE & THROAT

Rank	Hospital	U.S. News score	Survival score (10=best)	Patient safety score (9=best)	Number of patients	Nurse staffing score (higher is better)	A Nurse Magnet hospital	Patient services score (8=best)	Trauma center	Intensivists	% of specialists recommending hospital
1	U. of Michigan Hospitals-Michigan Medicine, Ann Arbor	100.0	9	7	343	2.7	Yes	8	Yes	Yes	12.0%
2	Stanford Health Care-Stanford Hospital, Stanford, Calif.	99.9	10	5	322	2.5	Yes	8	Yes	Yes	10.4%
3	University of Iowa Hospitals and Clinics, Iowa City	99.5	10	5	214	1.8	Yes	8	Yes	Yes	12.7%
4	Ohio State University Wexner Medical Center, Columbus	97.7	10	5	467	2.1	Yes	8	Yes	Yes	6.5%
5	Mayo Clinic, Rochester, Minn.	97.3	8	5	396	2.8	Yes	8	Yes	Yes	12.5%
6	Massachusetts Eye & Ear Infirmary, Mass. Gen. Hosp., Boston	94.4	7	5	355	2.4	Yes	8	Yes	Yes	21.2%
7	UCSF Medical Center, San Francisco	93.8	10	6	224	2.1	Yes	8	Yes	Yes	7.7%
8	Johns Hopkins Hospital, Baltimore	93.5	7	4	195	2.1	Yes	8	Yes	Yes	24.3%
9	UCLA Medical Center, Los Angeles	91.1	8	5	488	3.0	Yes	8	Yes	Yes	6.4%
10	University of North Carolina Hospitals, Chapel Hill	90.5	10	5	247	1.8	Yes	8	Yes	Yes	4.5%
11	Cleveland Clinic	90.4	10	6	257	2.1	Yes	8	No	Yes	10.2%
12	MUSC Health-University Medical Center, Charleston, S.C.	90.0	9	5	234	2.3	Yes	8	Yes	Yes	7.6%
13	Hosps. of the U. of Pennsylvania-Penn Presby., Philadelphia	88.6	7	6	432	2.4	Yes	8	Yes	Yes	8.6%
14	University of Texas MD Anderson Cancer Center, Houston	86.6	7	5	670	2.0	Yes	8	No	Yes	9.4%
15	Jefferson Health-Thomas Jefferson U. Hospitals, Philadelphia	85.5	9	5	456	2.2	Yes	8	Yes	Yes	2.6%
16	University Hospitals Cleveland Medical Center	81.9	9	5	244	2.6	Yes	8	Yes	Yes	1.9%
17	Memorial Sloan-Kettering Cancer Center, New York	81.3	9	5	363	2.1	Yes	8	No	Yes	3.3%
18	University of Virginia Medical Center, Charlottesville	80.5	9	5	115	2.1	Yes	8	Yes	Yes	3.9%
19	Memorial Hermann-Texas Medical Center, Houston	80.3	10	5	81	2.2	Yes	8	Yes	Yes	0.3%
20	University of California, Davis Medical Center, Sacramento	80.1	9	5	183	2.8	Yes	8	Yes	Yes	1.2%
21	New York-Presbyterian Hospital-Columbia and Cornell, N.Y.	79.9	9	4	294	2.9	No	8	Yes	Yes	3.2%
22	Barnes-Jewish Hospital, St. Louis	79.8	7	5	311	2.2	Yes	8	Yes	Yes	7.0%
23	Henry Ford Hospital, Detroit	79.7	10	5	130	2.1	No	8	Yes	Yes	0.7%
24	Rush University Medical Center, Chicago	79.6	10	5	156	2.2	Yes	8	Yes	Yes	1.0%
25	Ochsner Medical Center, New Orleans	78.8	10	5	192	1.9	Yes	8	Yes	Yes	1.0%
25	OHSU Hospital, Portland, Ore.	78.8	8	5	318	2.0	Yes	8	Yes	Yes	2.4%
27	Yale New Haven Hospital, New Haven, Conn.	78.5	9	4	353	2.0	Yes	8	Yes	Yes	1.2%
28	Mayo Clinic-Phoenix	78.0	8	6	241	2.9	Yes	8	No	Yes	2.1%
29	University of Alabama at Birmingham Hospital	77.6	7	6	499	1.8	Yes	8	Yes	Yes	2.0%
30	Wake Forest Baptist Medical Center, Winston-Salem, N.C.	77.3	8	5	386	1.6	Yes	8	Yes	Yes	2.1%
31	University of Utah Hospital, Salt Lake City	77.0	10	5	152	1.8	No	8	Yes	Yes	1.6%
32	UPMC Presbyterian Shadyside, Pittsburgh	76.3	5	5	493	1.9	Yes	8	Yes	Yes	9.2%
33	Vanderbilt University Medical Center, Nashville, Tenn.	75.6	4	6	359	2.5	Yes	8	Yes	Yes	10.8%
34	University of Cincinnati Medical Center	74.9	9	5	256	1.7	No	8	Yes	Yes	5.0%
35	Beaumont Hospital-Troy, Mich.	74.7	9	8	120	2.0	Yes	8	Yes	Yes	0.1%
35	Cedars-Sinai Medical Center, Los Angeles	74.7	8	5	171	2.6	Yes	8	Yes	Yes	0.6%
37	Mount Sinai Hospital, New York	74.2	6	6	326	1.9	Yes	8	Yes	Yes	5.7%
37	University of Washington Medical Center, Seattle	74.2	7	5	179	2.0	Yes	8	No	Yes	7.0%
39	University of Maryland Medical Center, Baltimore	74.0	8	3	219	2.9	Yes	8	Yes	Yes	1.2%
40	Baylor University Medical Center, Dallas	73.8	10	5	183	1.5	Yes	8	Yes	Yes	0.6%
41	University of Miami Hospital and Clinics-UHealth Tower	73.5	10	4	612	1.4	No	8	Yes	Yes	1.1%
42	Via Christi Hospital on St. Francis, Wichita, Kan.	72.0	10	5	73	1.8	No	6	Yes	Yes	0.0%
43	Strong Memorial Hosp. of U. of Rochester, Rochester, N.Y.	71.5	8	5	189	1.8	Yes	8	Yes	Yes	0.6%
44	New York Eye and Ear Infirmary of Mount Sinai, N.Y.	71.3	10	5	<11	1.4	Yes	8	No	Yes	1.8%
45	U. of Kentucky Albert B. Chandler Hospital, Lexington	71.0	8	5	186	1.9	Yes	8	Yes	Yes	0.4%
46	Vidant Medical Center, Greenville, N.C.	70.7	9	6	118	2.0	Yes	8	Yes	Yes	0.0%
47	Froedtert Hosp. and the Medical College of Wis., Milwaukee	69.6	8	5	116	1.8	Yes	8	Yes	Yes	1.1%
47	Reading Hospital, West Reading, Pa.	69.6	10	5	109	1.1	Yes	4	Yes	Yes	0.0%
49	Northwestern Memorial Hospital, Chicago	68.9	8	5	105	1.8	Yes	8	Yes	Yes	2.1%
50	Porter Adventist Hospital, Denver	68.5	9	3	195	1.9	Yes	8	No	Yes	0.4%

Terms are explained on Page 102.

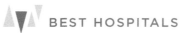
GASTROENTEROLOGY & GI SURGERY

Rank	Hospital	U.S. News score	Survival score (10=best)	Patient safety score (9=best)	Number of patients	Nurse staffing score (higher is better)	A Nurse Magnet hospital	Technology score (7=best)	Patient services score (8=best)	Trauma center	Intensivists	% of specialists recommending hospital
1	Mayo Clinic, Rochester, Minn.	100.0	10	5	7,802	2.8	Yes	7	8	Yes	Yes	43.8%
2	Cleveland Clinic	89.1	10	6	5,702	2.1	Yes	7	8	No	Yes	28.3%
3	Cedars-Sinai Medical Center, Los Angeles	81.3	10	5	7,176	2.6	Yes	7	8	Yes	Yes	9.0%
4	Johns Hopkins Hospital, Baltimore	81.2	10	4	3,196	2.1	Yes	7	8	Yes	Yes	19.0%
5	Mayo Clinic-Phoenix	78.9	10	6	3,550	2.9	Yes	7	8	No	Yes	5.6%
6	U. of Michigan Hospitals-Michigan Medicine, Ann Arbor	76.6	10	7	3,874	2.7	Yes	7	8	Yes	Yes	7.5%
7	UCLA Medical Center, Los Angeles	75.3	9	5	4,019	3.0	Yes	7	8	Yes	Yes	10.7%
8	Massachusetts General Hospital, Boston	74.2	7	5	4,958	2.4	Yes	7	8	Yes	Yes	15.2%
9	Mount Sinai Hospital, New York	73.1	8	6	4,615	1.9	Yes	7	8	Yes	Yes	11.6%
10	UPMC Presbyterian Shadyside, Pittsburgh	72.5	9	5	6,986	1.9	Yes	7	8	Yes	Yes	6.9%
11	Hosps. of the U. of Pennsylvania-Penn Presby., Philadelphia	71.0	8	6	3,995	2.4	Yes	7	8	Yes	Yes	7.7%
12	Mayo Clinic Jacksonville, Fla.	70.7	10	6	2,324	2.1	Yes	7	8	No	Yes	5.2%
13	Scripps La Jolla Hospitals, La Jolla, Calif.	70.1	10	5	2,764	3.1	Yes	7	8	Yes	Yes	0.6%
13	UCSF Medical Center, San Francisco	70.1	9	6	2,498	2.1	Yes	7	8	Yes	Yes	5.8%
15	Houston Methodist Hospital	70.0	10	5	4,740	2.0	Yes	7	8	No	Yes	1.3%
16	New York-Presbyterian Hospital-Columbia and Cornell, N.Y.	69.7	9	4	7,777	2.9	No	7	8	Yes	Yes	6.3%
17	NYU Langone Hospitals, New York, N.Y.	69.6	10	5	4,121	2.3	Yes	7	8	Yes	Yes	3.9%
18	Beaumont Hospital-Royal Oak, Mich.	68.7	10	6	5,836	1.9	Yes	7	8	Yes	Yes	0.8%
19	Cleveland Clinic Fairview Hospital, Cleveland	68.6	10	6	2,146	1.9	Yes	6	8	Yes	Yes	0.1%
20	University Hospitals Cleveland Medical Center	68.4	10	5	2,517	2.6	Yes	7	8	Yes	Yes	1.5%
20	University of North Carolina Hospitals, Chapel Hill	68.4	10	5	2,440	1.8	Yes	7	8	Yes	Yes	5.3%
22	Indiana University Health Medical Center, Indianapolis	68.2	10	5	4,139	2.0	Yes	7	8	Yes	Yes	2.8%
23	Hoag Memorial Hospital Presbyterian, Newport Beach, Calif.	67.7	10	7	4,692	2.4	Yes	6	8	No	Yes	0.0%
24	Ochsner Medical Center, New Orleans	67.5	10	5	4,301	1.9	Yes	7	8	Yes	Yes	1.7%
25	Cleveland Clinic Florida, Weston	67.2	10	5	2,090	2.5	No	7	8	No	Yes	4.3%
25	Tampa General Hospital	67.2	10	3	2,878	2.1	Yes	7	8	Yes	Yes	1.1%
27	Mission Hospital, Orange, Calif.	66.9	10	6	2,277	2.0	Yes	6	8	Yes	Yes	0.0%
27	Stanford Health Care-Stanford Hospital, Stanford, Calif.	66.9	9	5	3,324	2.5	Yes	7	8	Yes	Yes	2.2%
27	University of Colorado Hospital, Aurora	66.9	10	5	3,193	1.9	Yes	7	8	Yes	Yes	1.9%
30	Northwestern Memorial Hospital, Chicago	66.8	9	5	2,906	1.8	Yes	7	8	Yes	Yes	4.0%
31	Barnes-Jewish Hospital, St. Louis	66.5	7	5	4,971	2.2	Yes	7	8	Yes	Yes	4.4%
32	Jefferson Health-Thomas Jefferson U. Hospitals, Philadelphia	66.3	8	5	4,472	2.2	Yes	7	8	Yes	Yes	3.3%
33	Vanderbilt University Medical Center, Nashville, Tenn.	66.2	8	6	3,286	2.5	Yes	7	8	Yes	Yes	2.4%
34	Memorial Hermann-Texas Medical Center, Houston	66.1	10	5	1,164	2.2	Yes	7	8	Yes	Yes	0.5%
35	Advocate Good Samaritan Hospital, Downers Grove, Ill.	65.8	10	7	1,624	2.0	Yes	6	8	Yes	Yes	0.0%
36	Penn State Health Milton S. Hershey Medical Center, Hershey	65.6	10	6	2,499	1.7	Yes	7	8	Yes	Yes	0.7%
37	Loyola University Medical Center, Maywood, Ill.	65.1	10	5	2,075	2.4	Yes	7	8	Yes	Yes	0.2%
38	Baylor St. Luke's Medical Center, Houston	64.7	10	5	2,639	1.6	Yes	7	7	No	Yes	1.0%
39	Christiana Care Hospitals, Newark, Del.	64.6	10	5	5,224	2.0	Yes	6	8	Yes	Yes	0.3%
39	Duke University Hospital, Durham, N.C.	64.6	5	6	3,082	2.1	Yes	7	8	Yes	Yes	6.6%
39	Yale New Haven Hospital, New Haven, Conn.	64.6	8	4	5,440	2.0	Yes	7	8	Yes	Yes	2.4%
42	Baylor University Medical Center, Dallas	64.5	9	5	4,019	1.5	Yes	7	8	Yes	Yes	3.0%
42	Kaiser Permanente Los Angeles Medical Center	64.5	10	5	1,624	2.7	No	6	8	No	Yes	0.1%
42	University of Kansas Hospital, Kansas City	64.5	10	5	2,548	2.1	Yes	7	8	Yes	Yes	0.5%
42	University of Wisconsin Hospitals, Madison	64.5	10	5	2,604	2.1	Yes	7	8	Yes	Yes	0.5%
46	UF Health Shands Hospital, Gainesville, Fla.	64.4	9	5	2,251	1.9	Yes	7	8	Yes	Yes	2.1%
47	University of Chicago Medical Center	64.2	7	7	2,157	2.4	No	7	8	Yes	Yes	7.7%
48	Morristown Medical Center, Morristown, N.J.	64.1	10	5	2,953	2.1	Yes	6	8	Yes	Yes	0.0%
48	Sanford USD Medical Center, Sioux Falls, S.D.	64.1	10	5	2,389	2.4	Yes	6	8	Yes	Yes	0.0%
50	Emory University Hospital, Atlanta	64.0	10	5	2,497	1.9	Yes	7	8	No	Yes	2.5%

Terms are explained on Page 102.

GERIATRICS

Rank	Hospital	U.S. News score	Survival score (10=best)	Patient safety score (9=best)	Number of patients	Nurse staffing score (higher is better)	A Nurse Magnet hospital	NIA Alzheimer's center	Patient services score (9=best)	Intensivists	% of specialists recommending hospital
1	Mayo Clinic, Rochester, Minn.	100.0	10	5	32,095	2.8	Yes	Yes	9	Yes	12.3%
2	Johns Hopkins Hospital, Baltimore	97.5	10	4	8,640	2.1	Yes	Yes	9	Yes	19.2%
3	Mount Sinai Hospital, New York	94.5	10	6	21,549	1.9	Yes	Yes	9	Yes	22.8%
4	UCLA Medical Center, Los Angeles	90.0	10	5	19,365	3.0	Yes	No	9	Yes	24.5%
5	Cleveland Clinic	87.5	10	6	20,167	2.1	Yes	No	9	Yes	7.2%
6	Mayo Clinic-Phoenix	87.4	10	6	14,223	2.9	Yes	Yes	9	Yes	1.1%
7	U. of Michigan Hospitals-Michigan Medicine, Ann Arbor	86.8	10	7	11,941	2.7	Yes	Yes	9	Yes	4.7%
8	UCSF Medical Center, San Francisco	85.9	10	6	9,635	2.1	Yes	Yes	9	Yes	9.6%
9	Northwestern Memorial Hospital, Chicago	83.7	10	5	12,237	1.8	Yes	Yes	9	Yes	2.5%
10	Massachusetts General Hospital, Boston	82.9	10	5	22,725	2.4	Yes	Yes	9	Yes	4.4%
11	New York-Presbyterian Hospital-Columbia and Cornell, N.Y.	82.6	10	4	42,595	2.9	No	Yes	9	Yes	5.1%
12	UPMC Presbyterian Shadyside, Pittsburgh	81.8	9	5	26,646	1.9	Yes	Yes	9	Yes	8.7%
13	Hosps. of the U. of Pennsylvania-Penn Presby., Philadelphia	81.7	10	6	16,298	2.4	Yes	Yes	9	Yes	3.2%
14	NYU Langone Hospitals, New York, N.Y.	81.4	10	5	24,663	2.3	Yes	Yes	9	Yes	3.4%
14	Rush University Medical Center, Chicago	81.4	10	5	8,461	2.2	Yes	Yes	9	Yes	2.6%
16	Barnes-Jewish Hospital, St. Louis	81.0	10	5	17,621	2.2	Yes	Yes	9	Yes	3.0%
17	Keck Hospital of USC, Los Angeles	79.3	10	6	5,780	2.4	No	Yes	9	Yes	1.1%
18	UT Southwestern Medical Center, Dallas	78.9	10	5	7,084	2.3	Yes	Yes	9	Yes	1.0%
19	Banner University Medical Center Phoenix	78.7	10	5	7,863	2.3	Yes	Yes	9	Yes	0.5%
20	Cedars-Sinai Medical Center, Los Angeles	78.5	10	5	37,049	2.6	Yes	No	8	Yes	1.3%
21	University of California, Davis Medical Center, Sacramento	78.3	10	5	10,832	2.8	Yes	Yes	9	Yes	0.6%
22	University of Washington Medical Center, Seattle	78.1	10	5	4,920	2.0	Yes	Yes	9	Yes	2.0%
23	University of Kansas Hospital, Kansas City	77.9	10	5	9,595	2.1	Yes	Yes	9	Yes	0.9%
23	Yale New Haven Hospital, New Haven, Conn.	77.9	8	4	30,662	2.0	Yes	Yes	9	Yes	5.4%
25	Stanford Health Care-Stanford Hospital, Stanford, Calif.	76.1	10	5	13,968	2.5	Yes	Yes	9	Yes	1.3%
26	Mayo Clinic Jacksonville, Fla.	75.3	10	6	8,379	2.1	Yes	Yes	9	Yes	2.5%
27	University of Wisconsin Hospitals, Madison	74.8	10	5	9,494	2.1	Yes	Yes	9	Yes	2.0%
28	Indiana University Health Medical Center, Indianapolis	74.6	10	5	12,368	2.0	Yes	Yes	9	Yes	1.9%
29	Houston Methodist Hospital	74.2	10	5	21,216	2.0	Yes	No	9	Yes	0.9%
30	Beaumont Hospital-Royal Oak, Mich.	73.8	10	6	33,094	1.9	Yes	No	9	Yes	1.1%
31	Wake Forest Baptist Medical Center, Winston-Salem, N.C.	73.5	9	5	17,743	1.6	Yes	Yes	9	Yes	3.7%
32	UF Health Shands Hospital, Gainesville, Fla.	72.4	9	5	10,426	1.9	Yes	Yes	9	Yes	1.2%
33	Emory University Hospital at Wesley Woods, Atlanta	71.8	9	5	9,700	1.9	Yes	Yes	9	Yes	1.8%
34	OHSU Hospital, Portland, Ore.	71.3	10	5	7,984	2.0	Yes	Yes	9	Yes	0.3%
35	Scripps La Jolla Hospitals, La Jolla, Calif.	70.8	10	6	16,196	3.1	Yes	No	7	Yes	0.8%
36	UC San Diego Health-Jacobs Medical Center, Calif.	70.6	9	5	9,433	2.0	Yes	Yes	9	Yes	0.6%
37	University of Colorado Hospital, Aurora	70.5	10	5	11,546	1.9	Yes	No	9	Yes	1.7%
38	Abbott Northwestern Hospital, Minneapolis	70.2	10	5	24,574	2.4	Yes	No	9	Yes	0.0%
39	Duke University Hospital, Durham, N.C.	70.1	8	6	12,194	2.1	Yes	No	9	Yes	9.5%
40	Jefferson Health-Thomas Jefferson U. Hospitals, Philadelphia	69.8	10	5	16,927	2.2	Yes	No	9	Yes	3.1%
40	University Hospitals Cleveland Medical Center	69.8	10	5	11,146	2.6	Yes	No	9	Yes	0.7%
42	University of Alabama at Birmingham Hospital	69.1	10	6	14,077	1.8	Yes	No	8	Yes	3.7%
43	Brigham and Women's Hospital, Boston	69.0	10	5	14,618	2.3	No	Yes	9	Yes	0.7%
44	St. Cloud Hospital, St. Cloud, Minn.	68.8	10	5	24,112	2.2	Yes	No	8	Yes	0.0%
45	Cleveland Clinic Fairview Hospital, Cleveland	67.9	10	6	11,106	1.9	Yes	No	9	Yes	0.1%
46	Beth Israel Deaconess Medical Center, Boston	67.7	9	5	13,948	1.6	No	Yes	9	Yes	3.1%
46	DMC Harper University Hospital, Detroit	67.7	10	5	5,413	1.7	Yes	No	8	Yes	0.0%
46	Ohio State University Wexner Medical Center, Columbus	67.7	10	5	15,115	2.1	Yes	No	9	Yes	0.5%
49	Hoag Memorial Hospital Presbyterian, Newport Beach, Calif.	66.7	9	7	24,646	2.4	Yes	No	9	Yes	0.0%
50	Aurora St. Luke's Medical Center, Milwaukee	66.3	10	3	23,212	2.2	Yes	No	9	Yes	0.7%

Terms are explained on Page 102.

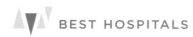

GYNECOLOGY

Rank	Hospital	U.S. News score	Survival score (10=best)	Patient safety score (9=best)	Number of patients	Nurse staffing score (higher is better)	A Nurse Magnet hospital	Technology score (5=best)	Patient services score (9=best)	Intensivists	% of specialists recommending hospital
1	Mayo Clinic, Rochester, Minn.	100.0	10	5	475	2.8	Yes	5	9	Yes	13.5%
2	U. of Michigan Hospitals-Michigan Medicine, Ann Arbor	87.0	10	7	197	2.7	Yes	5	9	Yes	4.4%
3	Memorial Sloan-Kettering Cancer Center, New York	86.6	9	5	642	2.1	Yes	5	8	Yes	7.1%
4	Johns Hopkins Hospital, Baltimore	84.2	10	4	146	2.1	Yes	5	9	Yes	10.1%
5	Cleveland Clinic	83.8	9	6	239	2.1	Yes	5	9	Yes	10.4%
6	UCSF Medical Center, San Francisco	81.8	10	6	155	2.1	Yes	5	9	Yes	8.2%
7	Stanford Health Care-Stanford Hospital, Stanford, Calif.	81.5	10	5	192	2.5	Yes	5	9	Yes	3.4%
8	Vanderbilt University Medical Center, Nashville, Tenn.	79.0	10	6	127	2.5	Yes	5	9	Yes	2.8%
9	Massachusetts General Hospital, Boston	77.2	9	5	288	2.4	Yes	5	9	Yes	4.8%
10	University of Wisconsin Hospitals, Madison	77.0	10	5	344	2.1	Yes	5	9	Yes	0.5%
11	Scripps La Jolla Hospitals, La Jolla, Calif.	76.4	10	6	162	3.1	Yes	5	8	Yes	1.2%
12	Barnes-Jewish Hospital, St. Louis	75.9	8	5	561	2.2	Yes	5	9	Yes	3.6%
13	Northwestern Memorial Hospital, Chicago	75.6	10	5	96	1.8	Yes	5	9	Yes	5.9%
14	Medical City Dallas	75.3	10	6	130	2.0	Yes	5	8	Yes	0.1%
14	Pennsylvania Hospital, Philadelphia	75.3	10	5	87	1.8	Yes	5	9	Yes	0.7%
14	University of California, Davis Medical Center, Sacramento	75.3	9	5	244	2.8	Yes	5	9	Yes	1.0%
17	Brigham and Women's Hospital, Boston	75.1	9	5	326	2.3	No	5	9	Yes	12.8%
18	MUSC Health-University Medical Center, Charleston, S.C.	75.0	10	5	222	2.3	Yes	5	9	Yes	0.5%
19	St. Joseph's Hospital and Medical Center, Phoenix	74.8	10	6	140	2.1	No	5	8	Yes	0.1%
20	UC Irvine Medical Center, Orange, Calif.	74.4	10	5	190	2.1	Yes	5	8	Yes	1.6%
20	United Hospital, St. Paul, Minn.	74.4	10	6	128	2.4	No	5	7	Yes	0.1%
22	Nebraska Medicine-Nebraska Medical Center, Omaha	73.9	10	5	84	2.2	Yes	5	9	Yes	0.7%
23	Cedars-Sinai Medical Center, Los Angeles	73.8	9	5	331	2.6	Yes	5	9	Yes	2.9%
24	Mount Sinai Hospital, New York	73.7	9	6	275	1.9	Yes	5	9	Yes	2.8%
25	University Hospitals Cleveland Medical Center	73.1	9	5	264	2.6	Yes	5	9	Yes	1.6%
25	University of Alabama at Birmingham Hospital	73.1	8	6	470	1.8	Yes	5	9	Yes	3.1%
27	Abbott Northwestern Hospital, Minneapolis	73.0	9	5	321	2.4	Yes	5	9	Yes	0.1%
28	Hosps. of the U. of Pennsylvania-Penn Presby., Philadelphia	72.7	9	6	195	2.4	Yes	5	9	Yes	3.1%
29	Aurora St. Luke's Medical Center, Milwaukee	72.6	10	3	196	2.2	Yes	5	9	Yes	0.4%
30	Loma Linda University Medical Center, Loma Linda, Calif.	72.4	10	5	124	2.6	No	5	8	Yes	0.3%
30	University of Colorado Hospital, Aurora	72.4	9	5	271	1.9	Yes	5	9	Yes	1.5%
32	University of Utah Hospital, Salt Lake City	72.1	10	5	145	1.8	No	5	9	Yes	1.6%
33	Huntington Memorial Hospital, Pasadena, Calif.	71.9	10	6	104	2.6	Yes	4	9	Yes	0.7%
34	Mayo Clinic Jacksonville, Fla.	71.8	10	6	95	2.1	Yes	5	8	Yes	0.9%
35	Keck Hospital of USC, Los Angeles	71.4	10	6	69	2.4	No	5	9	Yes	1.6%
36	Banner University Medical Center Tucson, Ariz.	71.0	10	4	163	2.0	Yes	5	8	Yes	0.0%
36	Rush University Medical Center, Chicago	71.0	9	5	266	2.2	Yes	5	9	Yes	0.4%
38	West Virginia University Hospitals, Morgantown, W.Va.	70.9	10	6	77	2.8	Yes	5	9	Yes	0.0%
39	Avera McKennan Hosp. and U. Hlth. Ctr., Sioux Falls, S.D.	70.7	10	5	179	1.2	Yes	5	8	Intensivists	0.1%
40	H. Lee Moffitt Cancer Center and Research Institute, Tampa	70.4	10	4	300	1.2	Yes	5	8	Yes	0.1%
41	John Muir Health-Walnut Creek Med. Ctr., Walnut Creek, Calif.	70.3	9	5	283	2.3	Yes	5	8	Yes	0.0%
42	New York-Presbyterian Hospital-Columbia and Cornell, N.Y.	69.8	8	4	308	2.9	No	5	9	Yes	7.6%
43	Swedish Medical Center, Englewood, Colo.	69.7	10	5	280	1.8	No	5	9	Yes	0.1%
44	St. Luke's Hospital of Kansas City, Mo.	69.6	10	5	144	1.6	Yes	5	8	Yes	0.1%
45	Highland Hospital, Rochester N.Y.	68.9	10	5	159	1.4	Yes	5	9	Yes	0.0%
45	University of North Carolina Hospitals, Chapel Hill	68.9	8	5	247	1.8	Yes	5	9	Yes	4.8%
47	Dartmouth-Hitchcock Medical Center, Lebanon, N.H.	68.7	10	5	135	1.7	No	5	9	Yes	0.0%
47	University of Washington Medical Center, Seattle	68.7	9	5	214	2.0	Yes	5	9	Yes	1.9%
49	Wake Forest Baptist Medical Center, Winston-Salem, N.C.	68.4	9	5	267	1.6	Yes	5	9	Yes	1.2%
50	University of Iowa Hospitals and Clinics, Iowa City	67.9	9	5	251	1.8	Yes	5	9	Yes	1.5%

Terms are explained on Page 102.

More @ usnews.com/besthospitals

NEPHROLOGY

Rank	Hospital	U.S. News score	Survival score (10=best)	Patient safety score (9=best)	Number of patients	Nurse staffing score (higher is better)	A Nurse Magnet hospital	Technology score (7=best)	Patient services score (8=best)	Intensivists	% of specialists recommending hospital
1	Mayo Clinic, Rochester, Minn.	100.0	10	5	2,122	2.8	Yes	7	8	Yes	23.4%
2	Cleveland Clinic	93.6	10	6	2,056	2.1	Yes	7	8	Yes	18.0%
3	Johns Hopkins Hospital, Baltimore	93.4	10	4	1,123	2.1	Yes	7	8	Yes	15.2%
4	UCSF Medical Center, San Francisco	91.3	10	6	1,011	2.1	Yes	7	8	Yes	9.3%
5	UCLA Medical Center, Los Angeles	88.6	10	5	1,384	3.0	Yes	7	8	Yes	7.6%
6	New York-Presbyterian Hospital-Columbia and Cornell, N.Y.	86.2	9	4	3,073	2.9	No	7	8	Yes	17.7%
7	Vanderbilt University Medical Center, Nashville, Tenn.	85.1	10	6	1,497	2.5	Yes	7	8	Yes	9.8%
8	U. of Michigan Hospitals-Michigan Medicine, Ann Arbor	83.8	10	7	1,238	2.7	Yes	7	8	Yes	3.6%
9	Massachusetts General Hospital, Boston	83.6	9	5	1,514	2.4	Yes	7	8	Yes	11.2%
10	Stanford Health Care-Stanford Hospital, Stanford, Calif.	82.4	10	5	950	2.5	Yes	7	8	Yes	5.4%
11	Mayo Clinic-Phoenix	81.2	10	6	1,443	2.9	Yes	7	8	Yes	2.2%
12	Cedars-Sinai Medical Center, Los Angeles	80.6	10	5	2,212	2.6	Yes	7	8	Yes	3.0%
13	University of Alabama at Birmingham Hospital	80.2	10	6	1,257	1.8	Yes	7	8	Yes	6.2%
14	Barnes-Jewish Hospital, St. Louis	79.9	10	5	1,906	2.2	Yes	7	8	Yes	5.5%
14	Mount Sinai Hospital, New York	79.9	10	6	1,472	1.9	Yes	7	8	Yes	5.1%
16	Hosps. of the U. of Pennsylvania-Penn Presby., Philadelphia	79.7	9	6	1,195	2.4	Yes	7	8	Yes	7.6%
16	University of California, Davis Medical Center, Sacramento	79.7	10	5	1,157	2.8	Yes	7	8	Yes	1.4%
18	Tampa General Hospital	79.4	10	3	1,502	2.1	Yes	7	8	Yes	1.3%
19	Duke University Hospital, Durham, N.C.	79.2	9	6	1,114	2.1	Yes	7	8	Yes	6.7%
20	University Hospitals Cleveland Medical Center	78.7	10	5	844	2.6	Yes	7	8	Yes	1.6%
21	University of Colorado Hospital, Aurora	78.4	10	5	1,155	1.9	Yes	7	8	Yes	2.2%
22	Ohio State University Wexner Medical Center, Columbus	77.5	10	5	1,665	2.1	Yes	7	8	Yes	2.9%
23	Indiana University Health Medical Center, Indianapolis	77.1	10	5	1,631	2.0	Yes	7	8	Yes	2.2%
23	OHSU Hospital, Portland, Ore.	77.1	10	5	647	2.0	Yes	7	8	Yes	0.5%
25	UT Southwestern Medical Center, Dallas	76.8	10	5	1,141	2.3	Yes	7	8	Yes	2.0%
26	University of North Carolina Hospitals, Chapel Hill	76.0	9	5	902	1.8	Yes	7	8	Yes	5.3%
27	UF Health Shands Hospital, Gainesville, Fla.	75.9	10	5	1,131	1.9	Yes	7	8	Yes	1.9%
28	Brigham and Women's Hospital, Boston	75.5	8	5	1,095	2.3	No	7	8	Yes	13.8%
28	NYU Langone Hospitals, New York, N.Y.	75.5	10	5	1,528	2.3	Yes	7	8	Yes	1.5%
30	University of Wisconsin Hospitals, Madison	75.1	10	5	950	2.1	Yes	7	8	Yes	0.4%
31	Yale New Haven Hospital, New Haven, Conn.	74.6	9	4	2,500	2.0	Yes	7	8	Yes	3.3%
32	Banner University Medical Center Phoenix	74.5	10	5	604	2.3	Yes	7	8	Yes	0.4%
32	VCU Medical Center, Richmond, Va.	74.5	10	5	562	2.4	Yes	7	8	Yes	0.4%
34	Rush University Medical Center, Chicago	74.3	10	5	745	2.2	Yes	7	8	Yes	2.4%
35	Houston Methodist Hospital	74.0	10	5	1,640	2.0	Yes	7	8	Yes	1.2%
35	Keck Hospital of USC, Los Angeles	74.0	10	6	1,374	2.4	No	7	8	Yes	0.9%
35	Northwestern Memorial Hospital, Chicago	74.0	9	5	1,399	1.8	Yes	7	8	Yes	2.7%
38	Wake Forest Baptist Medical Center, Winston-Salem, N.C.	73.7	9	5	1,858	1.6	Yes	7	8	Yes	3.2%
39	University of Kansas Hospital, Kansas City	73.5	10	5	1,210	2.1	Yes	7	8	Yes	0.4%
40	Beaumont Hospital-Royal Oak, Mich.	73.3	10	6	2,223	1.9	Yes	7	8	Yes	0.1%
41	University of Washington Medical Center, Seattle	72.8	10	5	668	2.0	Yes	7	8	Yes	3.5%
42	University of Virginia Medical Center, Charlottesville	72.5	10	5	622	2.1	Yes	7	8	Yes	1.1%
43	Jefferson Health-Thomas Jefferson U. Hospitals, Philadelphia	72.3	10	5	1,251	2.2	Yes	7	8	Yes	0.8%
44	Strong Memorial Hosp. of U. of Rochester, Rochester, N.Y.	72.1	10	5	1,135	1.8	Yes	7	8	Yes	0.1%
45	DMC Harper University Hospital, Detroit	71.9	10	5	806	1.7	Yes	7	8	Yes	0.0%
46	Kaiser Permanente Santa Clara Med. Ctr., Santa Clara, Calif.	71.7	10	5	551	2.5	No	6	8	Yes	0.0%
46	MUSC Health-University Medical Center, Charleston, S.C.	71.7	10	5	781	2.3	Yes	7	8	Yes	0.8%
48	Miami Valley Hospital, Dayton, Ohio	71.5	10	5	1,392	2.5	Yes	6	8	Yes	0.0%
48	Sentara Norfolk General Hospital, Norfolk, Va.	71.5	10	5	870	1.6	Yes	7	8	Yes	0.2%
50	Banner University Medical Center Tucson, Ariz.	71.1	10	4	543	2.0	Yes	7	7	Yes	1.4%
50	Froedtert Hosp. and the Medical College of Wis., Milwaukee	71.1	10	5	778	1.8	Yes	7	8	Yes	1.5%

Terms are explained on Page 102.

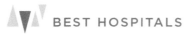

NEUROLOGY & NEUROSURGERY

Rank	Hospital	U.S. News score	Survival score (10=best)	Patient safety score (9=best)	Number of patients	Nurse staffing score (higher is better)	A Nurse Magnet hospital	NAEC epilepsy center	Technology score (5=best)	Patient services score (9=best)	Intensivists	% of specialists recommending hospital
1	Mayo Clinic, Rochester, Minn.	100.0	10	5	5,123	2.8	Yes	Yes	5	9	Yes	38.5%
2	Johns Hopkins Hospital, Baltimore	95.7	10	4	2,418	2.1	Yes	Yes	5	9	Yes	27.5%
3	UCSF Medical Center, San Francisco	89.1	9	6	2,682	2.1	Yes	Yes	5	9	Yes	21.8%
4	Cleveland Clinic	88.5	10	6	3,886	2.1	Yes	Yes	5	9	Yes	19.1%
5	New York-Presbyterian Hospital-Columbia and Cornell, N.Y.	87.4	10	4	6,759	2.9	No	Yes	5	9	Yes	18.0%
6	Massachusetts General Hospital, Boston	86.0	6	5	4,826	2.4	Yes	Yes	5	9	Yes	25.9%
7	Barnes-Jewish Hospital, St. Louis	82.4	10	5	4,713	2.2	Yes	Yes	5	9	Yes	8.4%
8	Northwestern Memorial Hospital, Chicago	81.9	10	5	2,330	1.8	Yes	Yes	5	9	Yes	2.4%
9	U. of Michigan Hospitals-Michigan Medicine, Ann Arbor	81.1	10	7	2,357	2.7	Yes	Yes	5	9	Yes	5.7%
10	UCLA Medical Center, Los Angeles	80.8	10	5	3,478	3.0	Yes	Yes	5	9	Yes	9.8%
11	Rush University Medical Center, Chicago	80.5	10	5	2,343	2.2	Yes	Yes	5	9	Yes	2.4%
12	NYU Langone Hospitals, New York, N.Y.	78.4	10	5	3,571	2.3	Yes	Yes	5	9	Yes	4.4%
13	Hosps. of the U. of Pennsylvania-Penn Presby., Philadelphia	77.1	8	6	3,392	2.4	Yes	Yes	5	9	Yes	8.7%
14	Stanford Health Care-Stanford Hospital, Stanford, Calif.	76.6	9	5	2,610	2.5	Yes	Yes	5	9	Yes	6.0%
15	St. Joseph's Hospital and Medical Center, Phoenix	76.0	10	6	4,446	2.1	No	Yes	5	9	Yes	6.0%
16	Cedars-Sinai Medical Center, Los Angeles	75.8	10	5	4,899	2.6	Yes	Yes	5	9	Yes	1.6%
17	Mount Sinai Hospital, New York	74.6	10	6	2,710	1.9	Yes	Yes	5	9	Yes	2.4%
18	University Hospitals Cleveland Medical Center	74.4	10	5	2,977	2.6	Yes	Yes	5	9	Yes	1.7%
19	Jefferson Health-Thomas Jefferson U. Hospitals, Philadelphia	74.3	10	5	5,174	2.2	Yes	Yes	5	9	Yes	3.2%
20	Brigham and Women's Hospital, Boston	73.2	9	5	3,397	2.3	No	Yes	5	9	Yes	6.6%
21	UT Southwestern Medical Center, Dallas	73.1	10	5	1,825	2.3	Yes	Yes	5	9	Yes	2.3%
22	Ohio State University Wexner Medical Center, Columbus	72.8	10	5	3,775	2.1	Yes	Yes	5	9	Yes	1.8%
23	Mayo Clinic-Phoenix	71.7	9	6	2,273	2.9	Yes	Yes	5	9	Yes	3.3%
24	Houston Methodist Hospital	71.6	10	5	3,942	2.0	Yes	Yes	5	9	Yes	2.6%
25	Beaumont Hospital-Royal Oak, Mich.	70.0	10	6	4,509	1.9	Yes	Yes	5	9	Yes	0.0%
26	Keck Hospital of USC, Los Angeles	69.4	10	6	1,075	2.4	No	Yes	5	9	Yes	1.1%
27	Indiana University Health Medical Center, Indianapolis	68.7	9	5	3,149	2.0	Yes	Yes	5	9	Yes	0.8%
28	University of California, Davis Medical Center, Sacramento	68.6	9	5	2,135	2.8	Yes	Yes	5	9	Yes	0.7%
29	DMC Harper University Hospital, Detroit	68.3	10	5	640	1.7	Yes	Yes	5	8	Yes	0.1%
30	University of Colorado Hospital, Aurora	68.2	10	5	2,393	1.9	Yes	Yes	5	9	Yes	1.3%
31	University of Kansas Hospital, Kansas City	68.0	8	5	2,286	2.1	Yes	Yes	5	9	Yes	1.7%
32	Duke University Hospital, Durham, N.C.	67.9	8	6	2,715	2.1	Yes	Yes	5	9	Yes	5.5%
32	UF Health Shands Hospital, Gainesville, Fla.	67.9	7	5	2,867	1.9	Yes	Yes	5	9	Yes	2.8%
34	Baylor St. Luke's Medical Center, Houston	67.7	10	5	2,038	1.6	Yes	Yes	5	8	Yes	3.0%
35	UPMC Presbyterian Shadyside, Pittsburgh	67.5	4	5	7,187	1.9	Yes	Yes	5	9	Yes	3.0%
36	University of Alabama at Birmingham Hospital	67.3	9	6	4,058	1.8	Yes	Yes	5	8	Yes	1.2%
37	Loyola University Medical Center, Maywood, Ill.	67.0	10	5	1,461	2.4	Yes	Yes	5	9	Yes	1.0%
38	Emory University Hospital, Atlanta	66.8	8	5	2,254	1.9	Yes	Yes	5	9	Yes	3.1%
38	Ochsner Medical Center, New Orleans	66.8	10	5	3,454	1.9	Yes	Yes	5	9	Intensivists	0.5%
40	Yale New Haven Hospital, New Haven, Conn.	66.5	7	4	4,295	2.0	Yes	Yes	5	9	Yes	2.2%
41	Mayo Clinic Jacksonville, Fla.	65.8	6	6	1,583	2.1	Yes	Yes	5	9	Yes	4.3%
42	Abbott Northwestern Hospital, Minneapolis	65.7	10	5	4,284	2.4	Yes	Yes	5	9	Yes	0.4%
43	Vanderbilt University Medical Center, Nashville, Tenn.	65.4	7	6	4,017	2.5	Yes	Yes	5	9	Yes	2.8%
44	St. Luke's Hospital of Kansas City, Mo.	64.4	9	5	3,303	1.6	Yes	Yes	5	9	Yes	0.6%
45	OhioHealth Riverside Methodist Hospital, Columbus	64.2	8	5	6,512	2.1	Yes	Yes	5	9	Yes	0.3%
46	UC San Diego Health-Jacobs Medical Center, Calif.	64.1	7	5	1,830	2.0	Yes	Yes	5	9	Yes	1.6%
47	Wake Forest Baptist Medical Center, Winston-Salem, N.C.	63.6	5	5	4,202	1.6	Yes	Yes	5	9	Yes	1.7%
48	Banner Heart Hospital, Mesa, Ariz.	63.5	10	5	306	2.1	No	No	5	9	Yes	0.0%
49	University of Wisconsin Hospitals, Madison	63.3	7	5	2,311	2.1	Yes	Yes	5	9	Yes	0.6%
50	Banner University Medical Center Phoenix	63.1	9	5	2,117	2.3	Yes	No	5	9	Yes	0.2%

Terms are explained on Page 102.

More @ usnews.com/besthospitals

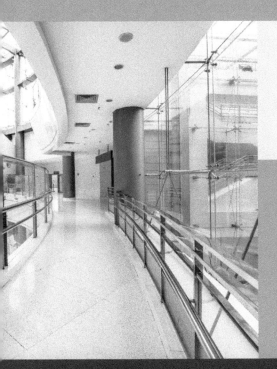
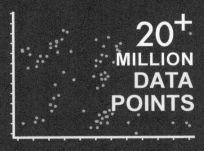

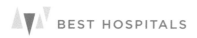
ORTHOPEDICS

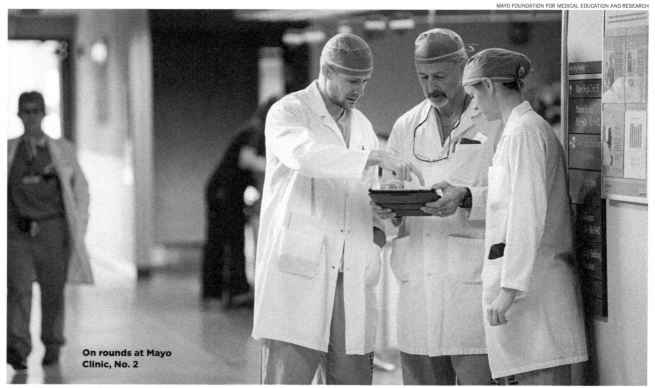

MAYO FOUNDATION FOR MEDICAL EDUCATION AND RESEARCH

On rounds at Mayo Clinic, No. 2

Rank	Hospital	U.S. News score	Survival score (10=best)	Patient safety score (9=best)	Number of patients	Nurse staffing score (higher is better)	A Nurse Magnet hospital	Technology score (2=best)	Patient services score (7=best)	Intensivists	% of specialists recommending hospital
1	Hospital for Special Surgery, New York	100.0	10	9	14,987	3.6	Yes	2	7	Yes	32.8%
2	Mayo Clinic, Rochester, Minn.	83.2	10	5	9,011	2.8	Yes	2	7	Yes	27.4%
3	Cleveland Clinic	71.4	10	6	3,360	2.1	Yes	2	7	Yes	15.0%
4	Rothman Institute at Thomas Jefferson U. Hosp., Philadelphia	69.1	10	5	5,746	2.2	Yes	2	7	Yes	7.9%
4	Rush University Medical Center, Chicago	69.1	10	5	3,130	2.2	Yes	2	7	Yes	7.8%
6	Massachusetts General Hospital, Boston	67.5	10	5	3,490	2.4	Yes	2	7	Yes	10.2%
7	UCSF Medical Center, San Francisco	66.9	10	6	3,003	2.1	Yes	2	7	Yes	3.1%
8	NYU Langone Orthopedic Hospital, New York	66.6	10	5	6,206	2.3	Yes	2	7	Yes	6.6%
9	Cedars-Sinai Medical Center, Los Angeles	66.3	10	5	6,637	2.6	Yes	2	7	Yes	1.9%
10	Johns Hopkins Hospital, Baltimore	66.2	10	4	1,191	2.1	Yes	2	7	Yes	6.3%
11	Duke University Hospital, Durham, N.C.	66.0	10	6	2,649	2.1	Yes	2	7	Yes	6.6%
12	Northwestern Memorial Hospital, Chicago	64.7	10	5	3,003	1.8	Yes	2	7	Yes	3.3%
13	Stanford Health Care-Stanford Hospital, Stanford, Calif.	64.2	10	5	4,422	2.5	Yes	2	7	Yes	3.5%
14	Barnes-Jewish Hospital, St. Louis	64.0	10	5	4,347	2.2	Yes	2	7	Yes	5.9%
14	University of Iowa Hospitals and Clinics, Iowa City	64.0	10	5	2,032	1.8	Yes	2	7	Yes	5.5%
16	UPMC Presbyterian Shadyside, Pittsburgh	63.9	9	5	4,928	1.9	Yes	2	7	Yes	7.2%
17	Mayo Clinic-Phoenix	62.8	10	6	3,697	2.9	Yes	2	7	Yes	1.4%
18	UCLA Medical Center, Los Angeles	62.5	10	5	2,378	3.0	Yes	2	7	Yes	2.8%
19	Hosps. of the U. of Pennsylvania-Penn Presby., Philadelphia	62.1	10	6	2,561	2.4	Yes	2	7	Yes	2.8%
20	University of Colorado Hospital, Aurora	61.8	10	5	2,678	1.9	Yes	2	7	Yes	1.2%
21	U. of Michigan Hospitals-Michigan Medicine, Ann Arbor	61.2	10	7	1,770	2.7	Yes	2	7	Yes	2.0%
22	Keck Hospital of USC, Los Angeles	60.9	10	6	2,270	2.4	No	2	7	Yes	2.0%
23	Pennsylvania Hospital, Philadelphia	60.5	10	5	1,631	1.8	Yes	2	7	Yes	0.6%
24	Beaumont Hospital-Royal Oak, Mich.	60.4	10	6	5,908	1.9	Yes	2	7	Yes	1.2%

(CONTINUED ON PAGE 126)

Terms are explained on Page 102.

More @ usnews.com/besthospitals

HOW YOU MOVE IS WHY WE'RE HERE.

AGAIN.

For the past nine years, HSS has been ranked #1 in the nation for orthopedics. That's because our world-class physicians are dedicated to providing the most personalized care and innovative treatment options. When it comes to your quality of life, we understand that how you move is everything. Learn more about our approach, our commitment to progress, and our leadership in orthopedics and rheumatology at **HSS.edu**

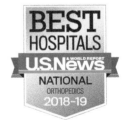

HOSPITAL FOR SPECIAL SURGERY

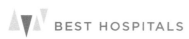

ORTHOPEDICS (CONTINUED)

Rank	Hospital	U.S. News score	Survival score (10=best)	Patient safety score (9=best)	Number of patients	Nurse staffing score (higher is better)	A Nurse Magnet hospital	Technology score (2=best)	Patient services score (7=best)	Intensivists	% of specialists recommending hospital
24	New England Baptist Hospital, Boston	60.4	10	6	4,969	2.5	No	2	7	Yes	1.0%
26	Abbott Northwestern Hospital, Minneapolis	60.1	10	5	6,951	2.4	Yes	2	7	Yes	0.1%
26	Houston Methodist Hospital	60.1	10	5	4,605	2.0	Yes	2	7	Yes	2.1%
28	Scripps La Jolla Hospitals, La Jolla, Calif.	59.9	9	6	4,147	3.1	Yes	2	6	Yes	1.0%
29	University of Washington Medical Center, Seattle	59.6	10	5	797	2.0	Yes	2	7	Yes	2.5%
30	Vanderbilt University Medical Center, Nashville, Tenn.	59.5	9	6	2,542	2.5	Yes	2	7	Yes	3.2%
31	Hoag Orthopedic Institute, Newport Beach, Calif.	59.1	10	7	7,110	2.4	Yes	2	7	Yes	0.4%
32	Northwestern Medicine Central DuPage Hosp., Winfield, Ill.	59.0	10	5	2,587	2.1	Yes	2	7	Yes	0.2%
33	Ohio State University Wexner Medical Center, Columbus	58.9	10	5	1,978	2.1	Yes	2	7	Yes	1.0%
34	VCU Medical Center, Richmond, Va.	58.8	10	5	1,575	2.4	Yes	2	7	Yes	0.6%
35	Penn State Health Milton S. Hershey Medical Center, Hershey	58.7	10	6	1,963	1.7	Yes	2	7	Yes	0.4%
36	Loyola University Medical Center, Maywood, Ill.	58.2	10	5	1,220	2.4	Yes	2	7	Yes	1.0%
37	MUSC Health-University Medical Center, Charleston, S.C.	58.1	10	5	1,470	2.3	Yes	2	7	Yes	0.8%
37	University of California, Davis Medical Center, Sacramento	58.1	10	5	2,198	2.8	Yes	2	7	Yes	0.7%
39	Tampa General Hospital	57.9	10	3	4,120	2.1	Yes	2	6	Yes	1.2%
40	Mount Sinai Hospital, New York	57.8	10	6	2,447	1.9	Yes	2	7	Yes	0.9%
41	Carolinas Medical Center, Charlotte, N.C.	57.7	9	5	5,224	1.6	Yes	2	7	Yes	2.7%
42	Cleveland Clinic Florida, Weston	57.6	10	5	1,269	2.5	No	2	7	Yes	0.5%
43	MemorialCare Long Beach Medical Center, Long Beach, Calif.	57.4	10	5	1,770	2.5	Yes	2	7	Yes	0.1%
44	Hackensack University Medical Center, Hackensack, N.J.	56.7	10	5	2,317	2.4	Yes	2	7	Yes	0.4%
45	Mercy Medical Center, Baltimore	56.6	10	5	2,783	1.4	Yes	2	6	Yes	0.0%
45	U. of Kentucky Albert B. Chandler Hospital, Lexington	56.6	10	5	1,738	1.9	Yes	2	7	Yes	0.9%
45	University of Minnesota Medical Center, Minneapolis	56.6	10	5	2,104	2.0	No	2	7	Yes	0.7%
45	University of Wisconsin Hospitals, Madison	56.6	10	5	1,910	2.1	Yes	2	7	Yes	0.9%
49	Porter Adventist Hospital, Denver	56.2	10	3	3,903	1.9	Yes	2	6	Yes	0.3%
49	UC San Diego Health-Jacobs Medical Center, Calif.	56.2	9	5	1,974	2.0	Yes	2	7	Yes	1.4%
49	UT Southwestern Medical Center, Dallas	56.2	10	5	1,305	2.3	Yes	1	7	Yes	0.4%

Terms are explained on Page 102.

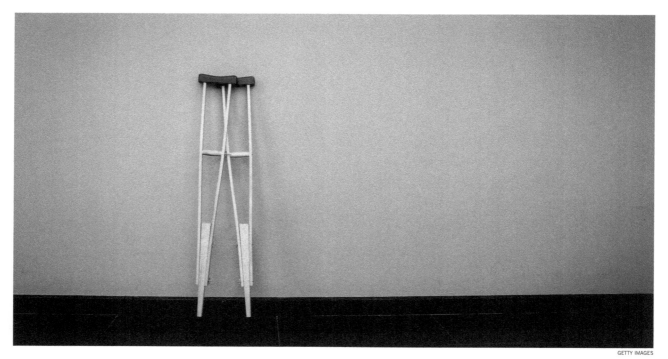

GETTY IMAGES

More @ usnews.com/besthospitals

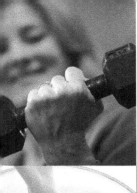

OUTSTANDING HOSPITALS DON'T SIMPLY TREAT FRAGILITY FRACTURES—
THEY PREVENT FRACTURES FROM RECURRING

THE BEST HOSPITALS AND PRACTICES OWN THE BONE

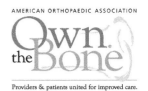

AMERICAN ORTHOPAEDIC ASSOCIATION

Own. the Bone

Providers & patients united for improved care.

The American Orthopaedic Association applauds the following institutions for their achievements and participation in the Own the Bone® quality improvement program:

STAR PERFORMERS

Institutions are recognized for at least 75% compliance on 5 of the 10 recommended secondary fracture prevention measures over the last year.

Akron General Medical Center - Akron, OH

Baptist Health – Mission Trail - San Antonio, TX

Buffalo Hospital – part of Allina Health - Buffalo, MN

^Christiana Care Health System – Christiana Hosptial - Newark, DE

^Christiana Care Health System – Wilmington Hospital - Wilmington, DE

Coastal Fracture Prevention Center - Sebastian, FL

Colorado Spine Institute PLLC - Johnstown, CO

Concord Hospital - Concord, NH

Cooper Health System - Camden, NJ

Crystal Clinic Orthopaedic Center - Akron, OH

Department of Orthopedics, Anne Arundel Medical Group, Anne Arundel Medical Center - Annapolis, MD

DHR Health - Edinburg, TX

Florida Hospital Flagler Orthopedics & Sports Medicine - Palm Coast, FL

^Greenville Health System/University Medical Center- Greenville, SC

Heiden Orthopedics - Cottonwood Heights, UT

Herrin Hospital - Herrin, IL

Huntington Hospital - Northwell Health - Huntington, NY

Illinois Bone & Joint Institute, LLC - Morton Grove, IL

Jefferson Hospital – Allegheny Health Network - Pittsburgh, PA

JPS Health Network - Fort Worth, TX

Lahey Hospital & Medical Center - Burlington, MA

LewisGale Medical Center - Salem, VA

MaineGeneral Orthopaedic Surgery - Augusta, ME

Marshfield Clinic Health System - Marshfield, WI

Medical City Arlington - Arlington, TX

Medical University of South Carolina Center for Osteoporosis and Bone Health - Charleston, SC

Memorial Regional Hospital - Hollywood, FL

Mendelson Kornblum Orthopedic & Spine Specialists - Warren, MI

Mercy Regional Medical Center - Durango, CO

Michigan Medicine, University of Michigan - Ann Arbor, MI

Newton Medical Center - Newton, KS

Northwell Health – Lenox Hill Hospital - Manhasset, NY

Northwest Orthopedic Specialists - Spokane, WA

Norton Women's and Children's Hospital - Louisville, KY

Novant Health Forsyth Medical Center - Winston - Salem, NC

NYU Langone Orthopedic Hospital - New York, NY

NYU Winthrop Hospital - Mineola, NY

OhioHealth Grant Medical Center - Columbus, OH

Orthopaedic Associates of Michigan - Grand Rapids, MI

Paramount Care, Inc. - Maumee, OH

Peninsula Regional Medical Center - Salisbury, MD

^Penrose – St. Francis Health Services - Colorado Springs, CO

ProMedica Toledo Hospital - Toledo, OH

Regions Hospital/HealthPartners Orthopaedic and Sports Medicine - Minneapolis, MN

^Sanford Medical Center Fargo - Fargo, ND

Southeast Georgia Health System - Brunswick, GA

St. Luke's Health System - Boise, ID

St. Luke's University Hospital and Health Network - Bethlehem, PA

St. Vincent's Medical Center - Bridgeport, CT

Sturgis Orthopedics - Sturgis, MI

Tahoe Forest Hospital District - Truckee, CA

Tallahassee Memorial HealthCare - Tallahassee, FL

The CORE Institute - Arizona - Phoenix, AZ

The Methodist Hospitals Ortho Spine Center - Merrillville, IN

^The Queen's Medical Center - Honolulu, HI

^The University of Vermont Health Network – Central Vermont Medical Center - Berlin, VT

TRIA Orthopaedic Center - Bloomington, MN

University Hospital - San Antonio, TX

University of Wisconsin Hospitals and Clinics - Madison, WI

UT Health East Texas Orthopedic Institute - Tyler, TX

UW Medicine/Northwest Hospital and Medical Center - Seattle, WA

Western Reserve Hospital - Cuyahoga Falls, OH

^WVU Medicine – Department of Orthopaedics - Morgantown, WV

NEWLY ENROLLED INSTITUTIONS

Anchorage Fracture & Orthopedic Clinic - Anchorage, AK

*ClinTech-Center for Spine Health - Johnstown, CO

Crisp Regional Hospital - Cordele, GA

Fairchild Medical Clinic - Yreka, CA

Florida Hospital Orthopedic Institute - Orlando, FL

*Florida Hospital Zephyrhills - Zephyrhills, FL

*Froedtert & The Medical College of Wisconsin - Milwaukee, WI

*Henry Ford Health System - Detroit, MI

Memorial Medical Center - Las Cruces, NM

Mercy Health – St. Vincent Medical Center - Toledo, OH

Oregon Health & Science University Department of Orthopaedics and Rehabilitation - Portland, OR

Sauk Prairie Healthcare - Prairie du Sac, WI

*St. Francis Orthopaedic Institute - Columbus, GA

St. Joseph's Hospital North - Lutz, FL

The Christ Hospital Health Network - Cincinnati, OH

*Wake Forest Baptist Health - Winston-Salem, NC

The AOA recognizes **Amgen** and **DePuy Synthes** for their 2018 Educational Alliance support.

^First in State to enroll in Own the Bone®

*Also a Star Performer

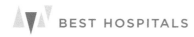

PULMONOLOGY

Rank	Hospital	U.S. News score	Survival score (10=best)	Patient safety score (9=best)	Number of patients	Nurse staffing score (higher is better)	A Nurse Magnet hospital	Technology score (6=best)	Patient services score (8=best)	Intensivists	% of specialists recom-mending hospital
1	National Jewish Health, Denver-U. of Colorado Hosp., Aurora	100.0	10	5	4,723	1.9	Yes	6	8	Yes	47.2%
2	Mayo Clinic, Rochester, Minn.	96.3	10	5	8,734	2.8	Yes	6	8	Yes	29.0%
3	Cleveland Clinic	88.5	10	6	5,246	2.1	Yes	6	8	Yes	24.4%
4	Massachusetts General Hospital, Boston	82.8	9	5	6,446	2.4	Yes	6	8	Yes	14.6%
5	Mayo Clinic-Phoenix	80.8	10	6	5,613	2.9	Yes	5	8	Yes	2.6%
5	U. of Michigan Hospitals-Michigan Medicine, Ann Arbor	80.8	10	7	3,897	2.7	Yes	6	8	Yes	6.3%
7	UCSF Medical Center, San Francisco	79.2	8	6	3,749	2.1	Yes	6	8	Yes	12.6%
8	UPMC Presbyterian Shadyside, Pittsburgh	78.8	8	5	7,818	1.9	Yes	6	8	Yes	11.5%
9	UCLA Medical Center, Los Angeles	78.6	9	5	7,481	3.0	Yes	6	8	Yes	6.7%
10	Barnes-Jewish Hospital, St. Louis	78.0	9	5	5,748	2.2	Yes	6	8	Yes	9.8%
11	Hosps. of the U. of Pennsylvania-Penn Presby., Philadelphia	77.6	7	6	5,889	2.4	Yes	6	8	Yes	10.6%
12	Johns Hopkins Hospital, Baltimore	77.2	7	4	2,720	2.1	Yes	6	8	Yes	16.3%
13	Scripps La Jolla Hospitals, La Jolla, Calif.	75.5	10	6	4,671	3.1	Yes	5	8	Yes	0.1%
14	Cedars-Sinai Medical Center, Los Angeles	75.3	9	5	11,321	2.6	Yes	6	8	Yes	1.2%
15	Vanderbilt University Medical Center, Nashville, Tenn.	74.9	8	6	4,620	2.5	Yes	6	8	Yes	6.5%
16	University of Alabama at Birmingham Hospital	74.8	10	6	5,910	1.8	Yes	6	8	Yes	2.6%
17	Duke University Hospital, Durham, N.C.	74.1	6	6	4,697	2.1	Yes	6	8	Yes	10.6%
17	UC San Diego Health-Jacobs Medical Center, Calif.	74.1	8	5	3,798	2.0	Yes	6	8	Yes	7.4%
19	Beaumont Hospital-Royal Oak, Mich.	73.9	10	6	9,498	1.9	Yes	5	8	Yes	0.8%
20	Ohio State University Wexner Medical Center, Columbus	73.4	10	5	6,392	2.1	Yes	6	8	Yes	1.2%
21	New York-Presbyterian Hospital-Columbia and Cornell, N.Y.	73.2	7	4	11,572	2.9	No	6	8	Yes	8.9%
22	UF Health Shands Hospital, Gainesville, Fla.	72.8	10	5	4,019	1.9	Yes	6	8	Yes	1.9%
23	Houston Methodist Hospital	72.7	10	5	6,447	2.0	Yes	6	8	Yes	0.9%
23	Yale New Haven Hospital, New Haven, Conn.	72.7	8	4	11,061	2.0	Yes	5	8	Yes	4.2%
25	Northwestern Memorial Hospital, Chicago	72.6	10	5	3,877	1.8	Yes	6	8	Yes	2.5%
26	University of California, Davis Medical Center, Sacramento	72.5	10	5	4,543	2.8	Yes	5	8	Yes	0.7%
27	Cleveland Clinic Fairview Hospital, Cleveland	72.2	10	6	3,769	1.9	Yes	5	8	Yes	0.2%
28	Miami Valley Hospital, Dayton, Ohio	72.0	10	5	6,027	2.5	Yes	5	8	Yes	0.5%
29	University of Wisconsin Hospitals, Madison	71.6	10	5	3,164	2.1	Yes	6	8	Yes	2.5%
30	St. Cloud Hospital, St. Cloud, Minn.	71.5	10	5	7,491	2.2	Yes	4	8	Yes	0.0%
31	Banner University Medical Center Phoenix	71.2	10	5	2,470	2.3	Yes	5	8	Yes	0.6%
32	Beaumont Hospital-Troy, Mich.	70.8	9	8	7,209	2.0	Yes	5	8	Yes	0.0%
32	NYU Langone Hospitals, New York, N.Y.	70.8	9	5	7,943	2.3	Yes	5	8	Yes	2.2%
34	St. Luke's Regional Medical Center, Boise, Idaho	70.7	10	6	5,620	2.1	Yes	5	6	Yes	0.0%
35	Mission Hospital, Orange, Calif.	70.3	10	6	5,083	2.0	Yes	5	8	Yes	0.0%
35	Parker Adventist Hospital, Colo.	70.3	10	5	1,483	2.2	Yes	5	8	Yes	0.0%
37	Stanford Health Care-Stanford Hospital, Stanford, Calif.	69.5	7	5	4,564	2.5	Yes	6	8	Yes	4.1%
38	Brigham and Women's Hospital, Boston	69.2	7	5	5,025	2.3	No	6	8	Yes	8.8%
39	Indiana University Health Medical Center, Indianapolis	69.1	9	5	4,998	2.0	Yes	6	8	Yes	0.5%
39	University of Iowa Hospitals and Clinics, Iowa City	69.1	9	5	2,554	1.8	Yes	6	8	Yes	1.9%
41	University of Kansas Hospital, Kansas City	69.0	10	5	3,727	2.1	Yes	5	8	Yes	0.7%
41	Wake Forest Baptist Medical Center, Winston-Salem, N.C.	69.0	9	5	7,306	1.6	Yes	5	8	Yes	1.1%
43	UT Southwestern Medical Center, Dallas	68.9	10	5	2,623	2.3	Yes	6	8	Yes	1.8%
44	University of Washington Medical Center, Seattle	68.8	9	5	1,804	2.0	Yes	6	8	Yes	5.4%
45	Froedtert Hosp. and the Medical College of Wis., Milwaukee	68.7	10	5	3,810	1.8	Yes	6	8	Yes	0.6%
46	Tampa General Hospital	68.4	10	3	4,009	2.1	Yes	6	8	Yes	1.0%
47	Abbott Northwestern Hospital, Minneapolis	68.3	10	5	6,043	2.4	Yes	5	8	Yes	0.1%
47	Cleveland Clinic Akron General, Ohio	68.3	10	5	5,082	1.2	Yes	5	8	Yes	0.1%
49	Banner University Medical Center Tucson, Ariz.	68.0	10	4	2,955	2.0	Yes	6	7	Yes	0.3%
49	Loyola University Medical Center, Maywood, Ill.	68.0	9	5	2,455	2.4	Yes	6	8	Yes	1.3%

Terms are explained on Page 102.

More @ usnews.com/besthospitals

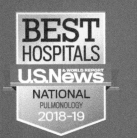

Breathing Science is Life.®

It's easy to take breathing for granted — until you can't.
At National Jewish Health in Denver, the nation's leading respiratory hospital, we help people who struggle to breathe get back to living the life they enjoy. For 119 years, our groundbreaking research and personalized care have transformed millions of lives. We breathe science, so you can breathe life. **To make an appointment, call 800.621.0505 or visit njhealth.org.**

BEST HOSPITALS
U.S.News & WORLD REPORT
NATIONAL
PULMONOLOGY
2018-19

National Jewish Health®

#1 in Respiratory Care

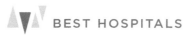 BEST HOSPITALS

UROLOGY

Rank	Hospital	U.S. News score	Survival score (10=best)	Patient safety score (9=best)	Number of patients	Nurse staffing score (higher is better)	A Nurse Magnet hospital	Technology score (6=best)	Patient services score (9=best)	Intensivists	% of specialists recommending hospital
1	Cleveland Clinic	100.0	10	6	1,015	2.1	Yes	6	9	Yes	39.0%
2	Johns Hopkins Hospital, Baltimore	99.9	10	4	665	2.1	Yes	6	9	Yes	30.5%
2	Mayo Clinic, Rochester, Minn.	99.9	10	5	1,323	2.8	Yes	6	9	Yes	23.9%
4	UCSF Medical Center, San Francisco	88.5	10	6	689	2.1	Yes	6	9	Yes	11.0%
5	U. of Michigan Hospitals-Michigan Medicine, Ann Arbor	88.3	10	7	813	2.7	Yes	6	9	Yes	6.9%
6	Vanderbilt University Medical Center, Nashville, Tenn.	86.2	9	6	931	2.5	Yes	6	9	Yes	11.2%
7	UCLA Medical Center, Los Angeles	85.2	7	5	629	3.0	Yes	6	9	Yes	13.6%
8	Memorial Sloan-Kettering Cancer Center, New York	82.5	9	5	1,058	2.1	Yes	6	8	Yes	10.2%
9	Keck Hospital of USC, Los Angeles	80.9	9	6	1,156	2.4	No	6	9	Yes	8.1%
10	NYU Langone Hospitals, New York, N.Y.	80.7	9	5	656	2.3	Yes	6	9	Yes	5.5%
11	New York-Presbyterian Hospital-Columbia and Cornell, N.Y.	80.6	9	4	1,333	2.9	No	6	9	Yes	7.2%
12	Duke University Hospital, Durham, N.C.	80.2	9	6	611	2.1	Yes	6	9	Yes	7.1%
13	Cedars-Sinai Medical Center, Los Angeles	80.1	10	5	1,183	2.6	Yes	6	9	Yes	0.8%
14	Mayo Clinic-Phoenix	79.6	10	6	915	2.9	Yes	6	8	Yes	2.7%
15	Barnes-Jewish Hospital, St. Louis	79.2	10	5	734	2.2	Yes	6	9	Yes	3.4%
16	Huntington Memorial Hospital, Pasadena, Calif.	79.0	10	6	306	2.6	Yes	6	9	Yes	0.2%
17	Stanford Health Care-Stanford Hospital, Stanford, Calif.	78.9	9	5	552	2.5	Yes	6	9	Yes	4.2%
18	Massachusetts General Hospital, Boston	78.1	9	5	669	2.4	Yes	6	9	Yes	4.8%
19	University of California, Davis Medical Center, Sacramento	77.8	10	5	579	2.8	Yes	6	9	Yes	0.5%
20	VCU Medical Center, Richmond, Va.	77.6	10	5	224	2.4	Yes	6	9	Yes	0.8%
21	University of Wisconsin Hospitals, Madison	77.5	10	5	417	2.1	Yes	6	9	Yes	2.1%
22	West Virginia University Hospitals, Morgantown, W.Va.	77.2	10	6	185	2.8	Yes	6	9	Yes	0.5%
23	University of Kansas Hospital, Kansas City	76.8	10	5	495	2.1	Yes	6	9	Yes	1.3%
23	University of Maryland Medical Center, Baltimore	76.8	10	3	283	2.9	Yes	6	9	Yes	0.7%
25	Hosps. of the U. of Pennsylvania-Penn Presby., Philadelphia	76.6	8	6	737	2.4	Yes	6	9	Yes	3.1%
26	Beaumont Hospital-Royal Oak, Mich.	76.4	9	6	866	1.9	Yes	6	9	Yes	1.7%
26	Northwestern Memorial Hospital, Chicago	76.4	9	5	552	1.8	Yes	6	9	Yes	4.7%
28	Tampa General Hospital	76.2	10	3	629	2.1	Yes	6	9	Yes	1.2%
29	UPMC Presbyterian Shadyside, Pittsburgh	76.0	9	5	814	1.9	Yes	6	9	Yes	3.2%
30	University of Virginia Medical Center, Charlottesville	75.4	10	5	247	2.1	Yes	6	9	Yes	2.2%
31	Loyola University Medical Center, Maywood, Ill.	74.9	10	5	453	2.4	Yes	6	8	Yes	1.5%
32	UW Medicine/Harborview Medical Center, Seattle	74.4	10	6	81	2.5	No	6	9	Yes	0.0%
33	UC Irvine Medical Center, Orange, Calif.	74.3	10	5	254	2.1	Yes	6	8	Yes	1.5%
34	UT Southwestern Medical Center, Dallas	74.0	8	5	685	2.3	Yes	6	9	Yes	4.6%
34	University of Alabama at Birmingham Hospital	74.0	9	6	494	1.8	Yes	6	9	Yes	1.4%
34	University of Iowa Hospitals and Clinics, Iowa City	74.0	10	5	334	1.8	Yes	6	9	Yes	1.3%
37	University of Colorado Hospital, Aurora	73.8	10	5	602	1.9	Yes	6	9	Yes	0.7%
38	Mount Sinai Hospital, New York	73.4	7	6	786	1.9	Yes	6	9	Yes	2.8%
39	Hahnemann University Hospital, Philadelphia	73.1	10	5	127	1.8	Yes	6	9	No	0.1%
40	Yale New Haven Hospital, New Haven, Conn.	72.9	9	4	992	2.0	Yes	6	9	Yes	1.0%
41	Hoag Memorial Hospital Presbyterian, Newport Beach, Calif.	72.8	9	7	752	2.4	Yes	6	9	Yes	0.0%
42	University Hospital, San Antonio	72.7	10	5	101	1.6	Yes	6	9	Yes	0.2%
43	Jefferson Health-Thomas Jefferson U. Hospitals, Philadelphia	72.5	7	5	747	2.2	Yes	6	9	Yes	2.8%
43	Ohio State University Wexner Medical Center, Columbus	72.5	9	5	644	2.1	Yes	6	9	Yes	0.9%
45	Parker Adventist Hospital, Colo.	72.2	10	5	80	2.2	Yes	6	8	Yes	0.0%
45	University of Chicago Medical Center	72.2	9	7	560	2.4	No	6	9	Yes	2.2%
47	Advocate Good Samaritan Hospital, Downers Grove, Ill.	72.1	10	7	205	2.0	Yes	6	8	Yes	0.0%
48	Emory University Hospital, Atlanta	72.0	10	5	574	1.9	Yes	6	9	Yes	1.6%
48	Vidant Medical Center, Greenville, N.C.	72.0	9	6	606	2.0	Yes	6	9	Yes	0.1%
50	Abbott Northwestern Hospital, Minneapolis	71.6	10	5	519	2.4	Yes	6	9	Yes	0.5%
50	University Hospitals Cleveland Medical Center	71.6	7	5	387	2.6	Yes	6	9	Yes	1.9%

Terms are explained on Page 102.

More @ usnews.com/besthospitals

U.S. NEWS APPOINTMENT BOOKING

usnews.com/health | A Booking Service from *U.S. News & World Report*

From U.S. News to Your Office

Appointment Booking lets U.S. News visitors request or book appointments with your providers directly from our website.

Why Appointment Booking?

- 5 million monthly website visitors
- 85% of those surveyed use Find a Doctor to research or book an appointment
- Shared Analytics for Trackable ROI

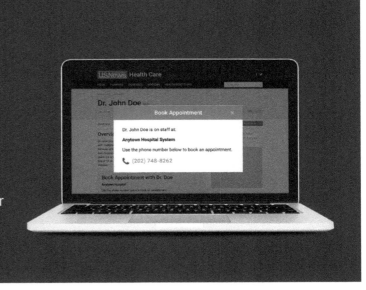

January Weekly Appointment Booking Calls

Week	Calls
January 1-7	733
January 8-14	780
January 15-21	683
January 22-28	871

Steps to Success

1. Select your Physicians
2. Update your Physician Profiles
3. Choose where to route your calls
4. See new patients

For more information or to request a demo, contact us

Kayla Devon
Product Manager, Health

✉ kdevon@usnews.com
☎ Phone: 202-955-2151

Manny Plummer
Sales Associate

✉ mplummer@usnews.com
☎ Phone: 202-823-4832

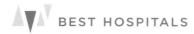 BEST HOSPITALS

These hospitals are among the best in their specialty

for particularly challenging patients, in the view of at least 5 percent of medical specialists surveyed by U.S. News over the past three years.

OPHTHALMOLOGY

Rank	Hospital	% of specialists recommending hospital
1	Bascom Palmer Eye Institute-University of Miami	54.7%
2	Wills Eye Hosp., Thomas Jefferson U. Hosp., Philadelphia	50.3%
3	Wilmer Eye Institute, Johns Hopkins Hospital, Baltimore	39.2%
4	Massachusetts Eye & Ear Infirmary, Mass. Gen. Hosp., Boston	27.0%
5	Stein and Doheny Eye Institutes, UCLA Med. Ctr., Los Angeles	22.6%
6	Duke University Hospital, Durham, N.C.	14.1%
7	University of Iowa Hospitals and Clinics, Iowa City	13.2%
8	U. of Michigan Hospitals-Michigan Medicine, Ann Arbor	8.9%
9	Cole Eye Institute, Cleveland Clinic	8.1%
10	UCSF Medical Center, San Francisco	7.7%
11	New York Eye and Ear Infirmary of Mount Sinai, N.Y.	6.8%
12	USC Roski Eye Institute, Los Angeles	5.9%

PSYCHIATRY

Rank	Hospital	% of specialists recommending hospital
1	McLean Hospital, Belmont, Mass.	22.7%
2	Massachusetts General Hospital, Boston	19.7%
3	New York-Presbyterian Hospital-Columbia and Cornell, N.Y.	15.0%
4	Johns Hopkins Hospital, Baltimore	14.0%
5	Menninger Clinic, Houston	13.7%
6	Sheppard Pratt Hospital, Baltimore	12.4%
7	Mayo Clinic, Rochester, Minn.	11.9%
8	Resnick Neuropsychiatric Hospital at UCLA, Los Angeles	10.2%
9	Yale New Haven Hospital, New Haven, Conn.	6.5%
10	Austen Riggs Center, Stockbridge, Mass.	5.9%
11	UCSF Medical Center, San Francisco	5.7%

REHABILITATION

Rank	Hospital	% of specialists recommending hospital
1	Shirley Ryan AbilityLab, Chicago	35.2%
2	Spaulding Rehab. Hosp., Massachusetts Gen. Hosp., Boston	19.9%
3	TIRR Memorial Hermann, Houston	19.5%
4	Kessler Institute for Rehabilitation, West Orange, N.J.	19.0%
5	University of Washington Medical Center, Seattle	16.7%
6	Mayo Clinic, Rochester, Minn.	14.6%
7	Rusk Rehabilitation at NYU Langone Hospitals, New York	13.7%
8	Craig Hospital, Englewood, Colo.	12.5%
9	Shepherd Center, Atlanta	11.6%
10	MossRehab, Elkins Park, Pa.	7.2%
11	New York-Presbyterian Hospital-Columbia and Cornell, N.Y.	6.4%
12	UPMC Presbyterian Shadyside, Pittsburgh	6.3%
13	Magee Rehabilitation Hospital-Jefferson Health, Philadelphia	5.3%

RHEUMATOLOGY

Rank	Hospital	% of specialists recommending hospital
1	Johns Hopkins Hospital, Baltimore	40.2%
2	Cleveland Clinic	39.6%
3	Hosp. for Special Surgery, New York-Presbyterian Hosp., N.Y.	37.1%
4	Mayo Clinic, Rochester, Minn.	33.8%
5	Brigham and Women's Hospital, Boston	24.1%
6	Massachusetts General Hospital, Boston	15.1%
7	UCSF Medical Center, San Francisco	15.0%
8	UCLA Medical Center, Los Angeles	14.5%
9	NYU Langone Orthopedic Hospital, New York	13.9%
10	University of Alabama at Birmingham Hospital	9.8%
11	U. of Michigan Hospitals-Michigan Medicine, Ann Arbor	7.8%
12	Duke University Hospital, Durham, N.C.	6.5%
13	UPMC Presbyterian Shadyside, Pittsburgh	6.0%

More @ usnews.com/besthospitals

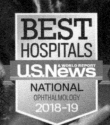

From pupils to pioneers.

Empathic doctors. Innovators in ophthalmology. It's easy to see why America's ophthalmologists named us the nation's #1 residency program.* And as one of the very best in eye care according to *U.S. News & World Report*, sharing our knowledge is more than an honor—it's a responsibility.

*Doximity 2018-2019 clinical reputation survey

WillsEye Hospital | Believing is Seeing

willseye.org
877.289.4557
840 Walnut Street
Philadelphia, PA 19107

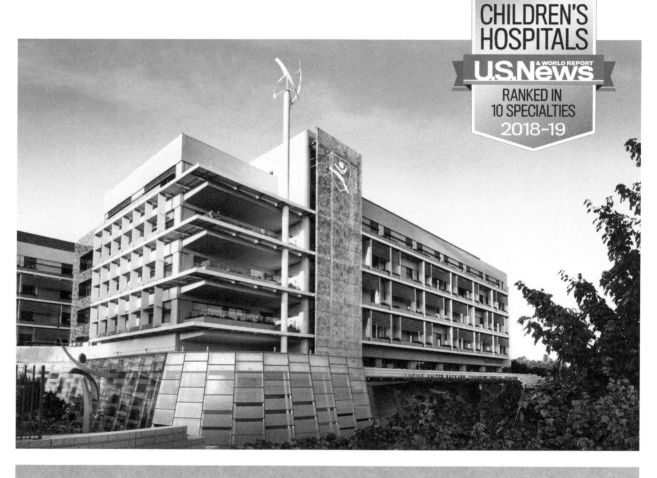
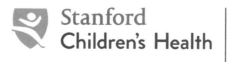

CHAPTER 4

144

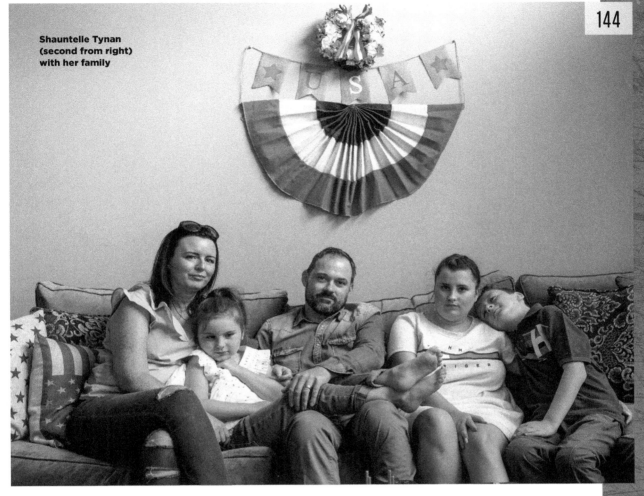

Shauntelle Tynan
(second from right)
with her family

Children's
Health

Getting Kids Help in Time

Rising rates of mental health and behavioral issues are prompting worry – and action

by **Lindsay Cates**

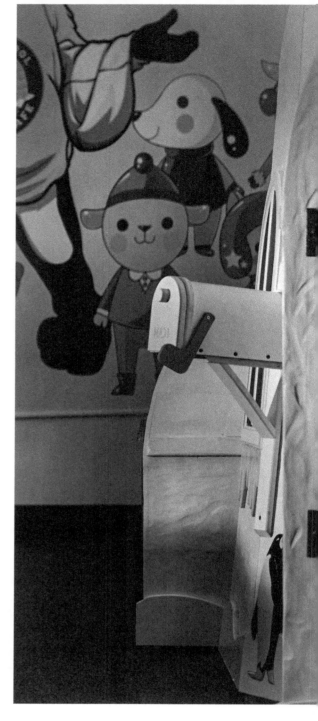

Three-year-old Nasiah was hitting other kids and doing nothing the teacher asked, says his mother, Shannon, who requested their last names remain private. His aggressive outbursts continued in kindergarten, where he showed little improvement even after working with school behavioral aides. Frustrated, Shannon sometimes wondered if she should "give up" on seeking help. She blamed herself, thinking: "What am I doing wrong?" When Nasiah's behavior continued to decline, school staff recommended he switch to nearby Edgewood Primary School, where students needing help with mental health and behavioral issues could access a special on-site program run by the University of Pittsburgh Medical Center's Western Psychiatric Institute and Clinic in partnership with the Pittsburgh Penguins Foundation.

Now, every morning before the school day starts, a trained C.O.O.L. Zone (short for "children overcoming obstacles and limits") therapist checks in with Nasiah, who attends weekly sessions in the program's dedicated therapeutic room – complete with an igloo-shaped playhouse – to learn coping skills. Diagnosed with attention deficit hyperactivity disorder, Nasiah, now age 7, can retreat to the igloo when he gets upset, pull out some play dough, and calm himself down. If an incident occurs beyond the C.O.O.L. Zone classroom, a trained pro is there to help. "They found things that worked for him," Shannon says. Today, he can go months without incident.

Launched as part of an effort to expand UPMC's psychiatric

services to more kids, the program additionally aims to help equip schools with integrated, full-service behavioral health teams. It's also an example of how health systems are responding to a growing problem. "I think every school should have it, and not just in elementary," says Dreahma Marshall, whose son Darius Turner, 8, joined the Edgewood program as a kindergartener when he was having trouble sitting still and would get up and "talk to everybody." When the family moved recently, Marshall was relieved to find a C.O.O.L. Zone at her son's new school.

Nearly 1 in 5 kids in the U.S. experiences a mental, emotional or behavioral disorder like ADHD in a given year. Sometimes the issues are mild and temporary; increasingly they are serious and even

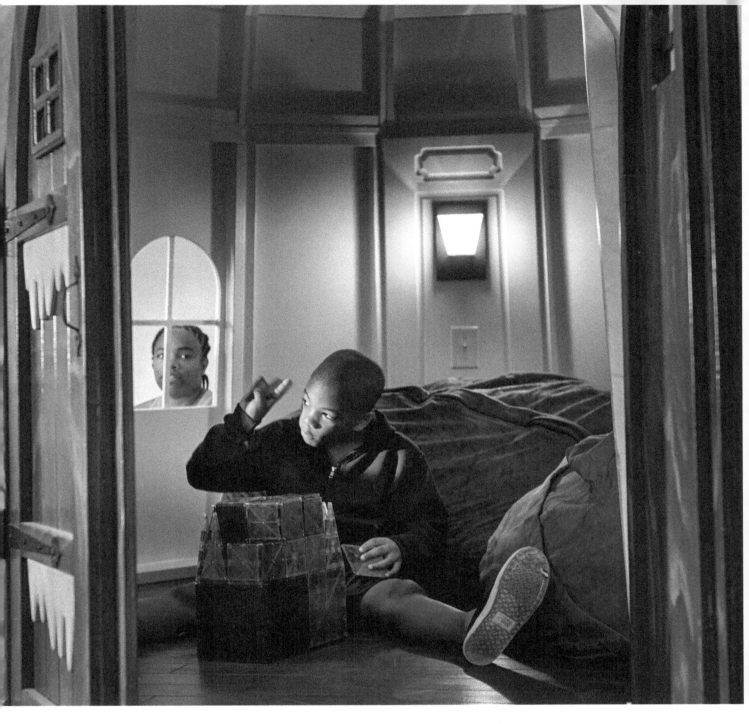

Darius Turner (with his mom at rear), in the "igloo" where kids can calm down during school

life-threatening. Yet regardless of severity, most kids don't receive any specialized treatment. Hospitals are aiming their efforts at early interventions while also scrambling to manage an influx of youth walking through their doors seeking mental and behavioral health care. "It's really a major public health problem," says David Axelson, chief of psychiatry and medical director of behavioral health at Nationwide Children's Hospital in Ohio.

The country's uptick in youth suicides is especially alarming. The number of kids ages 5 to 17 hospitalized for suicidal thoughts or suicide attempts has more than doubled since 2008, according to a recent Vanderbilt-led study analyzing data from 2008 to 2015. And rising rates of anxiety, autism spectrum disorder, and aggression are also worrisome.

A severe shortage of child and adolescent psychiatrists nationwide sometimes means monthslong wait times for families seeking specialty care. According to a recent survey by the American Academy of Child and Adolescent Psychiatry, there is a median of 11 child and adolescent psychiatrists per 100,000 kids across the U.S. Many rural counties have no such specialists. And pediatricians are often ill-equipped to manage mental and behavioral health issues, experts say. In turn, emergency rooms are filling up with kids needing help, and some hospitals are struggling to handle the numbers.

At Monroe Carell Jr. Children's Hospital at Vanderbilt, kids in the ER who need further psychiatric hospitalization often

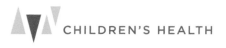

board in medical units for days because no beds are available in Tennessee psychiatric residential treatment facilities. "Eight years ago there was not nearly the same demand," and usually kids could be placed immediately, says Greg Plemmons, associate professor of clinical pediatrics at Vanderbilt University School of Medicine and lead author of the suicide-attempt study. This year, the hospital hired a nurse practitioner and dedicated an additional physician to help treat kids during the holding period, Plemmons says.

At the same time, children's hospitals are working to better train pediatric primary care

> "If a child or adolescent is **on the internet** more than two to three hours per day, that's a possible sign of depression."

providers to diagnose and treat mild cases of anxiety and depression. "The basics of primary care need to be different now," says Abigail Schlesinger, chief of the behavioral science division at UPMC Children's Hospital of Pittsburgh.

Children's Healthcare of Atlanta estimates that 25 percent of its primary care patients have mental and behavioral health concerns. In 2016, it established an educational program for pediatricians, which includes an online resource center, a phone support line staffed by a psychiatrist and psychologist, and a series of training videos on topics like youth depression. And when pediatricians need help, support systems are being put in place. Cincinnati Children's Hospital Medical Center now offers a program where any area physician can connect by phone with a specialist in minutes, with the opportunity for a direct consultation if needed. Pennsylvania's TiPS program, a phone-based psychiatric consultation service that Children's Hospital of Philadelphia helped launch with the state's human services department, assists providers and families as they navigate care and invites any child who can't be assisted by phone to a one-time appointment with a therapist. When Kate tried to get help for her 8-year-old daughter Clara, who'd become so paralyzed by fear after hearing tales of a "3 a.m. curse" that she would scream all night, their pediatrician brushed her off, saying the behavior would resolve when school started. It didn't. After calling back, Kate, who also requested anonymity, was given a list of community resources, including everything from marriage counseling to psychiatric hospitals; none seemed to fit Clara's needs. Discouraged, Kate tried a different pediatrician who suggested she call TiPS.

"I was really upset when I called them, and the TiPS folks were fabulous," Kate says. Her TiPS care coordinator recommended a psychiatrist who finally diagnosed Clara with high anxiety, noting she showed signs of obsessive compulsive behavior. TiPS kept following up to ensure Clara was getting the help she needed. Now, armed with strategies from a counselor who specializes in children's sleep and anxiety, Clara puts her fears into a "worry box" and has a designated "worry time" on days she needs it. She – and the rest of the family – can sleep through the night.

Pediatric primary care offices have also been called upon to step up their screening techniques. The American Academy of Pediatrics recently released new guidelines recommending depression screening for all kids starting at age 12, although experts say screening could begin as early as 6 if there is a concern. UPMC Children's Hospital of Pittsburgh has been working with its pediatricians to better screen for substance abuse. The National Institute of Mental Health classifies addiction to drugs or alcohol as a mental illness, pointing out that many with substance abuse problems also have an underlying mental illness, making treatment for each disorder more difficult. "It's really a pediatric problem just as much as, say, asthma," Schlesinger says.

In addition, training programs teaching the warning signs of mental health problems are popping up for the general public and professionals alike. For example, the Health Department and Community Health Center in Lake County, Illinois, have so far in 2018 held four full-day sessions for adults who work with youth on spotting red flags and getting kids help.

Some children's hospitals are creating spaces designed to manage the array – and severity – of behaviors seen daily. Nationwide Children's Hospital's nine-story Behavioral Health Pavilion, set to open in 2020, will eventually ramp up to include 48 inpatient beds, outpatient services and a psychiatric crisis center on the first floor. A dedicated emergency medical team will be on staff, ready to treat patients with medical complications from overdose attempts or self-harm. And there are plans to include a youth crisis stabilization unit specifically designed for suicidal patients who'd benefit from a short stay, Axelson says. The new pavilion is a huge expansion from Nationwide's current 16-bed inpatient unit and five-bed psychiatric emergency setup in the hospital's general medical emergency room. "There is a lot of overflow and no ability to do extended observation because the

> ❝Something as simple as **blowing bubbles** can help teach steady breathing to young kids.❞

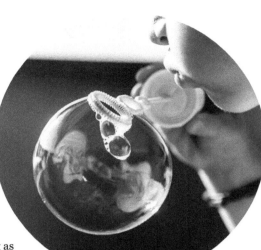

emergency room is overflowing as it is," Axelson says.

Facing similar capacity issues, Rady Children's Hospital in San Diego opted to create a psychiatric emergency center within its existing emergency department, which will open in 2019. The hospital went from seeing about 40 psychiatric emergency patients a month in 2012 to about 400 per month in the busiest months of 2017 and 2018. The new center will be staffed 24/7 with specialists trained in emergency psychiatric response.

Mental and behavioral health conditions are treatable, but finding the right resources can be a battle. Experts share advice for recognizing the warning signs and creating a safe, healthy and happy environment for your kids:

Find a pediatrician you trust. Look for a practice with a trained behavioral therapist, psychologist or psychiatrist on staff. Ensure your child is comfortable communicating with them, Schlesinger says. Allow young children to describe their chief complaint in their own words. By around age 12, kids should have time alone with their pediatrician to share concerns they may not wish to vocalize in front of parents.

Make your home safe. Most suicide attempts stem from firearms or overdoses, physicians say. Talk about gun safety with your children. If you have firearms, lock them away. Similarly, talk about safe use of prescription medications and store those securely.

Monitor screen time. If your child is on the internet more than two to three hours per day, that's a possible sign of depression, Plemmons says. Staying up late on a smartphone cuts into sleep hours and has been shown to increase anxiety. Some experts blame rising rates of youth mental health issues on social media, citing lack of face-to-face interaction compounded by a "fear of missing out"; others view it as a positive place to spread mental health awareness and get help for those whose posts may indicate quiet suffering.

Practice mindfulness. Mindfulness-based cognitive therapy is a proven way to curb sad thoughts. Apps like

Headspace and Happify walk teens through relaxation exercises and breathing techniques, or can target specific things like reducing worry and building relationships. Something as simple as blowing bubbles can help teach steady breathing to young kids, and yoga and meditation classes can help treat anxiety and depression.

Notice the warning signs. If school performance starts to sag or you observe a consistent pattern of sleeplessness, sadness, crying without cause, mood changes or appetite loss, it could be time to seek help. Teens are expected to change a bit, but not so much that you can't stand to be around them, Schlesinger says. In teens, withdrawing from activities they used to enjoy is a sign. Young kids may display more overt and drastic changes, like sudden new sleep habits.

Ask questions. Concerned? Spark a conversation. Many parents think they will plant the idea of suicide in their child by asking about it, but evidence shows that's not the case, Plemmons says. And after you ask, listen. Avoid the temptation to problem-solve.

Get connected with the right help. If there is no emergency, start with your pedia-

> ❝**Yoga and meditation** classes can help treat anxiety and depression.❞

trician or school, if it offers appropriate health services. They can often recommend preliminary strategies, or determine if a psychiatric evaluation is necessary. Already have a trusted psychiatrist or counselor? Go to them first. If there is a concern about immediate safety, get to the nearest emergency facility specializing in psychiatric assessment, even if it means a further drive, Axelson says.

Be persistent. If a certain specialist or strategy isn't working, don't hesitate to try something different or ask for more help, says Michael Sorter, director of the division of child and adolescent psychiatry at Cincinnati Children's. "A lot of times the squeaky wheel gets the grease." ●

On the Path to a Healthy Weight

Parents have a huge role to play in battling childhood obesity

by **Stacey Colino**

t's no secret: The U.S. is in the grip of a childhood obesity epidemic. While some reports have suggested that rates have stabilized, a February 2018 study in Pediatrics found no such plateau. In fact, the data for kids ages 2 to 19 from 1999 to 2016 revealed increases in obesity at all ages and a sharp uptick in severe obesity among those ages 2 to 5 and girls 16 to 19.

Far more than a cosmetic issue, obesity has been linked to an increased risk of just about every disease in the book, including Type 2 diabetes, heart disease, asthma, gastroesophageal reflux, sleep apnea, joint problems, fatty liver disease and gallstones. "For parents, it's not that hard to envision the long-term health risks associated with [a child's] obesity and the limitations on what a child can do because of the extra weight," says Meagan O'Neill, a pediatrician at Riley Children's Health in Indiana.

Meanwhile, the body positivity movement has been gaining momentum across the country, pumping out a steady drumbeat of messaging that promotes acceptance of different sizes and shapes and helps people feel comfortable in their skin regardless of weight. These are worthy goals, experts say, yet they may seem out of sync with efforts to curb obesity. Indeed, encouraging kids to achieve and

maintain a healthy weight – without triggering body insecurities – can feel like a delicate balancing act for parents. But if the right strategies are used, experts say kids can shed excess pounds and improve their health, energy, well-being and self-esteem. "We encourage a big focus on changing behaviors – those are things parents and kids have control over," says Brian Saelens, a child health psychologist and professor of pediatrics at the Seattle Children's Research Institute and the University of Washington.

Various innovative hospital-affiliated programs are helping kids adopt healthy habits. For example, researchers from Massachusetts General Hospital have introduced a one-hour before-school physical activity program called Build Our Kids' Success, or BOKS, in 24 schools; after 12 weeks, kids who participated three times a week saw improvements in their BMI as well as in their interest in schoolwork. Twice-weekly participants saw significant boosts to mood, vitality and energy.

At Seattle Children's, a program called Success in Health: Impacting Families Together, or SHIFT, has been convening parents and kids for weekly sessions that teach healthy eating and physical activity behaviors. In 2016, Heather Armstrong, 44, and her daughter Lauren, 11, joined

the five-month program because both had been struggling with their weight. By keeping a food journal and having weekly meetings with a counselor, "we really began to notice patterns between what we ate, how much physical activity we got, and our weight," says Armstrong, a teacher who lost 12 pounds on the program while her daughter lost 8. Armstrong was so impressed that she has volunteered as a peer counselor.

Even if your kids don't have access to such a program, they can still reap benefits from the lessons imparted. Here's how experts suggest fostering healthy habits in your kids, while promoting body positivity:

Banish negative body talk. Strike words like "fat" and "chubby" from your vocabulary. Making critical comments about your child's body or your own as a motivation tactic is "counterproductive," says Elsie Taveras, who co-authored the BOKS study and is chief of the division of general academic pediatrics at Mass General and a professor of pediatrics at Harvard Medical School. "It's almost a form of bullying. Some language that may be thought of as endearing can be demeaning and hurtful – 'my big girl' or references to love handles or baby fat."

Instead, adopt a family policy nixing the practice of commenting on the shape of people's bodies. "Body shaming creates more negative emotions and diminishes self-esteem, and many times children will turn to food to cope," says Kevin C. Sloan, psychology department supervisor for the division of nutrition and preventive medicine at Beaumont Health in Royal Oak, Michigan.

Meanwhile, make an effort to promote a positive body image from the inside out. As a family, adopt a vocabulary that focuses primarily on how bodies feel and function. "Body image is competency-based – it's about 'this is what my body can do for me,'" Saelens says. "Encourage kids to think about what their body can do, rather than how it looks." As a parent, you can model this behavior by commenting on how strong your legs felt while you were running or that you felt like a superhero when you hoisted your carry-on bag into the overhead bin.

Describe food as fuel. Draw a parallel between a high-performance car and your child's body by discussing the importance of putting the right amount of high-octane fuel (food) into the tank and giving the engine proper maintenance with regular physical activity. That analogy sets you up to educate about "what types of foods we should be eating to enhance performance," says Kristi King, spokesperson for the Academy of Nutri-

tion and Dietetics and a senior pediatric dietitian at Texas Children's Hospital in Houston. "Come up with a family definition of healthy foods," she advises, and shop accordingly. It helps to distinguish between high-octane fuel (fruits, vegetables, whole grains, dairy, nuts and seeds, and lean proteins) and once-in-a-while foods like chips and cookies. "Don't criminalize certain foods or make restricted foods rewards," Taveras says. Doing so could lead kids to sneak, hoard or binge on forbidden items.

Promote the perks of healthier habits. When working with an overweight child, registered dietitian Sandra Arevalo, director of nutrition services and community outreach at Community Pediatrics, a program at Montefiore Medical Center in New York, will often say things like, "Wouldn't you like to be able to run faster, breathe easier or be less tired in P.E. class?" The response? "They say yes! That opens the door for them to focus on the health benefits of changing their behavior," she says. Parents can initiate similar conversations with their kids.

Lead the way. "You are your child's first example for how to live a healthy life and take care of your body," O'Neill says. "If you're concerned about your child's weight, you have to change your eating and activity patterns, too." Con-

sider changes you can make together, whether it's ditching sugar-sweetened beverages or avoiding fast food. And aim to have at least one family meal each day, King advises. "Focus on getting back to basics: planning meals and snacks and doing prep work with kids, so they have healthy foods like fruit, vegetables, nuts and seeds ready to grab when they're on the go." According to a recent study, for kids ages 2 to 5, snacking eats up 28 percent of total calorie intake. And snack times account for 47 percent of beverages consumed per day. So it's important to make snacking count nutritionally.

Make movement a family affair. Set a weekly physical-activity goal, O'Neill suggests. This could include family walks, bike rides, games of soccer or Frisbee, or anything else your kids like. If they're into video games, find one that's dance-based or involves some other movement-oriented activity everyone can enjoy. To get families exercising together, Riley Children's Health has teamed up with The Children's Museum of Indianapolis to open a center offering 12 outdoor and three indoor interactive sports experiences and physical activity exhibits, including soccer, basketball and tennis. Look for similar facilities near you.

Beyond the family time, it helps if

kids can make physical activity part of the school routine, Taveras says.

"We have to look for ways to increase physical activity in places where kids spend their time," she says. UCLA Health's Sound Body Sound Mind program, for example, has installed state-of-the-art fitness centers – with weight machines, Spin bikes, cardio machines, agility ladders, a variety of resistance-training equipment and circuit-based exercise templates – in 141 middle and high schools, mostly in the Los Angeles area.

"We want to see this generation of kids who have been plagued by the childhood obesity epidemic and the physical inactivity epidemic take personal ownership over their fitness journeys," says Matthew Flesock, executive director of the program. Before the curriculum was offered in 12 schools that received fitness centers during the 2016-17 academic year, only 38 percent of those students passed California's state-mandated fitness test; after eight weeks on the program, 57 percent of those students passed. The program "has affected how I eat – it makes me not want to eat as much junk food as I used to; it makes me want to take care of my body more and

> The **body positivity movement** has been gaining momentum across the country, pumping out a steady drumbeat of messaging that promotes acceptance of different sizes and shapes and helps people feel comfortable in their skin regardless of weight.

Original Barbie has been joined by a "curvy" version.

stay healthy," says Byron Ruvalcaba, 16, a junior at Benjamin Franklin High School in Highland Park, California.

Give kudos for their efforts. Rather than focusing on results of the changes your child is making, "give positive feedback about how hard they're trying," O'Neill says. "Even teenagers are desperate for positive affirmation from their parents." Remember: Sometimes the goal isn't so much to see the numbers on the scale drop but to either stop rapid weight gain as kids grow or hold their weight steady so their height can catch up, Saelens notes. Meantime, focusing on the good care they're taking of their bodies will help strengthen their resolve.

Stay on top of social media. Numerous studies report potentially strong negative associations between social media exposure and kids' body image. But 2017 research found that positive parental influence and a supportive school environment go a long way toward mitigating harmful effects among girls ages 12 to 14. So talk openly with your kids about what they're seeing on their feeds. "Ask them who their friends are on social media and whether they've experienced negative encounters or comments that bothered them," Sloan advises.

If they have, discuss these issues and help your kids put them into perspective, perhaps by emphasizing their positive qualities to help them view body type as just one component of their makeup. Also, encourage kids to "engage in social networks that are going to be helpful and self-affirming, such as groups that cater toward artistic or musical interests if that appeals to your child," Sloan suggests.

If diet changes and fitness programs don't sufficiently help an obese teen shed excess weight, bariatric surgery, particularly sleeve gastrectomy (in which the stomach is surgically reduced to about a quarter of its original size), may be an option. This is especially true if the teen has Type 2 diabetes, sleep apnea or severe fatty liver disease. Even then, the focus is on improving health, rather than looks. "I talk about the surgery as a means to better health and longevity," says Thomas Inge, director of pediatric surgery and adolescent bariatric surgery at Children's Hospital Colorado and a professor of surgery and pediatrics at the University of Colorado–Denver. "For kids and teenagers, weight is a really big deal in terms of their quality of life. It affects their family and peer relationships, physical and mental health, their self-esteem and social competence. When they come back to see me a month or two after the surgery, there are often tears of joy in their eyes." •

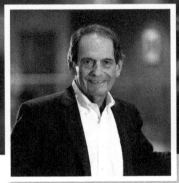

DELIVERING HOPE THROUGH GENE THERAPY

Jerry R. Mendell, MD

Children with devastating neuromuscular disorders are finding hope through precise gene-based therapies.

A case in point: Dr. Jerry Mendell's gene replacement therapy for spinal muscular atrophy type 1, a progressive muscle-weakening disease that typically results in death by age 2.

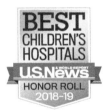

The SMA gene therapy, developed at Nationwide Children's, harnesses the ability of a viral vector to deliver missing genetic material to a cell. Results from the Phase 1 clinical trial show infants with SMA Type 1 reaching milestones and living longer than ever seen in the natural progression of the disease.

Learn more about this 2017 Science Breakthrough of the Year at NationwideChildrens.org/specialties/spinal-muscular-atrophy-clinic.

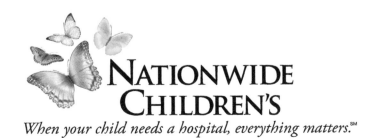

When your child needs a hospital, everything matters.^{SM}

W25416

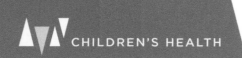
A Long Journey to Health

How six kids with serious medical challenges are receiving cutting-edge care and beating the odds

Courage. Grit. And a big dose of personality. That's what these kids are made of. Each has faced a life-altering health issue, at times when those around them are experiencing their first heartbeat, learning long division, going to prom. While they hail from different parts of the country, and globe, these youngsters are united by a dogged drive to survive and supported by families who have been relentless in getting them to the best treatments available. All were patients at a pediatric center that earned a spot on the 2018-19 U.S. News Best Children's Hospitals Honor Roll. Here are their stories.

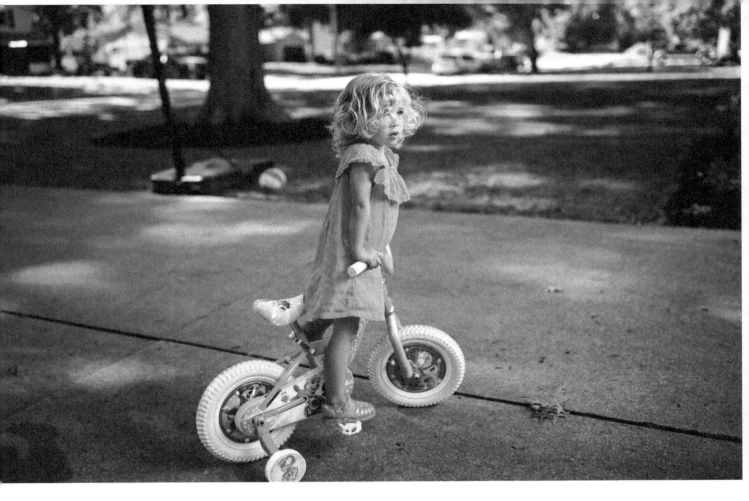

Maeve Seabold • 3 years old

About halfway through their second pregnancy, Kelly and Dan Seabold, both in their 30s, headed to their ultrasound appointment with confidence. As experienced nurses and parents of twin boys, they knew what to expect. Or so they thought. When the ultrasound technician spotted a mass protruding from the base of their baby's spine, everything changed. The doctor diagnosed it as a sacrococcygeal teratoma or SCT. The rare tumor develops in the womb, occurring in 1 out of every 35,000 to 40,000 live births. At only 21 weeks gestation, their daughter Maeve was growing, but so was her tumor. And it was hoarding the blood flow and nutrients she needed, putting strain on her tiny heart.

Kelly and Dan immediately set to work researching Maeve's condition. They combed through medical journals, noting that most of the relevant articles were authored by researchers at Children's Hospital of Philadelphia. "I was scared," Kelly says. "I could look at the journals and the outcomes and see that, you know, babies with vascular SCTs don't do well." So they asked to be referred to CHOP. The couple placed their sons in the protection of close family. Then, they traveled from their Avon Lake, Ohio, home to Pennsylvania. After an exhaustive day of tests, Kelly and Dan learned that the noncancerous teratoma, now the size of a rutabaga, had caused a dangerous buildup of fluid that was putting Maeve at high risk of heart failure. Kelly's health was deteriorating, too. The fluid buildup endangering Maeve was also settling around her mother's heart

Her Challenge:
A rare tumor

Hospital:
Children's Hospital of Philadelphia

Fun Fact:
Loves licking cookie batter from the spatula

and soon, Kelly was experiencing signs of maternal mirror syndrome, a rare condition that can occur in high-risk fetal diagnoses, causing the mother to develop symptoms that mimic the baby's.

Joined by a team of experts, Scott Adzick, CHOP's surgeon in chief and a leader in fetal surgery for SCT, presented the couple with their options, which were limited. Do nothing, and Maeve could die in the womb. Or undergo emergency fetal surgery the next day to remove the tumor, and face the possibility of a premature delivery. If the tumor ruptured before surgeons could reach it, Maeve also might not make it. The procedure, he explained, would involve making an incision in the uterus to reach Maeve, removing the external portion of her tumor, and then returning Maeve to the womb for the rest of the pregnancy. After birth, Maeve would need a second surgery to extract the internal portion of the teratoma. Kelly and Dan opted for surgery to give Maeve the best chance.

When Adzick began to operate, he discovered a worst-case-scenario complication: Maeve's tumor had ruptured overnight. The surgical team worked quickly to prevent Maeve from bleeding out and to remove the teratoma, which was slightly bigger than Maeve. Her heart stopped three times during the procedure, but Adzick carefully administered CPR with his index finger and was able to stabilize Maeve before returning her to the womb. "I had to use virtually every trick, every fetal surgery trick I've ever learned in doing this over 30 years for this particular case," Adzick says.

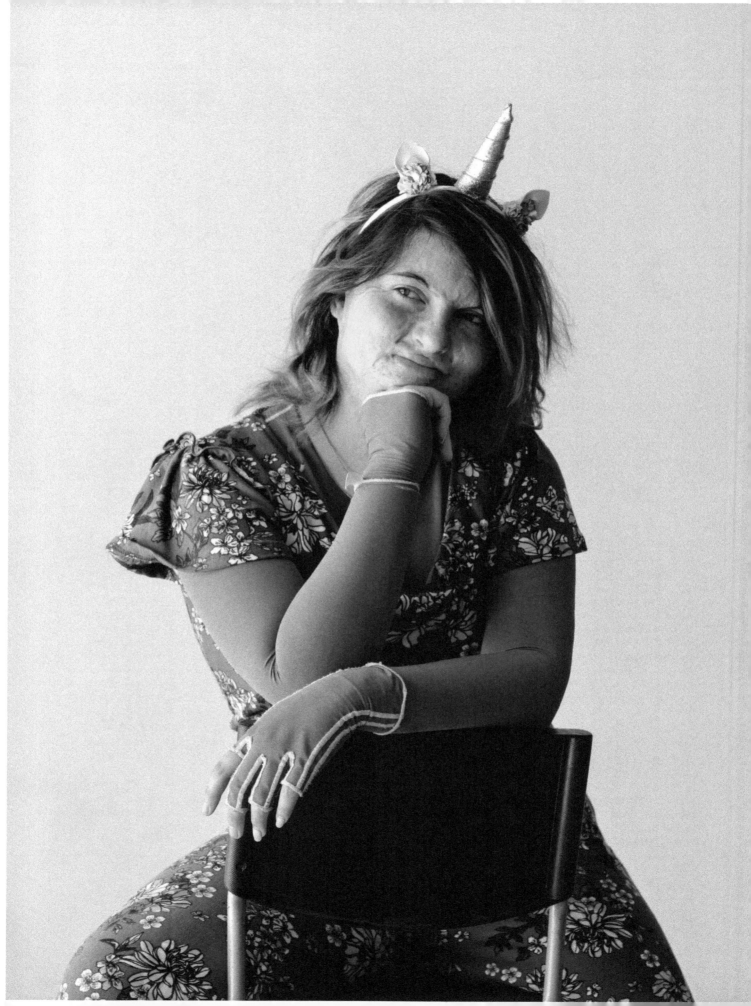

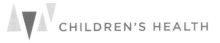
Hours later, the ultrasound showed that Maeve's heart was functioning normally. She was already healing, and Kelly's mirror syndrome resolved. "It was really amazing," Dan says. "It started to seem real that we were going to have success." Because the tumor was so large, necessitating a significant incision in Kelly's uterus, Kelly was at risk of preterm labor. So the couple stayed at CHOP to be monitored for the rest of the pregnancy. Their family brought their twin sons to visit, but the extended separation and the stress of Maeve's ordeal weighed heavily on them. Maeve's steady improvement gave them hope.

Julie Moldenhauer, a member of the team and medical director of the Garbose Family Special Delivery Unit, oversaw their recovery. To avoid additional complications, she delivered Maeve prematurely by cesarean section at 32 weeks. Maeve came into the world screaming and full of life. In the neonatal intensive care unit, she continued to show the same resilience. Shortly thereafter, Adzick removed the internal portion of her tumor, ensuring nothing was left behind (important, since it's possible for these tumors to regrow and become cancerous if not completely excised) and worked to reconstruct her backside. After about six weeks, Maeve healed enough to leave intensive care and go home.

Today, the little girl's enthusiasm is infectious. A happy, healthy toddler, Maeve enjoys roller coasters and chasing after her older brothers. And she's completely tumor-free. –*Ann Claire Carnahan*

Trinity Larson • 14 years old

Life can change in a second – sometimes with just a shift in the wind. Trinity learned that painful lesson in 2017, when at age 12, she was huddling with friends around a bonfire in the mountain town of Granby, Colorado. When a flammable mixture was shaken onto the fire, Trinity was accidentally splattered. As flames burst and the breeze picked up, she was engulfed.

She was airlifted to Children's Hospital Colorado in Aurora, the state's only pediatric burn center. Kim Wiebers, her mother, was upwards of 30 miles away when she got the call. She rushed to the hospital, where she anxiously waited for Trinity to arrive. "It was the hardest thing to see," she recalls. Her energetic, fun-loving daughter lay helpless, with burns on her face, ears, neck, left arm, left side, right arm, stomach and thighs. Thankfully, her eyes and throat escaped harm.

Along with "full-thickness" burns that destroyed both skin layers covering 25 percent of her body, Trinity suffered damage to her lungs from smoke inhalation and was placed on a ventilator.

She underwent a series of skin grafts over the next few weeks, making multiple trips to the operating room, says Steve Moulton, director of the pediatric trauma and burn programs at CHC. "Obviously, her burn injuries were very painful. They're disfiguring. She's required a fair amount of laser therapy and steroid injections to deal with the scarring." She has undergone 13 operations so far. "It takes a couple of years to get the end result," Moulton says. "It's a process."

Trinity doesn't remember much about her month in intensive care, where she required heavy medication. "I slept a lot because of the drugs," she says. "I dreamed I was in Hawaii the whole time."

Next, she moved to the burn recovery unit. That was more difficult in some ways as she became aware of pain. "People were making me move, sitting up and standing, to get me better," she says. "But it hurt my back, because I was lying in bed for so long." Still, she worked hard to recover. Child life specialists helped her feel more like a kid and less like a patient. She played games, colored and took up quilting. Almost two months to the day after the accident, she was finally discharged.

Her Challenge:
Burn survivor

Hospital:
Children's Hospital Colorado

Fun Fact:
Rocks out to Panic! at the Disco

Helping patients like Trinity recover from such extensive injuries requires coordinated care. "You've got ICU doctors helping to manage the ventilator," Moulton says. "You've got pulmonary doctors who can insert a scope down the airway and help suck out all the soot. You have a burn surgeon and a plastic surgeon. You have therapists, including physical and occupational therapists, who deal with the burns and eventual scars of the legs, arms, hands and face."

Pediatric nurses and nutritionists with burn expertise closely monitor and provide daily care for these kids.

Burn psychologist Brad Jackson has helped Trinity address the significant emotional toll. Severe, disfiguring burns can be "devastating" for young patients, Moulton says, adding: "She's actually done exceptionally well." Burn camps offered by the hospital and directed by pediatric occupational therapist Trudy Boulter let kids like Trinity have fun outdoors and meet other burn survivors. "The idea is to help them understand that their burn does not define them," Moulton says.

Trinity doesn't dwell on the circumstances of her injury. "She's got such a good heart about the whole situation," Wiebers says. "When she was ready to talk about it, she said, 'Mom, I'm not mad. It was an accident – it's not anybody's fault.'"

She wears soft, stretchy pressure garments and custom masks to help her burns heal. She wears a clear mask in public. Sometimes, she and her mother disagree over just how long she needs to keep it on (the goal: at least six hours daily). As an active girl, she would rather ditch the mask and just hang out with her friends or her little sister. "The mask gets hot," Trinity says. "Moisture builds up, and it's itchy." Wearing it in public can make her self-conscious. "People never used to stare directly at me before," she says. "But now they stare when I wear my mask or garments, and it makes me feel a little weird." Even so, that doesn't stop her from speaking up and telling her story when asked to at school or public events.

Trinity is grateful for all the care she's received. What helps her the most? "All the support I get from family and friends," she says. "Just that they're there and showing me they care and encouraging me to do this." –*Lisa Esposito*

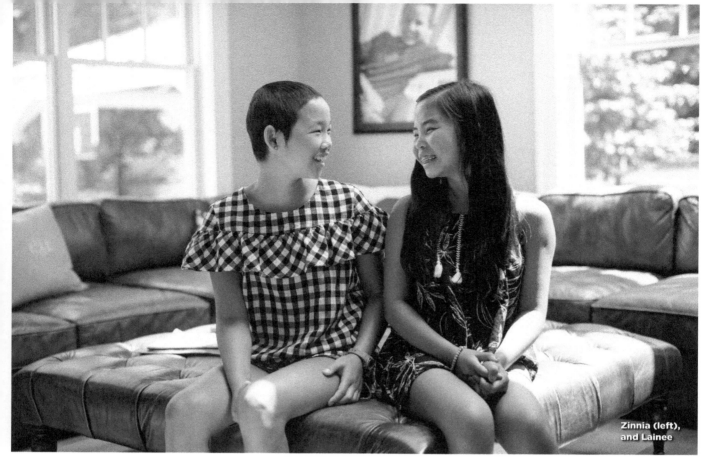

Zinnia (left), and Lainee

Zinnia and Lainee Jones • 13 and 12 years old

Lainee and Zinnia Jones are not related by blood, but they are united by it. In 2011, the best friends became sisters when they were both adopted from an orphanage in China by Laura and Chris Jones of Wheaton, Illinois. Before bringing them home, Mom and Dad also learned that both girls have beta thalassemia, a genetic blood disorder that prevents them from producing enough hemoglobin, a protein in red blood cells that moves oxygen through the body. About 100,000 children worldwide are born each year with severe forms of the condition, according to the National Human Genome Research Institute, and they suffer from fatigue, anemia and often other deeper issues, such as organ damage and bone deformities.

For Lainee and Zinnia, managing thalassemia has meant blood transfusions every two to three weeks to cycle in healthy, hemoglobin-rich blood, plus chelation medications to prevent iron buildup in their bodies (a side effect of the transfusions). The transfusions help curb the girls' frequent exhaustion, but they also carry risks of future liver and heart damage from iron overload. Plus, "it just really runs our lives," Laura says. "Every vacation, every school event, we just always have to think, 'What about blood? Where are you going to get blood?'"

The girls' treatment plan was developed at Ann and Robert H. Lurie Children's Hospital of Chicago, which has a comprehensive thalassemia program that is the largest in the Midwest. About three years ago, Alexis Thompson, the girls' doctor and the director of that program, told the family about an emerging gene therapy called LentiGlobin that had been showing promise for

Their Challenge: A genetic blood disorder

Hospital: Ann and Robert H. Lurie Children's Hospital of Chicago

Fun Fact: They have six siblings

people with thalassemia in clinical trials. Doctors harvest stem cells from the blood of a person with thalassemia and introduce a functional version of the gene that produces hemoglobin before returning it to the patient (related story, Page 20). "In an ideal world, you'd love to fix only what's broken," says Thompson, hematology section head and chair for childhood cancer and blood disorders at Lurie Children's. This targeted gene therapy allows for a laser-focused approach, giving clinicians the ability "to just take the single gene that's abnormal and to add the capacity to then make a protein that previously the patients lacked," Thompson says. She was lead author of an analysis of two trials, published in April 2018 in the New England Journal of Medicine, in which 22 patients ages 12 to 35 with transfusion-dependent beta thalassemia received the therapy. After a median span of about two years, 15 of them no longer needed transfusions, and others required them much less often. "It really is a real fundamental advancement for the future for children," Thompson says. The next phase of trials is enrolling kids as young as 5.

In May of 2017, the family learned that Zinnia had been accepted into a clinical trial. Doctors collected her stem cells over several days. Those cells were then sent to a lab where researchers introduced the targeted LentiGlobin, thereby inserting the healthy gene.

Zinnia returned to the hospital in early 2018, where she was given chemotherapy to prepare her body to accept the new cells. Doctors infused the modified stem cells back into her body, and she spent about seven weeks in the hospital healing. Zinnia had

Best Children's Hospital
9 years in a row

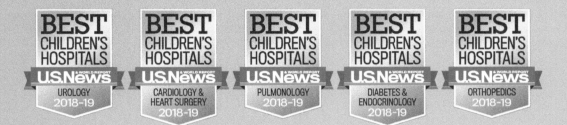

For the ninth year in a row, Orlando Health Arnold Palmer Hospital for Children has been recognized as a "Best Children's Hospital," as ranked by *U.S. News & World Report*. When it comes to the best care for your kids, choose a national leader, that's right in your own backyard.

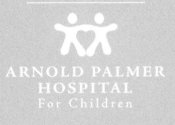

ORLANDO
HEALTH®

ARNOLD PALMER
HOSPITAL
For Children

Healthier *Kids,*
Stronger *Families.*

ArnoldPalmerHospital.com

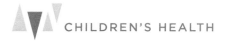

CHILDREN'S HEALTH

her last blood transfusion in February. Her hemoglobin levels have been normal ever since. "I'm doing great," she says. "I'm just loving it because I don't have to go back to the hospital every two weeks, and I have energy." Because the chemotherapy and prep for the stem cell transplant can impact fertility, Zinnia and her parents also elected to have Lurie Children's doctors remove one of her ovaries and preserve it in case she wants to have kids of her own someday.

Lainee, who has a slightly different genetic subtype of thalassemia that has also responded well to the gene therapy, is hoping to receive the treatment soon – once iron levels in her liver come down and doctors determine that the organ is healthy enough. For Zinnia, "it was the hardest thing she's ever gone through," Laura says, but "she has a new sense of freedom, I think, that she's never felt before." *–Michael Morella*

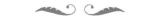

Justin Hittle • 16 years old

magine the odds of being struck by lightning while walking from your car to your front door. That's about as unlikely a scenario as what happened to Justin Hittle in 2017, says Johns Hopkins pediatric surgeon Eric Jelin. While playing lacrosse with friends during an impromptu practice session in the backyard, Justin, then 15, was struck by the ball in the chest, causing his heart to stop. He collapsed and wasn't breathing. His panicked sister reached their dad and a friend called 911. Two neighbors rushed over to administer CPR until paramedics arrived eight minutes later. Justin was raced to Johns Hopkins Bayview Medical Center, where he was stabilized, placed on a ventilator and had chest tubes inserted to prevent a collapsed lung. He underwent various tests, which revealed the diagnosis: commotio cordis – a rare and often deadly change to a heart's rhythm following chest trauma.

The condition occurs when a "very specific part of the heart is struck with a particular kind of object at a particular speed," says Jelin, the physician who was on-call at the time of the accident and who, along with a team of experts, treated Justin at the Johns Hopkins Children's Center, where he was transferred and stayed for 10 days. When the ball hit Justin, his cardiac cycle was immediately disrupted. It made impact during the precise window of time – a matter of milliseconds – when his heart was susceptible. According to the American Heart Association, only about 10 to 20 cases of commotio cordis are reported annually, typically in baseball, hockey and lacrosse players. A national commotio cordis registry was not established until the mid-1990s, and information about the condition is still being discovered. While CPR helped save Justin's life, it also caused damage to his lungs, creating new complications.

His Challenge:
Freak accident

Hospital:
Johns Hopkins
Children's Center

Fun Fact: He's a
skateboarding ace

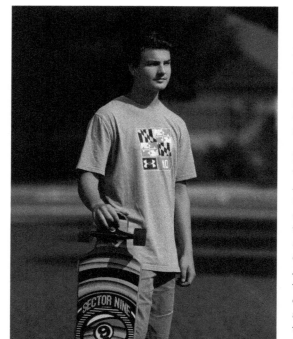

At Hopkins, Justin was given medication to help his heart pump blood more efficiently. Requiring maximum support to survive, he was monitored constantly. Doctors struggled to raise his oxygen levels. As a result of the trauma, Justin developed acute respiratory distress syndrome, a life-threatening complication that inhibited his breathing.

His prognosis was grim. "When we came to see him at the hospital initially, he was unconscious – he looked bad," his mother, Stacey, recalls. She was especially worried about Justin's brain because he had gone so long without oxygen in the yard. But her outlook brightened with a simple gesture. "I said something to him, and he looked at me and squeezed my hand," Stacey says.

Within a week, he was walking hospital halls and throwing a ball while standing on a balance board. A year later, Justin appears to have made a full recovery, though Jelin can't rule out the possibility of future complications. "Not a huge amount is known about recurrence of this sort of thing," Jelin says. Justin can no longer play lacrosse, which he took up at age 5. Actually, cardiologists have advised him to avoid any sport with a ball, due to the "worry of it happening again," Justin says. (Commercially available protection equipment isn't strong enough to prevent a potential repeat incident, Jelin adds.)

Justin spends his time in other ways. An honors student, he loves skateboarding and snowboarding. The family credits his rapid recovery to his strength, the expert care he received at Hopkins, and to their quick-thinking neighbors who did CPR – without which Justin may have died in the yard. To pay it forward, the Hittles have led a CPR training session for the community. That he has "no residual problems whatsoever," Stacey says, is "pretty amazing." *–Alison Murtagh*

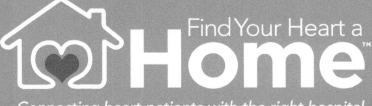

Find Your Heart a **Home**™

Connecting heart patients with the right hospital

Q | Is Your Heart In The Right Hands?

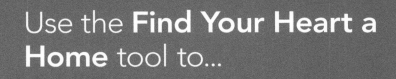
Use the **Find Your Heart a Home** tool to...

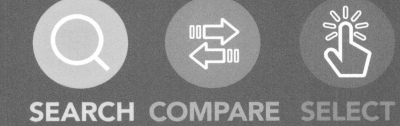

SEARCH   **COMPARE**   **SELECT**

...the **right hospital** for you or a loved one.

Get Started at *FindYourHeartaHome.org*

Powered by ACC's NCDR® and CardioSmart®

AMERICAN COLLEGE *of* CARDIOLOGY

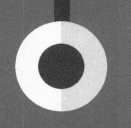

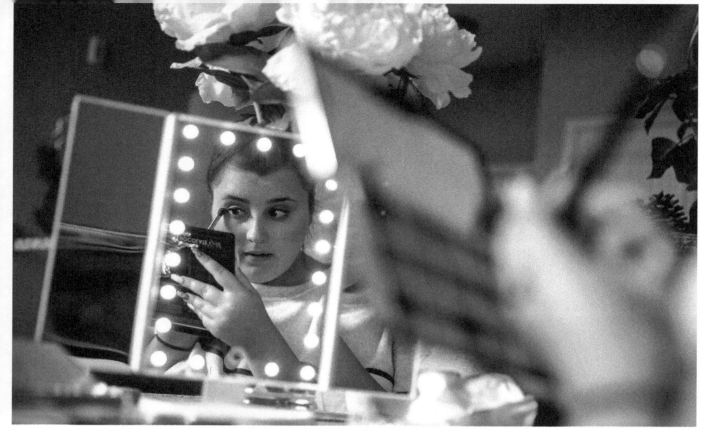

Shauntelle Tynan • 20 years old

Shauntelle Tynan had to travel more than 4,000 miles, from her home in Ireland to Houston, Texas, to get the right treatment for a rare blood cancer – undiagnosed since childhood. She had always been sickly: She suffered more than 100 ear infections that failed to respond to antibiotics. By age 12, she endured bouts of diarrhea and serious rashes, and was so parched that she'd drink about 6 gallons of water daily. Tests showed she didn't have diabetes, so a psychologist attributed her excessive thirst to anxiety.

Her symptoms worsened. By May 2015, when Shauntelle was 16, she was battling severe, ulcerated rashes that local doctors thought stemmed from a serious infection – but again, tests were negative. "I was constantly back and forth with the doctors, and they acted like we were crazy," says her mother, Leona.

Finally, the culprit was uncovered: Langerhans cell histiocytosis, or LCH, a cancer that strikes perhaps a dozen Irish children in a given year and affects about 600 Americans annually, experts say. The disease is caused by the overproduction of Langerhans cells, a type of white blood cell that fights infection but can form tumors or damage the liver, spleen, bone marrow and other organ systems. In Shauntelle's case, the cancer had invaded her pituitary gland, skin and gastrointestinal tract, explaining her mix of seemingly unrelated symptoms.

Even with a diagnosis, local doctors were stumped. Desperate, Leona scoured the internet until she found a leading expert in LCH, Kenneth McClain, clinical director of the histiocytosis program at Texas Children's Cancer and Hematology Centers. One morning, around 2 a.m., she fired off an email to McClain. "I didn't expect he would actually answer," Leona recalls. Forty min-

Her Challenge:
Rare blood cancer

Hospital:
Texas Children's Hospital in Houston

Fun Fact: Enjoys filming makeup tutorials

utes later, he responded. Within weeks, Mom and daughter were headed to see him. Throughout that summer and fall, McClain advised her doctors in Ireland on the initial treatment (various chemotherapies), and Shauntelle and her mom shuttled back and forth to Houston to be seen. The Tynans held fundraisers for the trips. But the teen continued to deteriorate. Worried Shauntelle's cancer would get to a stage of no return, McClain decided she needed to be in Houston full time. There, she could participate in a clinical trial for a promising chemotherapy called clofarabine, shown effective for patients who don't respond to other treatments, he says. But there was a huge catch. Shauntelle's insurance wouldn't cover care in Texas – and the price tag was more than $500,000. "It was a nightmare," Leona says. Help came from an unexpected source. Shauntelle regularly posted Facebook videos about her cancer fight to comfort other teens battling rare malignancies. When she heard about the hospital bill, she shared an emotional video explaining that going to Houston was her "last chance." The video went viral. Within 48 hours, Shauntelle had raised more than $694,000. In February 2017, Mom and daughter headed back to Houston, where they live in an apartment that an Irish charitable foundation paid for through the first year.

Shauntelle is improving and looks forward to returning home in October. "Everything seems to be clearing up," she says. McClain will closely monitor her for the next couple of years, and she will remain on oral chemo for at least a year. Once in Ireland, she plans to start college, although she's changed her major. "I'm abandoning medicine because I don't want to be in a hospital for the rest of my life," she says. "Now I'm leaning towards the law." –Linda Marsa

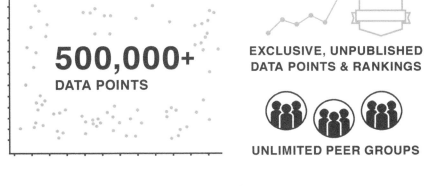
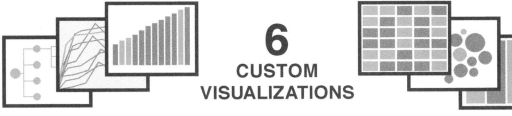
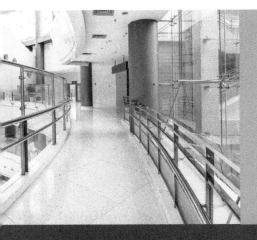

The Honor Roll

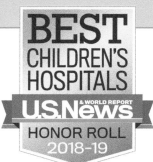

Hospitals on this elite list excelled in every pediatric specialty. For each specialty in which a hospital ranked among the 50 best, it received points toward the Honor Roll: 25 points for No. 1, 24 for No. 2 and so on, with hospitals ranked 21-50 receiving 5 points. The 10 hospitals with the most points defined the Honor Roll.

1 **Boston Children's Hospital**
238 points

2 **Cincinnati Children's Hospital Medical Center**
229 points

3 **Children's Hospital of Philadelphia**
225 points

4 **Texas Children's Hospital**
Houston, 196 points

5 **Children's National Medical Center**
Washington, D.C.
165 points

6 **Children's Hospital Los Angeles**
163 points

7 **Nationwide Children's Hospital**
Columbus, Ohio
147 points

8 **Johns Hopkins Children's Center**
Baltimore
139 points

9 **Children's Hospital Colorado**
Aurora
133 points

10 **Ann and Robert H. Lurie Children's Hospital of Chicago**
128 points

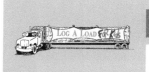

FOR 30 YEARS LOG A LOAD HAS DELIVERED MIRACLES TO KIDS ACROSS THE COUNTRY.

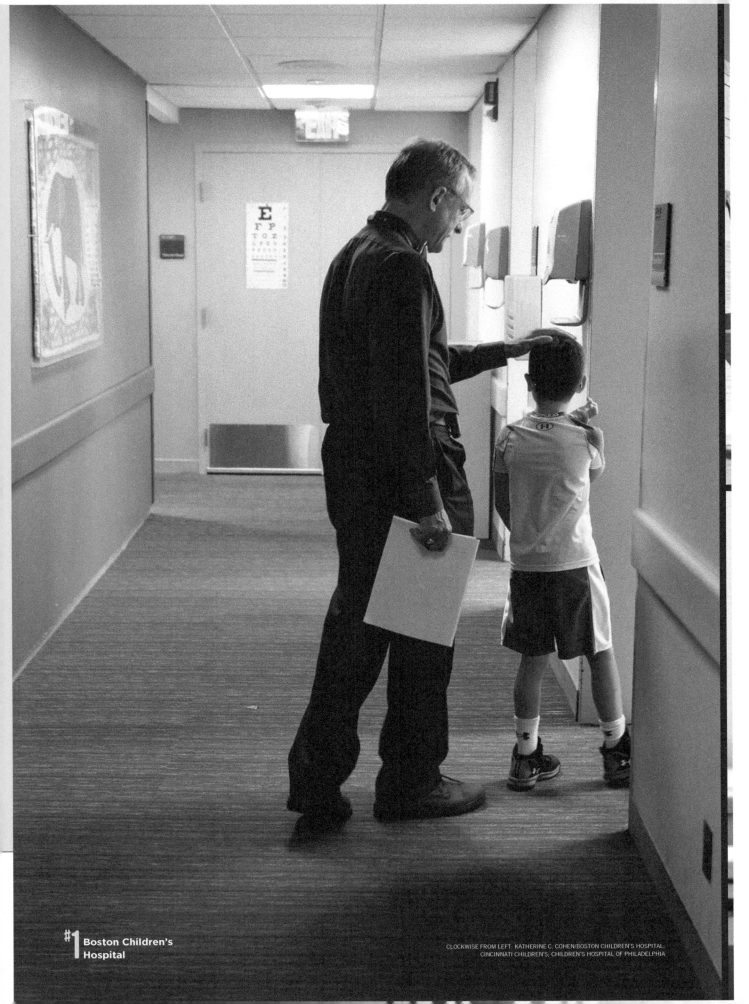

OUR BREAKTHROUGHS

TRANSFORM LIVES

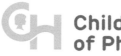

Children's Hospital of Philadelphia® | Breakthroughs.
Every day.®

Surgery before she was born changed Audrey's future.

— AND LIFETIMES

Breakthroughs come in all sizes.

From restoring the sight of children with a rare form of congenital blindness to restoring the soccer season for a teen with asthma, every day we relentlessly pursue ways to improve children's health and well-being.

We understand, whether big or small, every breakthrough matters to the people who matter the most to us: children.

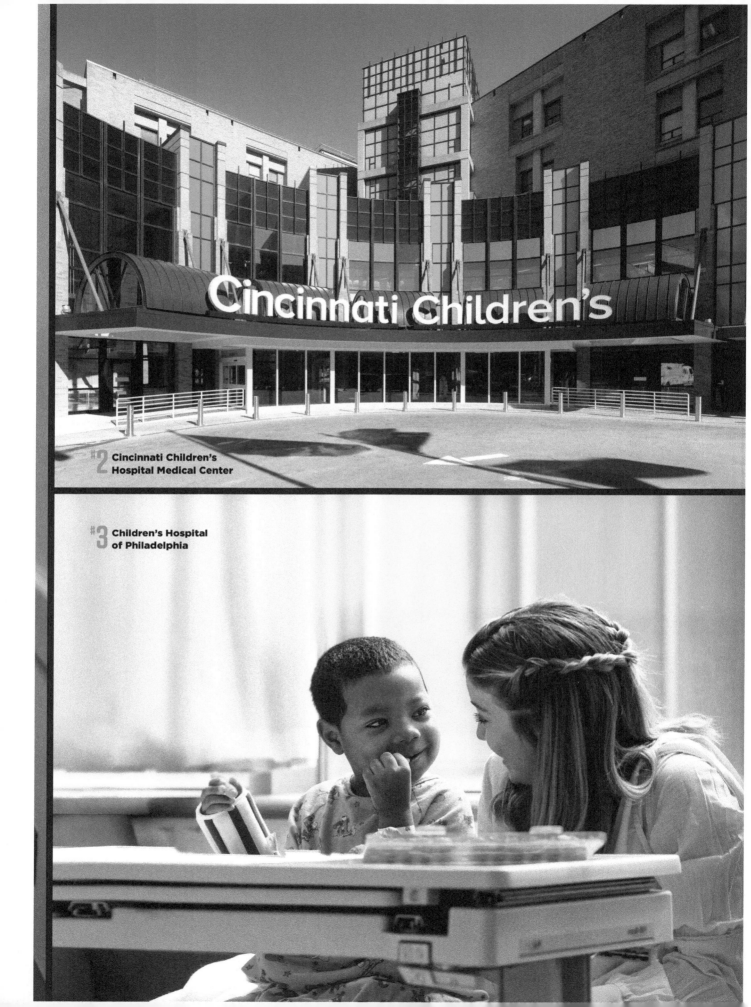

#2 **Cincinnati Children's Hospital Medical Center**

#3 **Children's Hospital of Philadelphia**

A Key to the Rankings

How we identified 86 outstanding hospitals in 10 specialties

by **Avery Comarow** and **Ben Harder**

Where should desperate parents take a newborn with a life-threatening heart defect, or find ongoing care for a child with failing kidneys or lung-clogging cystic fibrosis? The local hospital's pediatric department might see plenty of kids, but won't likely have the expertise to treat the sickest children. Even within the compact universe of fewer than 200 children's hospitals, some are better than others. U.S. News created the Best Children's Hospitals rankings to help parents, in consultation with their doctors, find the ones best suited to help their child.

The 2018-19 rankings highlight top children's centers in 10 specialties: cancer, cardiology and heart surgery, diabetes and endocrinology, gastroenterology and GI surgery, neonatology, nephrology, neurology and neurosurgery, orthopedics, pulmonology and urology. This year, 86 hospitals ranked in at least one specialty. These children's hospitals include both dedicated pediatric hospitals that treat only children and pediatric departments embedded within larger hospitals. The 2018-19 Honor Roll recognizes 10 standouts that scored near the top in all or most specialties.

Judging the excellence of children's hospitals is far more challenging than evaluating hospitals in adult care (as U.S. News has done since 1990 in Best Hospitals for high-risk patients in 16 specialties, page 96). Which information to collect and standards for interpreting it are constant sources of debate. Nor is there a pediatric version of the federal Medicare database that U.S. News draws on in ranking the adult hospitals.

Almost all of the medical data used in these rankings are therefore obtained by asking hospitals to complete a lengthy online survey. This year, 118 of the 189 hospitals surveyed by U.S. News provided enough data to be evaluated in at least

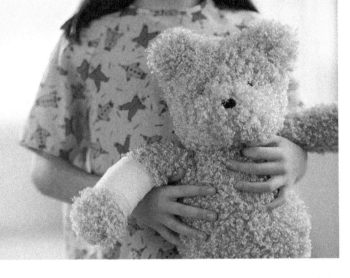

GETTY IMAGES

one specialty. Most surveyed hospitals are members of the Children's Hospital Association; a few are specialty centers or non-CHA hospitals that were previously ranked or were recommended by trusted sources.

This year's survey was updated with the help of 147 medical directors, clinical specialists and other pediatric experts who served as advisers on 12 U.S. News specialty task forces. RTI International, a North Carolina-based research and consulting firm, ran the survey and analyzed the findings.

Whether and how high an institution was ranked depended on three elements: its clinical outcomes (such as survival and surgical complications), its delivery of care (how well a hospital synchronizes all that must be done to treat patients effectively and keep them safe), and its resources (such as staffing and technology). A detailed FAQ about the rankings is available at usnews.com/aboutchildrens. Each element contributed one-third of a hospital's overall score in most specialties. Here are the basics:

Clinical outcomes. These reveal a hospital's success at keeping kids alive after their treatment or surgery, protecting them from infections and complications, and improving their quality of life.

Delivery of care. How well a hospital handles day-to-day care was determined in part by compliance with accepted "best practices," such as having a full-time infection preventionist and holding regular conferences to discuss unexpected deaths and complications. U.S. News also surveys pediatric specialists annually, asking them to identify up to 10 hospitals they consider best in their area of expertise for children with serious or difficult medical problems, ignoring distance and cost. Results from surveys in 2016, 2017 and 2018 were factored into a hospital's score. More than 4,000 physicians responded to the 2018 survey.

Resources. Surgical volume, nurse-patient ratio, clinics and programs for conditions such as asthma, and dozens of other measures were considered. ●

A Word on the Terms

USED IN MORE THAN ONE SPECIALTY

A Nurse Magnet hospital: hospital recognized by American Nurses Credentialing Center as meeting standards for nursing excellence.
Infection prevention score, ICU: ability to prevent central-line bloodstream infections in intensive care units.
Infection prevention score, overall: ability to prevent infections through measures such as hand hygiene and vaccination.
No. of best practices: how well hospital adheres to recommended ways of diagnosing and treating patients, such as documenting blood sugar levels for a high percentage of outpatients (diabetes & endocrinology) and conducting hip exams with ultrasound specialists (orthopedics).
Nurse-patient ratio: balance of full-time registered nurses to inpatients.
Patient volume score: relative number of patients in past year with specified disorders.
% of specialists recommending hospital: percentage of physician specialists responding to surveys in 2016, 2017 and 2018 who named hospital among best for very challenging patients.
Procedure volume score: relative number of tests and nonsurgical procedures in past one, two or three years, such as implanting radioactive seeds in a cancerous thyroid (diabetes & endocrinology) and using an endoscope for diagnosis (gastroenterology). Surgical procedures are included in orthopedics.
Surgery volume score: relative num-

ber of patients who had specified surgical procedures in past year.
Surgical complications prevention score: ability to prevent surgery-related complications and readmissions within 30 days (neurology & neurosurgery, orthopedics, urology).
U.S. News score: 0 to 100 summary of overall performance in specialty.
NA: not applicable; service not provided by hospital.
NR: data not reported or unavailable.

USED IN ONE SPECIALTY

CANCER
Bone marrow transplant survival score: survival of stem cell recipients at 100 days.
Five-year survival score: survival five years after treatment for acute lymphoblastic leukemia, acute myeloid leukemia, and neuroblastoma.
Palliative care score: how well program meets specified training and staffing standards for children with terminal or life-limiting conditions, and number of cancer patients referred to program.

CARDIOLOGY & HEART SURGERY
Catheter procedure volume score: relative number of specified catheter-based procedures in past year, such as inserting stents and treating heart rhythm problems.
Norwood/hybrid surgery survival score: survival at one year after the first in a series of reconstructive surgeries, evaluated over past four years.
Risk-adjusted surgical survival

score: survival in the hospital and 30 days from discharge after congenital heart surgery, adjusted for operative and patient risk, evaluated over past four years.

DIABETES & ENDOCRINOLOGY
Diabetes management score: ability to prevent serious problems in children with Type 1 diabetes and to keep blood sugar levels in check.
Hypothyroid management score: relative proportions of children treated for underactive thyroid who test normal and of infants who begin treatment by 3 weeks of age.

GASTROENTEROLOGY & GI SURGERY
Liver transplant survival score: One- and three-year survival after liver transplant.
Nonsurgical procedure volume score: relative number of tests and noninvasive procedures.
Selected treatments success score: shown, for example, by high remission rates for inflammatory bowel disease and few complications from endoscopic procedures.

NEONATOLOGY
Infection prevention score, NICU: ability to prevent central-line bloodstream infections in neonatal ICU.
Leaves NICU on breast milk score: relative percentage of infants discharged from NICU receiving some nutrition from breast milk.
Keeping breathing tube in place score: ability to minimize inappropriate breathing-tube removal in intubated infants.

NEPHROLOGY
Biopsy complications prevention score: ability to minimize complications after kidney biopsy.
Dialysis management score: relative

proportion of dialysis patients in past two years who tested normal.
Infection prevention score, dialysis: ability to minimize dialysis-related infection.
Kidney transplant survival score: based on patient survival and functioning kidney at one and three years.

NEUROLOGY & NEUROSURGERY
Clinic patient volume score: relative number of clinic patients in past year with specified disorders or procedures.
Epilepsy management score: ability to treat children with epilepsy.
Surgical survival score: survival at 30 days after complex surgery and procedures, such as those involving brain tumors, epilepsy and head trauma.

ORTHOPEDICS
Fracture repair score: ability to treat complex leg and forearm fractures efficiently.

PULMONOLOGY
Asthma inpatient care score: ability to minimize asthmatic children's asthma-related deaths, length of stay, and readmissions.
Cystic fibrosis management score: ability to improve lung function and nutritional status.
Lung transplant survival score: reflects number of transplants in past two years, one-year survival, and recognition by United Network for Organ Sharing.

UROLOGY
Minimally invasive volume score: relative number of patients in past year who had specified nonsurgical procedures.
Testicular torsion care score: promptness of emergency surgery to correct twisted spermatic cord.

KYLEE

Age 14, Osteogenesis Imperfecta

Born with Osteogenesis Imperfecta (Brittle Bone Disease), Kylee has had broken bones all her life. That's why her family turned to the orthopedic specialists at Children's—an expert team ensuring this amazing teen can reach her full potential.

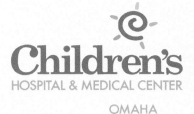

We know children.

Experienced, unparalleled care for a full spectrum of bone, joint and muscle disorders brings families from across the Midwest and the United States to Children's Hospital & Medical Center in Omaha. Our orthopedics program specializes in treatment for Osteogenesis Imperfecta, spinal irregularities and other congenital or acquired orthopedic conditions.

For a pediatric orthopedic specialist, call **1.800.833.3100** or visit **ChildrensOmaha.org/Orthopedics.**

BEST CHILDREN'S HOSPITALS
U.S.News & WORLD REPORT
ORTHOPEDICS
2018-19

CANCER

Rank	Hospital	U.S. News score	Five-year survival score (15=best)	Bone marrow transplant survival score (6=best)	Infection prevention score, overall (37=best)	Infection prevention score, ICU (15=best)	Patient volume score (21=best)	Nurse-patient ratio (higher is better)	A Nurse Magnet hospital	Palliative care score (8=best)	% of specialists recom-mending hospital
1	Cincinnati Children's Hospital Medical Center	100.0	15	4	36	13	21	4.5	Yes	8	49.5%
2	Children's Hospital of Philadelphia	99.7	14	5	34	10	20	3.7	Yes	8	62.6%
3	Dana-Farber/Boston Children's Cancer and Blood Disorders Center	97.8	14	5	33	8	21	4.3	Yes	8	59.9%
4	St. Jude Children's Research Hospital, Memphis, Tenn.	96.9	14	5	34	10	21	4.6	Yes	8	42.8%
5	Nationwide Children's Hospital, Columbus, Ohio	93.6	14	6	35	12	21	3.4	Yes	8	13.4%
6	Texas Children's Hospital, Houston	92.8	11	5	36	8	21	3.9	Yes	8	39.4%
7	Children's National Medical Center, Washington, D.C.	91.4	13	5	35	13	21	3.5	Yes	8	14.6%
8	Children's Hospital Colorado, Aurora	90.9	12	5	33	14	21	3.3	Yes	8	20.1%
9	Children's Hospital Los Angeles	90.5	13	5	34	10	19	3.7	Yes	8	29.2%
10	Johns Hopkins Children's Center, Baltimore	88.7	15	6	35	8	18	3.2	Yes	8	18.1%
11	Children's Healthcare of Atlanta	86.5	12	6	35	9	21	4.6	No	8	18.4%
12	Memorial Sloan Kettering Children's Cancer Center, New York	84.8	12	4	33	12	19	4.4	Yes	8	15.8%
13	UCSF Benioff Children's Hospitals, San Francisco and Oakland	83.2	13	5	34	9	18	3.9	Yes	7	12.4%
14	Monroe Carell Jr. Children's Hospital at Vanderbilt, Nashville, Tenn.	81.6	15	5	33	11	21	3.2	Yes	8	1.3%
15	Seattle Children's Hospital	80.8	11	5	32	7	20	3.3	Yes	8	35.3%
16	Nemours Alfred I. duPont Hosp. for Children, Wilmington, Del.	78.5	14	6	34	10	14	4.2	Yes	8	0.8%
17	Duke Children's Hospital and Health Center, Durham, N.C.	78.2	13	5	36	11	19	3.2	Yes	8	5.0%
18	Ann and Robert H. Lurie Children's Hospital of Chicago	77.4	11	4	33	9	21	3.3	Yes	8	16.4%
19	Children's Hospital of Wisconsin, Milwaukee	76.6	11	5	28	14	18	4.2	Yes	8	3.0%
20	Phoenix Children's Hospital	76.3	14	4	34	14	21	3.0	No	8	2.9%
21	Lucile Packard Children's Hospital Stanford, Palo Alto, Calif.	76.2	13	6	34	7	21	3.7	No	6	7.4%
22	Rainbow Babies and Children's Hospital, Cleveland	75.8	10	5	29	13	13	2.7	Yes	8	4.2%
23	Cleveland Clinic Children's Hospital	75.7	8	6	34	11	15	3.4	Yes	8	0.9%
24	C.S. Mott Children's Hospital-Michigan Medicine, Ann Arbor	75.0	12	4	34	12	12	3.7	Yes	8	3.8%
25	MUSC Health-Children's Hospital, Charleston, S.C.	74.7	13	6	34	13	9	3.0	Yes	8	0.4%
26	Mayo Clinic Children's Center, Rochester, Minn.	74.4	11	6	32	10	9	4.0	Yes	8	1.0%
27	Primary Children's Hospital, Salt Lake City	73.7	13	6	35	7	18	4.2	No	8	1.4%
28	Children's Medical Center Dallas	73.6	9	3	34	12	21	3.1	Yes	8	6.2%
29	Children's Cancer Hosp.-U. of Texas M.D. Anderson Cancer Ctr., Houston	73.2	6	5	31	15	17	2.9	Yes	8	6.7%
30	Rady Children's Hospital, San Diego	73.0	12	6	30	10	11	3.1	Yes	8	2.4%
31	Levine Children's Hospital, Charlotte, N.C.	72.6	13	6	34	12	7	3.1	Yes	8	0.3%
32	NY-Presby. Morgan Stanley-Komansky Children's Hospital, N.Y.	72.0	12	4	33	13	21	3.2	No	8	4.9%
33	Children's Mercy Kansas City, Mo.	71.9	11	5	36	8	20	4.4	Yes	7	2.8%
34	Children's Hospital at Montefiore, New York	71.7	13	4	36	14	7	3.7	No	8	1.6%
35	North Carolina Children's Hospital at UNC, Chapel Hill	71.5	10	6	35	10	19	4.9	Yes	8	0.9%
36	UCLA Mattel Children's Hospital, Los Angeles	71.3	13	5	28	8	15	3.6	Yes	8	2.8%
36	University of Iowa Stead Family Children's Hospital, Iowa City	71.3	15	6	27	10	16	3.1	Yes	8	0.8%
38	Children's Hospital of Pittsburgh of UPMC	71.0	11	4	32	11	21	3.4	Yes	8	5.4%
39	American Family Children's Hospital, Madison, Wis.	70.4	13	5	31	11	7	4.0	Yes	5	0.7%
39	Children's Hospital of Alabama at UAB, Birmingham	70.4	12	5	30	11	19	3.6	No	8	1.7%
41	Doernbecher Children's Hospital, Portland, Ore.	69.7	13	3	32	11	11	3.8	Yes	8	2.4%
42	Spectrum Hlth. Helen DeVos Children's Hosp., Grand Rapids, Mich.	69.5	9	6	30	11	8	3.7	Yes	8	1.4%
43	Yale New Haven Children's Hospital, New Haven, Conn.	69.3	11	6	29	9	16	2.2	Yes	8	0.9%
44	Riley Hospital for Children at IU Health, Indianapolis	69.2	12	4	32	5	19	4.1	Yes	8	1.6%
45	Penn State Children's Hospital, Hershey, Pa.	68.7	11	6	27	9	14	3.5	Yes	8	1.4%
45	St. Louis Children's Hospital-Washington University	68.7	9	4	35	10	7	3.6	Yes	8	5.2%
47	Cook Children's Medical Center, Fort Worth	68.6	14	3	30	12	21	3.9	Yes	8	1.8%
48	Wolfson Children's Hospital, Jacksonville, Fla.	67.4	12	4	30	13	11	2.4	Yes	8	0.4%
49	UF Health Shands Children's Hospital, Gainesville, Fla.	67.1	12	6	28	10	9	2.7	Yes	8	0.8%
50	CHOC Children's Hospital, Orange, Calif.	67.0	13	4	35	8	9	3.7	Yes	8	1.9%

Terms are explained on Page 162.

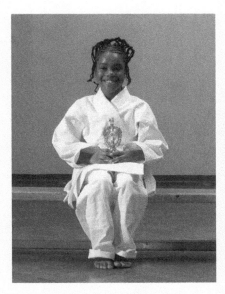
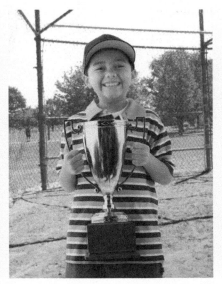
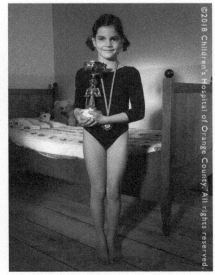
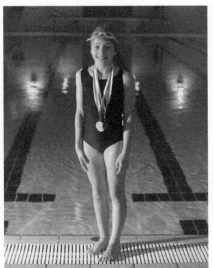

"IT IS AMAZING
WHAT YOU CAN
ACCOMPLISH IF
YOU DO NOT
CARE WHO GETS
THE CREDIT."

-HARRY TRUMAN

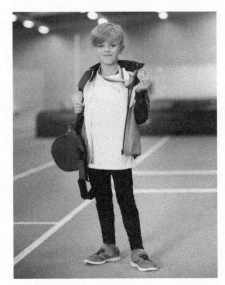
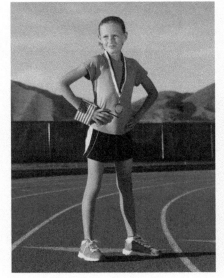
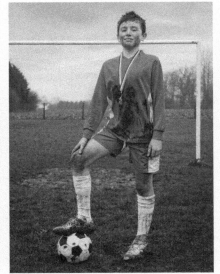
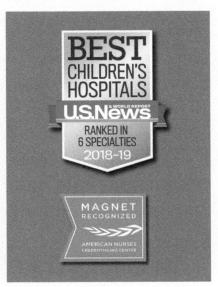

Since our founding, CHOC Children's has been striving to bring first-class care to every child in Southern California.
So on behalf of all the kids who make what we do so rewarding, we're honored to be named one of the nation's
best children's hospitals by U.S. News & World Report. Learn more at CHOC.org **CHOC** Children's.

CARDIOLOGY & HEART SURGERY

Rank	Hospital	U.S. News score	Risk-adjusted surgical survival score (10=best)	Norwood/ hybrid surgery survival score (12=best)	Infection prevention score, overall (42=best)	Infection prevention score, ICU (5=best)	Surgery volume score (12=best)	Catheter procedure volume score (33=best)	Nurse-patient ratio (higher is better)	A Nurse Magnet hospital	% of specialists recommending hospital
1	Texas Children's Hospital, Houston	100.0	10	9	41	2	10	33	3.9	Yes	51.3%
2	Boston Children's Hospital	94.4	8	8	38	2	12	33	4.3	Yes	75.0%
3	Ann and Robert H. Lurie Children's Hospital of Chicago	87.8	9	10	38	3	6	19	3.3	Yes	16.3%
4	C.S. Mott Children's Hospital-Michigan Medicine, Ann Arbor	87.4	8	9	39	4	11	30	3.7	Yes	40.3%
5	Children's Hospital Los Angeles	87.0	8	12	39	2	11	31	3.7	Yes	17.2%
6	Children's Hospital of Pittsburgh of UPMC	84.3	10	11	37	3	6	21	3.4	Yes	10.7%
7	Children's Medical Center Dallas	83.7	8	11	39	2	8	27	3.1	Yes	4.0%
8	Cincinnati Children's Hospital Medical Center	83.2	5	11	41	3	9	30	4.5	Yes	31.8%
9	Phoenix Children's Hospital	81.2	10	8	39	4	9	27	3.0	No	1.9%
10	Le Bonheur Children's Hospital, Memphis, Tenn.	80.7	10	10	39	2	6	21	3.1	Yes	2.4%
11	MUSC Children's Heart Network of South Carolina, Charleston	80.6	9	11	39	5	7	23	3.0	Yes	8.1%
12	Children's Hospital of Philadelphia	78.2	5	10	39	2	12	33	3.7	Yes	67.0%
13	Children's Mercy Kansas City, Mo.	77.1	8	10	41	2	8	27	4.4	Yes	3.4%
14	Children's Hospital of Wisconsin, Milwaukee	76.6	9	11	33	4	7	17	4.2	Yes	10.3%
15	Children's Hospital and Medical Center, Omaha	76.5	8	10	40	4	7	23	4.3	Yes	1.2%
16	Seattle Children's Hospital	76.3	7	9	39	1	9	27	3.3	Yes	14.2%
17	Lucile Packard Children's Hospital Stanford, Palo Alto, Calif.	76.0	5	9	41	1	11	30	3.7	No	43.4%
18	Children's Hospital Colorado, Aurora	75.9	5	9	38	4	9	29	3.3	Yes	12.3%
19	UF Health Shands Children's Hospital, Gainesville, Fla.	75.1	9	12	34	4	5	13	2.7	Yes	0.9%
20	NY-Presby. Morgan Stanley-Komansky Children's Hospital, N.Y.	74.2	5	11	38	3	10	32	3.2	No	18.9%
21	Riley Hospital for Children at IU Health, Indianapolis	72.8	8	9	36	1	8	23	4.1	Yes	2.6%
22	Levine Children's Hospital, Charlotte, N.C.	72.4	8	11	39	4	6	20	3.1	Yes	2.4%
23	Advocate Children's Heart Institute, Oak Lawn and Park Ridge, Ill.	72.0	9	11	36	2	8	25	4.0	Yes	2.0%
24	Penn State Children's Hospital, Hershey, Pa.	70.9	10	12	31	3	4	15	3.5	Yes	1.0%
25	Rady Children's Hospital, San Diego	70.4	7	12	36	4	7	30	3.1	Yes	4.7%
26	Cleveland Clinic Children's Hospital	69.7	6	11	39	3	4	22	3.4	Yes	2.2%
27	Mayo Clinic Children's Center, Rochester, Minn.	69.3	7	10	39	0	7	19	4.0	Yes	6.1%
28	Cook Children's Medical Center, Fort Worth	68.9	8	10	36	4	8	23	3.9	Yes	0.7%
29	Nationwide Children's Hospital, Columbus, Ohio	68.8	4	9	40	2	8	28	3.4	Yes	17.4%
30	Primary Children's Hospital, Salt Lake City	67.6	5	11	41	1	9	31	4.2	No	6.5%
31	St. Louis Children's Hospital-Washington University	67.0	4	8	40	4	6	31	3.6	Yes	4.3%
32	Children's Healthcare of Atlanta	66.5	4	7	40	3	12	33	4.6	No	27.4%
33	Johns Hopkins Children's Center, Baltimore	65.7	6	10	40	2	6	23	3.2	Yes	2.5%
34	UCSF Benioff Children's Hospitals, San Francisco and Oakland	65.2	7	9	40	3	6	28	3.9	Yes	8.6%
35	Children's National Medical Center, Washington, D.C.	64.3	3	9	40	5	6	28	3.5	Yes	11.6%
36	Arnold Palmer Hospital for Children, Orlando	63.8	9	12	33	5	4	17	3.7	Yes	0.6%
36	Duke Children's Hospital and Health Center, Durham, N.C.	63.8	3	10	41	5	6	26	3.2	Yes	3.7%
38	SSM Hlth. Cardinal Glennon Children's Hosp.-St. Louis U., St. Louis	62.5	7	11	39	1	6	14	3.1	No	0.6%
39	Spectrum Hlth. Helen DeVos Children's Hosp., Grand Rapids, Mich.	62.1	9	12	34	3	4	16	3.7	Yes	0.5%
40	Children's Hospital of Alabama at UAB, Birmingham	61.9	5	10	35	3	6	24	3.6	No	1.8%
41	University of Maryland Children's Hospital, Baltimore	61.3	8	8	32	3	4	13	3.0	Yes	0.4%
42	Monroe Carell Jr. Children's Hospital at Vanderbilt, Nashville, Tenn.	61.0	4	9	38	3	9	30	3.2	Yes	5.4%
43	University of Virginia Children's Hospital, Charlottesville	59.9	4	10	38	3	4	19	2.8	Yes	1.3%
44	Johns Hopkins All Children's Hospital, St. Petersburg, Fla.	58.8	5	9	39	4	6	23	3.3	No	1.6%
45	Children's Memorial Hermann Hospital, Houston	58.1	7	10	35	2	5	23	3.2	Yes	0.5%
46	American Family Children's Hospital, Madison, Wis.	56.7	6	12	37	3	4	19	4.0	Yes	0.7%
47	UCLA Mattel Children's Hospital, Los Angeles	56.4	4	8	33	4	5	30	3.6	Yes	4.9%
48	Nicklaus Children's Hospital, Miami	56.2	4	9	36	4	6	28	3.0	Yes	3.1%
49	Yale-New Haven/Connecticut Children's Medical Ctrs., New Haven	53.9	6	8	33	3	4	17	2.2	Yes	1.5%
50	Arkansas Children's Hospital, Little Rock	53.6	4	9	37	4	5	23	3.3	Yes	1.0%

Terms are explained on Page 162.

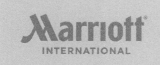

#9

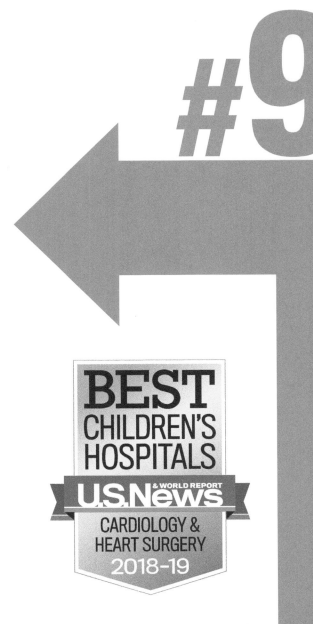

KIDS ARE AT THE HEART OF EVERYTHING WE DO

BEST CHILDREN'S HOSPITALS
U.S.News & WORLD REPORT
CARDIOLOGY & HEART SURGERY
2018-19

For us, this shield means we're helping kids do what they should be doing. Kids should be laughing, playing, and singing. Kids should be kids. That's the reason we are honored we earned this shield and the reason we'll never stop improving. For more info visit phoenixchildrens.org

PHOENIX CHILDREN'S ®

DIABETES & ENDOCRINOLOGY

Rank	Hospital	U.S. News score	Diabetes manage-ment score (42=best)	Hypothyroid manage-ment score (3=best)	Infection prevention score, overall (37=best)	Patient volume score (30=best)	Procedure volume score (26=best)	Nurse-patient ratio (higher is better)	A Nurse Magnet hospital	No. of best practices (108=best)	% of specialists recom-mending hospital
1	Children's Hospital of Philadelphia	100.0	35	3	34	30	26	3.7	Yes	106	61.1%
2	Boston Children's Hospital	93.2	30	3	32	30	26	4.3	Yes	102	56.7%
3	Cincinnati Children's Hospital Medical Center	91.0	29	3	35	30	23	4.5	Yes	106	33.2%
4	Children's Hospital of Pittsburgh of UPMC	90.1	34	3	30	30	23	3.4	Yes	104	26.7%
5	Children's Hospital Los Angeles	89.8	35	3	33	30	20	3.7	Yes	98	24.5%
6	Texas Children's Hospital, Houston	86.5	29	3	35	30	25	3.9	Yes	102	21.8%
7	Children's Hospital Colorado, Aurora	85.2	27	3	31	30	25	3.3	Yes	98	31.1%
8	Yale New Haven Children's Hospital, New Haven, Conn.	83.2	35	3	29	29	26	2.2	Yes	103	15.3%
9	Seattle Children's Hospital	83.0	30	3	33	30	26	3.3	Yes	103	12.9%
10	Children's National Medical Center, Washington, D.C.	82.0	32	3	35	30	26	3.5	Yes	107	4.9%
10	UCSF Benioff Children's Hospitals, San Francisco and Oakland	82.0	29	3	33	30	21	3.9	Yes	92	17.4%
12	North Carolina Children's Hospital at UNC, Chapel Hill	79.8	35	3	35	27	22	4.9	Yes	103	2.7%
13	Lucile Packard Children's Hospital Stanford, Palo Alto, Calif.	79.2	33	3	34	29	15	3.7	No	88	15.9%
14	Johns Hopkins Children's Center, Baltimore	78.9	30	3	35	22	13	3.2	Yes	102	13.5%
15	Mayo Clinic Children's Center, Rochester, Minn.	77.9	33	3	32	27	23	4.0	Yes	99	4.1%
16	Riley Hospital for Children at IU Health, Indianapolis	77.1	28	3	31	30	21	4.1	Yes	94	11.3%
17	St. Louis Children's Hospital-Washington University	76.3	29	3	33	28	20	3.6	Yes	95	3.9%
18	Nationwide Children's Hospital, Columbus, Ohio	76.2	24	3	34	30	25	3.4	Yes	101	8.7%
19	NY-Presby. Morgan Stanley-Komansky Children's Hospital, N.Y.	75.3	31	3	33	30	21	3.2	No	106	8.0%
20	Children's Mercy Kansas City, Mo.	74.3	26	3	34	30	22	4.4	Yes	97	3.8%
21	Rainbow Babies and Children's Hospital, Cleveland	74.0	28	3	31	28	20	2.7	Yes	105	5.2%
22	Children's Medical Center Dallas	73.3	25	3	32	29	26	3.1	Yes	88	8.8%
23	C.S. Mott Children's Hospital-Michigan Medicine, Ann Arbor	73.2	29	3	33	28	21	3.7	Yes	96	2.5%
24	MassGeneral Hospital for Children, Boston	72.6	29	3	25	27	23	3.9	Yes	100	5.3%
25	Mount Sinai Kravis Children's Hospital, New York	72.5	29	3	32	29	26	3.8	Yes	106	2.7%
26	Rady Children's Hospital, San Diego	72.4	29	3	29	30	26	3.1	Yes	97	2.3%
27	Children's Hospital of Wisconsin, Milwaukee	71.9	31	3	28	26	21	4.2	Yes	91	1.6%
27	UF Health Shands Children's Hospital, Gainesville, Fla.	71.9	28	3	27	24	15	2.7	Yes	95	9.0%
29	Ann and Robert H. Lurie Children's Hospital of Chicago	71.8	26	3	31	29	25	3.3	Yes	93	6.5%
30	Nemours Alfred I. duPont Hosp. for Children, Wilmington, Del.	71.0	29	3	33	27	21	4.2	Yes	91	0.9%
31	Monroe Carell Jr. Children's Hospital at Vanderbilt, Nashville, Tenn.	70.9	23	3	31	30	24	3.2	Yes	95	5.2%
32	Duke Children's Hospital and Health Center, Durham, N.C.	70.0	26	3	33	27	17	3.2	Yes	98	2.3%
33	University of Virginia Children's Hospital, Charlottesville	69.9	30	3	31	21	14	2.8	Yes	93	2.2%
34	Arnold Palmer Hospital for Children, Orlando	69.8	34	3	28	27	23	3.7	Yes	104	0.3%
35	Doernbecher Children's Hospital, Portland, Ore.	68.8	27	3	30	27	20	3.8	Yes	86	3.9%
35	Phoenix Children's Hospital	68.8	27	3	33	30	26	3.0	No	103	1.4%
37	Connecticut Children's Medical Center, Hartford	68.5	32	3	32	30	21	3.1	No	93	1.2%
38	Primary Children's Hospital, Salt Lake City	68.1	30	3	34	28	22	4.2	No	87	0.5%
39	Cleveland Clinic Children's Hospital	68.0	24	3	32	29	20	3.4	Yes	97	2.0%
40	Cohen Children's Medical Center, New Hyde Park, N.Y.	67.7	23	3	34	28	24	3.4	Yes	97	1.8%
41	NYU Winthrop Hospital Children's Medical Center, Mineola, N.Y.	67.6	31	3	33	24	8	2.1	Yes	103	1.1%
42	Children's Hospitals and Clinics of Minnesota, Minneapolis	67.4	31	3	30	29	22	3.3	Yes	86	1.0%
43	Holtz Children's Hosp. at UM-Jackson Memorial Med. Ctr., Miami	67.1	39	3	18	25	24	2.3	No	101	2.3%
44	Children's Healthcare of Atlanta	67.0	24	3	32	30	26	4.6	Yes	92	2.7%
44	Valley Children's Healthcare and Hospital, Madera, Calif.	67.0	31	3	34	27	19	3.0	Yes	92	0.8%
46	Cook Children's Medical Center, Fort Worth	66.7	26	3	29	25	19	3.9	Yes	100	3.8%
47	University of Minnesota Masonic Children's Hospital, Minneapolis	66.5	27	3	28	27	19	3.7	No	100	2.3%
48	Children's Hospital of Alabama at UAB, Birmingham	66.4	27	3	30	30	25	3.6	No	97	2.1%
49	Children's Hospital and Medical Center, Omaha	65.7	26	3	35	27	20	4.3	Yes	90	0.0%
49	Norton Children's Hospital, Louisville, Ky.	65.7	29	3	33	29	22	2.9	No	90	1.6%
49	University of Chicago Comer Children's Hospital	65.7	29	3	31	19	18	3.4	No	91	2.4%

Terms are explained on Page 162.

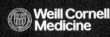

GASTROENTEROLOGY & GI SURGERY

Rank	Hospital	U.S. News score	Selected treatments success score (9=best)	Liver transplant survival score (6=best)	Infection prevention score, overall (43=best)	Infection prevention score, ICU (5=best)	Patient volume score (24=best)	Surgery volume score (14=best)	Nonsurgical procedure volume score (16=best)	Nurse-patient ratio (higher is better)	A Nurse Magnet hospital	% of specialists recommending hospital
1	Cincinnati Children's Hospital Medical Center	100.0	8	5	42	3	24	14	16	4.5	Yes	58.3%
2	Boston Children's Hospital	95.6	7	5	39	2	24	13	16	4.3	Yes	62.1%
3	Children's Hospital of Philadelphia	95.1	7	5	40	2	24	13	16	3.7	Yes	57.5%
4	Texas Children's Hospital, Houston	90.2	8	4	38	2	24	12	16	3.9	Yes	35.5%
5	Children's Hospital Los Angeles	89.1	9	6	40	2	22	12	16	3.7	Yes	14.4%
6	Children's Medical Center Dallas	86.3	9	6	39	2	23	14	16	3.1	Yes	9.1%
7	Children's Hospital Colorado, Aurora	86.0	6	4	39	4	23	14	16	3.3	Yes	33.1%
8	Ann and Robert H. Lurie Children's Hospital of Chicago	84.9	7	6	39	3	23	14	16	3.3	Yes	18.9%
9	Children's Hospital of Pittsburgh of UPMC	84.3	8	5	38	3	24	12	12	3.4	Yes	20.5%
10	Children's Healthcare of Atlanta	84.1	8	6	41	3	23	13	16	4.6	No	8.2%
11	Nationwide Children's Hospital, Columbus, Ohio	81.9	9	NR	40	2	23	13	15	3.4	Yes	42.2%
12	Children's National Medical Center, Washington, D.C.	81.4	7	5	41	5	23	13	15	3.5	Yes	3.7%
13	Seattle Children's Hospital	80.0	7	6	39	1	21	10	14	3.3	Yes	22.1%
14	Children's Hospital of Wisconsin, Milwaukee	79.9	7	6	34	4	18	9	16	4.2	Yes	6.2%
15	NY-Presby. Morgan Stanley-Komansky Children's Hospital, N.Y.	79.7	9	5	39	3	21	12	15	3.2	No	7.5%
16	Children's Hospital at Montefiore, New York	78.3	9	6	42	4	16	9	11	3.7	No	3.0%
17	Johns Hopkins Children's Center, Baltimore	78.0	9	3	41	2	24	14	15	3.2	Yes	7.5%
18	UCSF Benioff Children's Hospitals, San Francisco and Oakland	77.6	7	5	39	3	22	10	11	3.9	Yes	8.8%
19	C.S. Mott Children's Hospital-Michigan Medicine, Ann Arbor	77.0	7	5	40	4	23	13	14	3.7	Yes	4.0%
20	St. Louis Children's Hospital-Washington University	76.7	7	6	40	4	17	10	11	3.6	Yes	5.1%
21	Riley Hospital for Children at IU Health, Indianapolis	75.9	8	6	35	1	20	12	15	4.1	Yes	4.7%
22	Rady Children's Hospital, San Diego	74.8	8	6	35	4	22	9	13	3.1	Yes	2.9%
23	Cleveland Clinic Children's Hospital	73.0	6	5	38	3	22	13	16	3.4	Yes	4.0%
24	Monroe Carell Jr. Children's Hosp. at Vanderbilt, Nashville, Tenn.	72.4	8	3	39	3	22	11	16	3.2	Yes	4.1%
25	Children's Mercy Kansas City, Mo.	72.2	8	3	41	2	22	12	14	4.4	Yes	4.6%
26	Phoenix Children's Hospital	71.3	8	5	38	4	24	11	13	3.0	No	2.2%
27	Lucile Packard Children's Hospital Stanford, Palo Alto, Calif.	70.0	6	6	41	1	21	12	11	3.7	No	11.6%
28	Duke Children's Hospital and Health Center, Durham, N.C.	69.5	7	5	42	5	15	11	8	3.2	Yes	2.0%
29	MassGeneral Hospital for Children, Boston	68.3	6	6	32	2	19	8	12	3.9	Yes	4.9%
30	Le Bonheur Children's Hospital, Memphis, Tenn.	67.9	8	4	41	2	13	12	8	3.1	Yes	1.6%
31	Levine Children's Hospital, Charlotte, N.C.	67.1	7	4	39	4	17	13	13	3.1	Yes	1.0%
32	Children's Hospital of Michigan, Detroit	66.9	9	6	31	3	21	5	10	3.0	No	0.1%
33	Nemours Alfred I. duPont Hosp. for Children, Wilmington, Del.	66.3	7	4	40	2	14	10	9	4.2	Yes	1.0%
34	UCLA Mattel Children's Hospital, Los Angeles	66.1	6	3	34	4	18	6	11	3.6	Yes	6.7%
35	SSM Hlth. Cardinal Glennon Children's Hosp.-St. Louis U., St. Louis	62.9	8	6	40	1	12	6	8	3.1	No	0.4%
36	Mount Sinai Kravis Children's Hospital, New York	62.7	8	3	36	1	15	6	11	3.8	Yes	3.3%
37	University of Minnesota Masonic Children's Hosp., Minneapolis	62.0	6	6	35	2	19	10	12	3.7	No	0.4%
38	Children's Hospital and Medical Center, Omaha	61.5	9	NA	37	4	13	12	13	4.3	Yes	1.0%
39	Primary Children's Hospital, Salt Lake City	60.7	6	5	40	1	22	12	12	4.2	No	1.3%
40	Children's Hospital of Alabama at UAB, Birmingham	59.8	8	2	34	3	19	10	14	3.6	No	2.3%
41	American Family Children's Hospital, Madison, Wis.	59.6	6	6	37	3	8	5	10	4.0	Yes	0.2%
42	Cohen Children's Medical Center, New Hyde Park, N.Y.	59.2	8	NA	40	3	13	9	14	3.4	Yes	1.4%
43	Yale New Haven Children's Hospital, New Haven, Conn.	58.8	6	4	33	3	14	10	6	2.2	Yes	2.5%
44	Rainbow Babies and Children's Hospital, Cleveland	58.6	9	NA	37	3	17	6	12	2.7	Yes	1.8%
45	MUSC Health-Children's Hospital, Charleston, S.C.	58.4	4	4	37	5	17	10	15	3.0	Yes	0.8%
46	Valley Children's Healthcare and Hospital, Madera, Calif.	57.9	9	NA	41	3	17	9	16	3.0	Yes	1.0%
47	Ochsner Hospital for Children, New Orleans	56.6	6	5	33	5	10	4	12	2.7	Yes	0.4%
48	University of Virginia Children's Hospital, Charlottesville	55.6	6	6	34	3	10	7	7	2.8	Yes	1.0%
49	North Carolina Children's Hospital at UNC, Chapel Hill	53.9	6	3	41	0	14	11	11	4.9	Yes	1.3%
50	University of Chicago Comer Children's Hospital	52.6	3	4	37	5	16	12	11	3.4	No	2.3%

NA=not applicable. NR=not reported. Terms are explained on Page 162.

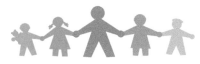

UCSF Benioff Children's Hospitals
Oakland | San Francisco

BEST CHILDREN'S HOSPITALS
U.S. News & WORLD REPORT
CANCER
2018-19

BEST CHILDREN'S HOSPITALS
U.S. News & WORLD REPORT
CARDIOLOGY &
HEART SURGERY
2018-19

BEST CHILDREN'S HOSPITALS
U.S. News & WORLD REPORT
DIABETES &
ENDOCRINOLOGY
2018-19

BEST CHILDREN'S HOSPITALS
U.S. News & WORLD REPORT
GASTROENTEROLOGY
& GI SURGERY
2018-19

BEST CHILDREN'S HOSPITALS
U.S. News & WORLD REPORT
NEONATOLOGY
2018-19

BEST CHILDREN'S HOSPITALS
U.S. News & WORLD REPORT
NEPHROLOGY
2018-19

BEST CHILDREN'S HOSPITALS
U.S. News & WORLD REPORT
NEUROLOGY &
NEUROSURGERY
2018-19

BEST CHILDREN'S HOSPITALS
U.S. News & WORLD REPORT
ORTHOPEDICS
2018-19

BEST CHILDREN'S HOSPITALS
U.S. News & WORLD REPORT
PULMONOLOGY
2018-19

BEST CHILDREN'S HOSPITALS
U.S. News & WORLD REPORT
UROLOGY
2018-19

UCSF Benioff Children's Hospitals rank among the country's best in all 10 specialties, and are recognized as best in Northern California in 6 specialties.

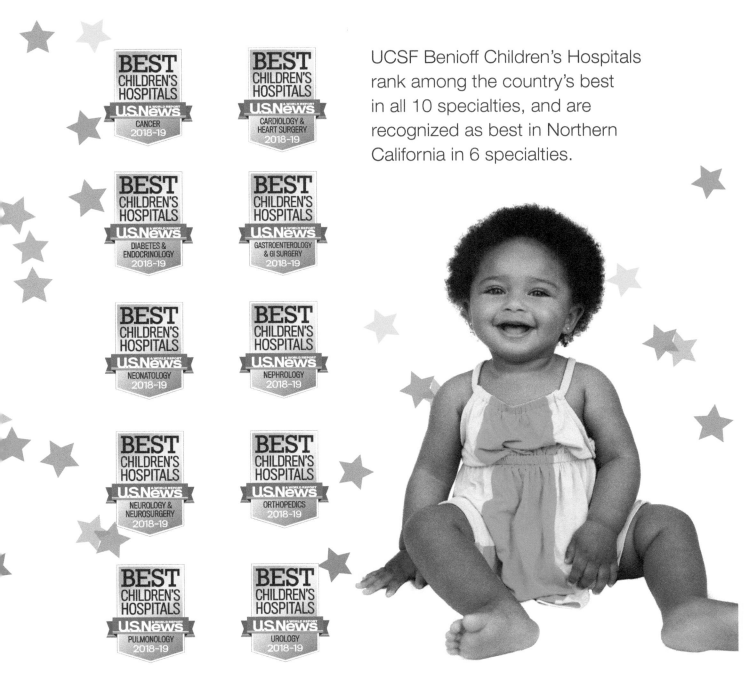

ucsfbenioffchildrens.org/usnews

NEONATOLOGY

Rank	Hospital	U.S. News score	Leaves NICU on breast milk score (3=best)	Keeping breathing tube in place score (5=best)	Infection prevention score, overall (38=best)	Infection prevention score, NICU (5=best)	Patient volume score (30=best)	Nurse-patient ratio (higher is better)	A Nurse Magnet hospital	No. of best practices (94=best)	% of specialists recom-mending hospital
1	Children's National Medical Center, Washington, D.C.	100.0	3	5	37	5	30	3.1	Yes	94	14.8%
2	Children's Hospital of Philadelphia	98.2	3	5	36	3	30	3.8	Yes	88	48.3%
3	Boston Children's Hospital	94.4	3	4	35	3	26	4.0	Yes	94	40.9%
4	Children's Hospital Colorado, Aurora	94.3	3	4	35	5	26	3.4	Yes	91	13.8%
5	Cincinnati Children's Hospital Medical Center	89.8	2	3	38	5	29	3.8	Yes	92	28.3%
6	Rainbow Babies and Children's Hospital, Cleveland	87.4	2	4	33	5	19	3.8	Yes	92	17.6%
7	UCSF Benioff Children's Hospitals, San Francisco and Oakland	85.4	2	5	37	4	25	3.3	Yes	90	11.9%
8	NY-Presby. Morgan Stanley-Komansky Children's Hospital, N.Y.	82.2	3	5	35	4	29	3.0	No	89	11.8%
9	St. Louis Children's Hospital-Washington University	80.8	2	4	37	4	26	3.3	Yes	93	8.9%
10	C.S. Mott Children's Hospital-Michigan Medicine, Ann Arbor	80.3	3	3	36	5	21	2.6	Yes	83	4.4%
11	Ann & Robert H. Lurie Children's Hosp.-Prentice Women's Hosp., Chicago	78.1	3	3	35	4	24	2.5	Yes	89	9.3%
12	Rady Children's Hospital, San Diego	77.7	3	4	33	4	23	2.9	Yes	87	5.1%
13	Mayo Clinic Children's Center, Rochester, Minn.	77.2	2	5	35	5	11	4.5	Yes	88	1.9%
14	Children's Hospital Los Angeles	76.1	2	5	36	3	28	3.7	Yes	91	10.0%
15	Nationwide Children's Hospital, Columbus, Ohio	75.7	2	2	37	4	26	2.6	Yes	89	15.1%
16	Johns Hopkins Children's Center, Baltimore	74.4	2	4	37	3	26	2.9	Yes	86	11.9%
17	Duke Children's Hospital and Health Center, Durham, N.C.	73.3	2	4	38	4	18	2.5	Yes	89	6.5%
18	Monroe Carell Jr. Children's Hospital at Vanderbilt, Nashville, Tenn.	72.8	2	3	35	4	25	2.8	Yes	90	7.1%
19	University of Virginia Children's Hospital, Charlottesville	72.6	2	4	35	5	17	2.3	Yes	87	1.7%
20	Seattle Children's Hospital	72.5	3	5	36	1	24	3.5	Yes	83	14.9%
21	CHOC Children's Hospital, Orange, Calif.	72.3	3	5	37	3	18	3.5	Yes	90	3.0%
21	Texas Children's Hospital, Houston	72.3	2	3	38	2	28	2.9	Yes	93	19.0%
23	Children's Healthcare of Atlanta	71.8	2	4	37	4	27	3.3	No	89	4.4%
24	Children's Medical Center Dallas-Parkland Memorial Hospital	70.8	2	4	35	4	21	2.6	Yes	87	4.2%
25	Connecticut Children's Medical Center, Hartford	70.5	3	5	34	5	20	2.4	No	90	0.8%
26	University of California Davis Children's Hospital, Sacramento	70.4	2	5	36	4	17	3.3	Yes	92	1.0%
27	Children's Hospital at Montefiore, New York	70.3	3	4	38	4	10	3.0	No	93	1.2%
28	Children's Hospital of Alabama at UAB, Birmingham	69.6	3	5	33	3	29	3.4	No	91	4.0%
29	Doernbecher Children's Hospital, Portland, Ore.	69.2	1	5	34	5	16	2.7	Yes	87	0.6%
30	Lucile Packard Children's Hospital Stanford, Palo Alto, Calif.	69.1	3	4	37	1	18	4.4	No	90	20.2%
31	Johns Hopkins All Children's Hospital, St. Petersburg, Fla.	67.3	2	4	36	5	19	2.5	No	90	1.3%
32	Cohen Children's Medical Center, New Hyde Park, N.Y.	66.8	3	3	36	3	21	2.8	Yes	93	1.7%
33	Valley Children's Healthcare and Hospital, Madera, Calif.	66.5	2	3	37	5	20	2.9	Yes	89	0.8%
34	Phoenix Children's Hospital	66.3	3	5	36	3	28	2.9	No	88	0.7%
35	Nicklaus Children's Hospital, Miami	66.2	3	5	33	4	11	2.8	Yes	84	2.0%
36	Yale New Haven Children's Hospital, New Haven, Conn.	66.1	2	5	30	4	15	2.4	Yes	87	2.6%
37	Primary Children's Hospital, Salt Lake City	65.2	2	4	38	3	30	3.9	No	89	2.2%
38	Advocate Children's Hospital-Park Ridge, Ill.	64.9	3	4	27	5	11	2.4	Yes	84	0.9%
39	UF Health Shands Children's Hospital, Gainesville, Fla.	64.3	2	5	28	4	17	2.8	Yes	87	0.8%
40	Inova Children's Hospital, Falls Church, Va.	64.0	3	2	36	5	20	2.7	No	87	2.0%
41	Children's Mercy Kansas City, Mo.	63.9	2	3	37	3	26	4.1	Yes	93	6.0%
42	Florida Hospital for Children, Orlando	63.8	2	5	31	5	14	2.2	Yes	83	0.5%
43	Children's Hospital of Pittsburgh of UPMC	63.3	3	3	34	1	23	3.0	Yes	93	9.3%
44	Akron Children's Hospital, Ohio	62.2	2	3	31	5	16	3.2	Yes	89	1.3%
45	Le Bonheur Children's Hospital, Memphis, Tenn.	61.8	2	3	37	3	18	2.7	Yes	92	1.2%
45	University of Minnesota Masonic Children's Hospital, Minneapolis	61.8	3	5	30	3	17	3.1	No	88	1.2%
47	SSM Hlth. Cardinal Glennon Children's Hosp.-St. Louis U., St. Louis	61.6	2	4	36	4	17	3.0	No	86	1.6%
48	UCLA Mattel Children's Hospital, Los Angeles	61.4	3	5	30	2	11	4.3	Yes	88	4.9%
49	University of Iowa Stead Family Children's Hospital, Iowa City	61.3	2	5	30	5	21	2.9	Yes	78	4.3%
50	Cleveland Clinic Children's Hospital	60.4	2	3	36	3	12	2.9	Yes	90	1.5%

Terms are explained on Page 162.

Here, this is
MENDING A BROKEN HEART

With a dedication to research and innovation, Children's Hospital Colorado offers expert pediatric care and leading outcomes in congenital cardiothoracic surgery–like survival rates higher than the national average for the most complex heart surgeries. Still, Dr. Jeff Jacot and Dr. James Jaggers of the Heart Institute want kids to not only survive, but thrive. Using a 3D printing innovation, they're weaving a baby's own stem cells into synthetic patches used to reconstruct a variety of heart malformations. The goal is to create a structure that grows with the child over time, which means fewer pediatric heart surgeries along the way. For babies born with HLHS, the future is bright.

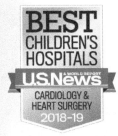
100%
Transplant
survival rate

500+
Heart surgeries
annually

50+
Cardiac trained
physicians

TOP 10%
For heart
surgery outcomes

Children's Hospital Colorado
Here, it's different.™

NEPHROLOGY

Rank	Hospital	U.S. News score	Kidney transplant survival score (24=best)	Biopsy complications prevention score (6=best)	Dialysis management score (12=best)	Infection prevention score, overall (60=best)	Infection prevention score, ICU (5=best)	Infection prevention score, dialysis (9=best)	Patient volume score (20=best)	Nurse-patient ratio (higher is better)	A Nurse Magnet hospital	% of specialists recommending hospital
1	Boston Children's Hospital	100.0	23	6	12	56	2	8	19	4.3	Yes	56.7%
2	Cincinnati Children's Hospital Medical Center	99.7	23	6	12	58	3	9	19	4.5	Yes	57.4%
3	Texas Children's Hospital, Houston	96.0	23	6	12	59	2	9	19	3.9	Yes	35.0%
4	Children's Hospital of Philadelphia	95.8	24	6	12	57	2	7	17	3.7	Yes	49.0%
5	Children's Mercy Kansas City, Mo.	92.9	24	6	12	59	2	9	20	4.4	Yes	25.1%
6	Children's National Medical Center, Washington, D.C.	90.3	23	6	12	58	5	8	19	3.5	Yes	9.1%
7	Children's Healthcare of Atlanta	90.1	23	6	12	58	3	8	19	4.6	No	26.2%
8	Seattle Children's Hospital	89.1	23	6	12	57	1	5	20	3.3	Yes	49.3%
9	Lucile Packard Children's Hospital Stanford, Palo Alto, Calif.	86.6	24	6	12	59	1	8	18	3.7	No	30.9%
10	Johns Hopkins Children's Center, Baltimore	86.4	23	6	12	58	2	8	13	3.2	Yes	18.5%
11	Nationwide Children's Hospital, Columbus, Ohio	85.0	22	5	11	58	2	8	17	3.4	Yes	22.9%
12	Ann and Robert H. Lurie Children's Hospital of Chicago	83.7	20	6	12	56	3	8	20	3.3	Yes	12.6%
12	UCLA Mattel Children's Hospital, Los Angeles	83.7	20	6	10	49	4	9	13	3.6	Yes	16.5%
14	UCSF Benioff Children's Hospitals, San Francisco and Oakland	82.7	22	6	11	57	3	9	14	3.9	Yes	7.4%
15	Children's Hospital of Pittsburgh of UPMC	81.1	24	6	12	55	3	6	15	3.4	Yes	9.6%
16	Children's Medical Center Dallas	80.3	24	6	10	53	2	9	17	3.1	Yes	8.3%
17	Duke Children's Hospital and Health Center, Durham, N.C.	80.0	24	6	12	59	5	8	15	3.2	Yes	4.4%
18	Children's Hospital Los Angeles	78.9	24	6	12	57	2	8	18	3.7	Yes	4.6%
19	C.S. Mott Children's Hospital-Michigan Medicine, Ann Arbor	78.5	23	4	12	55	4	6	12	3.7	Yes	11.5%
20	Levine Children's Hospital, Charlotte, N.C.	76.2	24	6	11	57	4	9	15	3.1	Yes	2.9%
21	St. Louis Children's Hospital-Washington University	76.0	23	5	12	58	4	7	14	3.6	Yes	4.8%
22	Children's Hospital of Wisconsin, Milwaukee	75.9	24	6	9	49	4	7	18	4.2	Yes	2.8%
23	Phoenix Children's Hospital	75.8	24	6	11	56	4	9	18	3.0	No	1.4%
24	Riley Hospital for Children at IU Health, Indianapolis	74.8	23	6	12	54	1	8	14	4.1	Yes	3.8%
25	Doernbecher Children's Hospital, Portland, Ore.	74.7	24	6	12	55	3	8	16	3.8	Yes	1.1%
26	Children's Hospital Colorado, Aurora	74.5	23	6	8	54	4	8	17	3.3	Yes	5.1%
27	Children's Hospital at Montefiore, New York	73.9	22	6	12	59	4	3	14	3.7	No	6.3%
28	University of Iowa Stead Family Children's Hospital, Iowa City	72.6	24	6	8	51	4	6	13	3.1	Yes	6.4%
29	MUSC Health-Children's Hospital, Charleston, S.C.	72.5	24	6	11	57	5	7	16	3.0	Yes	1.1%
30	Spectrum Hlth. Helen DeVos Children's Hosp., Grand Rapids, Mich.	72.0	24	6	12	53	3	8	15	3.7	Yes	0.8%
31	Nemours Alfred I. duPont Hosp. for Children, Wilmington, Del.	71.8	24	5	8	55	2	8	16	4.2	Yes	1.7%
31	NY-Presby. Morgan Stanley-Komansky Children's Hospital, N.Y.	71.8	23	6	12	56	3	7	20	3.2	No	3.2%
33	U. Minn. Masonic Children's Hosp.-Children's Minn., Minneapolis	70.7	22	6	12	52	2	6	14	3.7	No	5.3%
34	Rady Children's Hospital, San Diego	70.5	24	4	10	53	4	9	17	3.1	Yes	4.2%
35	University of California Davis Children's Hospital, Sacramento	70.2	20	6	11	57	3	6	11	5.4	Yes	1.5%
36	North Carolina Children's Hospital at UNC, Chapel Hill	69.8	24	6	12	56	0	8	12	4.9	Yes	1.9%
37	Children's Hospital of Michigan, Detroit	69.7	24	6	12	51	3	8	18	3.0	No	1.9%
38	Monroe Carell Jr. Children's Hosp. at Vanderbilt, Nashville, Tenn.	68.6	21	4	8	52	3	9	12	3.2	Yes	2.8%
39	Children's Hospital of Alabama at UAB, Birmingham	68.0	24	6	8	53	3	5	20	3.6	No	3.6%
40	Le Bonheur Children's Hospital, Memphis, Tenn.	67.3	22	5	8	57	2	7	15	3.1	Yes	4.7%
41	Children's Hospital of Richmond at VCU, Va.	67.1	16	6	12	46	4	8	14	2.2	Yes	0.9%
42	Arkansas Children's Hospital, Little Rock	67.0	21	6	11	54	4	9	9	3.3	Yes	0.9%
43	Rainbow Babies and Children's Hospital, Cleveland	66.3	19	6	12	54	3	7	18	2.7	Yes	0.7%
44	American Family Children's Hospital, Madison, Wis.	66.1	22	6	12	55	3	5	13	4.0	Yes	0.7%
45	Yale New Haven Children's Hospital, New Haven, Conn.	65.7	16	6	12	52	3	8	11	2.2	Yes	1.1%
46	Mount Sinai Kravis Children's Hospital, New York	65.3	22	6	8	54	1	8	9	3.8	Yes	3.0%
46	Penn State Children's Hospital, Hershey, Pa.	65.3	24	6	9	48	3	9	8	3.5	Yes	0.5%
48	Cohen Children's Medical Center, New Hyde Park, N.Y.	64.9	NR	6	12	57	3	8	13	3.4	Yes	0.6%
49	Cleveland Clinic Children's Hospital	64.7	10	6	10	57	3	8	13	3.4	Yes	1.8%
50	Johns Hopkins All Children's Hospital, St. Petersburg, Fla.	64.2	23	6	10	57	2	8	11	3.3	No	0.3%

NR=not reported. Terms are explained on Page 162.

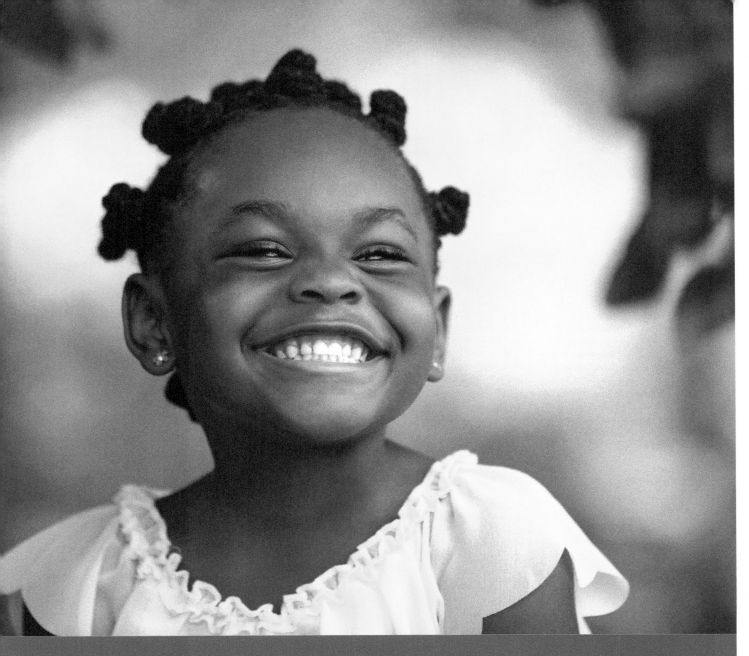

We have a history of transplant innovation.
So she can have a future full of promise.

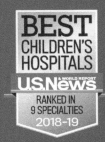

UPMC Children's Hospital of Pittsburgh has been at the forefront of pediatric transplant services since 1981. We are proud to be among the top centers in the nation for blood and marrow, heart, kidney, intestine, liver, and lung transplantation and cellular therapies. Our experience, expertise, and commitment to innovation and compassionate care are the reasons why. But what means the most to us is the hope we bring to our patients who are given a second chance at life. To learn more about our Transplant Services, visit CHP.edu/Transplant or call 412-692-3000.

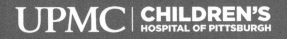

UPMC Children's Hospital of Pittsburgh is affiliated with the University of Pittsburgh School of Medicine and nationally ranked in nine clinical specialties by *U.S. News & World Report.*

NEUROLOGY & NEUROSURGERY

Rank	Hospital	U.S. News score	Surgical survival score (12=best)	Surgical complications prevention score (22=best)	Epilepsy management score (8=best)	Infection prevention score, overall (41=best)	Surgery volume score (42=best)	Nurse-patient ratio (higher is better)	A Nurse Magnet hospital	% of specialists recommending hospital
1	Boston Children's Hospital	100.0	12	22	8	37	39	4.3	Yes	61.3%
2	Cincinnati Children's Hospital Medical Center	95.0	12	21	8	40	37	4.5	Yes	29.6%
3	Texas Children's Hospital, Houston	94.9	12	20	8	40	39	3.9	Yes	34.5%
4	Johns Hopkins Children's Center, Baltimore	91.8	12	21	8	39	37	3.2	Yes	26.7%
5	Children's National Medical Center, Washington, D.C.	91.6	12	22	8	39	36	3.5	Yes	17.9%
6	Children's Hospital of Philadelphia	91.0	12	22	4	38	35	3.7	Yes	51.7%
7	Nationwide Children's Hospital, Columbus, Ohio	90.4	12	22	8	39	31	3.4	Yes	16.9%
8	St. Louis Children's Hospital-Washington University	87.5	12	19	7	39	36	3.6	Yes	22.6%
9	Children's Hospital Los Angeles	86.8	11	21	8	38	41	3.7	Yes	11.8%
10	Seattle Children's Hospital	85.9	12	20	7	38	28	3.3	Yes	22.8%
11	Nicklaus Children's Hospital, Miami	85.2	12	22	8	35	33	3.0	Yes	10.5%
12	Ann and Robert H. Lurie Children's Hospital of Chicago	84.9	12	22	6	36	39	3.3	Yes	16.8%
13	Children's Hospital Colorado, Aurora	83.6	10	16	8	37	37	3.3	Yes	21.1%
14	Children's Medical Center Dallas	82.6	12	22	7	38	40	3.1	Yes	4.7%
15	C.S. Mott Children's Hospital-Michigan Medicine, Ann Arbor	81.2	12	21	8	38	27	3.7	Yes	5.9%
16	Children's Hospital of Pittsburgh of UPMC	81.1	12	19	6	35	35	3.4	Yes	11.6%
17	NY-Presby. Morgan Stanley-Komansky Children's Hospital, N.Y.	80.8	12	22	8	37	27	3.2	No	7.7%
18	Primary Children's Hospital, Salt Lake City	80.7	12	20	7	40	31	4.2	No	8.9%
19	UCSF Benioff Children's Hospitals, San Francisco and Oakland	80.6	11	16	6	39	35	3.9	Yes	16.0%
20	Lucile Packard Children's Hospital Stanford, Palo Alto, Calif.	80.4	12	19	8	40	33	3.7	No	10.7%
21	Mayo Clinic Children's Center, Rochester, Minn.	79.8	12	16	8	37	28	4.0	Yes	6.5%
22	Rady Children's Hospital, San Diego	79.4	12	22	8	35	42	3.1	Yes	2.4%
23	UCLA Mattel Children's Hospital, Los Angeles	79.0	12	22	8	32	22	3.6	Yes	7.4%
24	Cleveland Clinic Children's Hospital	77.8	12	19	5	38	21	3.4	Yes	13.7%
25	Le Bonheur Children's Hospital, Memphis, Tenn.	76.9	12	15	7	39	28	3.1	Yes	6.6%
26	Children's Hospital at Montefiore, New York	76.6	12	21	6	40	27	3.7	No	4.8%
27	Cohen Children's Medical Center, New Hyde Park, N.Y.	76.5	12	22	6	38	31	3.4	Yes	2.4%
28	Phoenix Children's Hospital	76.0	12	19	7	37	40	3.0	No	3.6%
29	Cook Children's Medical Center, Fort Worth	75.8	12	21	8	35	31	3.9	Yes	2.1%
30	Monroe Carell Jr. Children's Hospital at Vanderbilt, Nashville, Tenn.	75.5	11	16	8	35	33	3.2	Yes	3.1%
31	Children's Mercy Kansas City, Mo.	75.0	10	16	8	39	28	4.4	Yes	2.6%
31	Riley Hospital for Children at IU Health, Indianapolis	75.0	12	18	6	36	38	4.1	Yes	2.9%
33	Mount Sinai Kravis Children's Hospital, New York	74.9	12	22	8	36	21	3.8	Yes	0.1%
34	Children's Hospital of Alabama at UAB, Birmingham	74.5	12	16	8	34	40	3.6	No	7.1%
35	Duke Children's Hospital and Health Center, Durham, N.C.	72.9	11	13	8	40	32	3.2	Yes	3.2%
36	Doernbecher Children's Hospital, Portland, Ore.	71.7	12	19	5	36	27	3.8	Yes	2.0%
37	Johns Hopkins All Children's Hospital, St. Petersburg, Fla.	70.2	12	21	7	38	29	3.3	No	0.8%
38	Children's Hospital of Wisconsin, Milwaukee	69.4	12	11	7	33	25	4.2	Yes	3.7%
39	CHOC Children's Hospital, Orange, Calif.	68.8	11	14	7	39	32	3.7	Yes	2.3%
39	Levine Children's Hospital, Charlotte, N.C.	68.8	11	20	6	38	26	3.1	Yes	0.8%
41	Children's Memorial Hermann Hospital, Houston	68.4	12	20	6	35	24	3.2	Yes	0.8%
41	University of Virginia Children's Hospital, Charlottesville	68.4	11	20	5	37	18	2.8	Yes	1.8%
43	Nemours Alfred I. duPont Hosp. for Children, Wilmington, Del.	68.3	12	11	8	38	18	4.2	Yes	0.4%
44	Akron Children's Hospital, Ohio	67.1	10	20	6	34	21	3.4	Yes	1.2%
45	Arkansas Children's Hospital, Little Rock	67.0	12	17	6	34	23	3.3	Yes	0.9%
46	Children's Healthcare of Atlanta	66.5	11	13	5	39	36	4.6	No	3.2%
47	Wolfson Children's Hospital, Jacksonville, Fla.	66.3	11	16	6	35	21	2.4	Yes	0.8%
48	Children's Hospital of Michigan, Detroit	65.9	12	13	8	31	23	3.0	No	0.5%
48	Yale New Haven Children's Hospital, New Haven, Conn.	65.9	12	20	5	33	19	2.2	Yes	1.0%
50	UF Health Shands Children's Hospital, Gainesville, Fla.	65.4	12	17	6	33	16	2.7	Yes	0.6%

Terms are explained on Page 162.

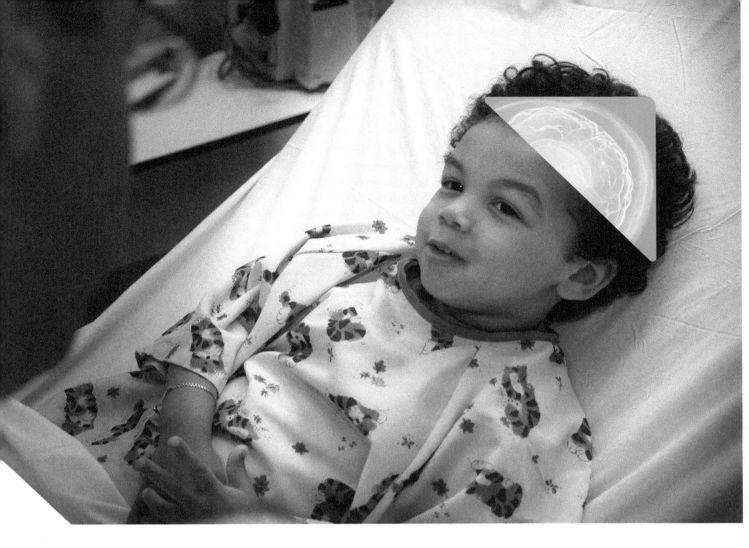

100% devoted to your child.

For the 12th consecutive year, Cohen Children's Medical Center was named one of the best children's hospitals in the nation with rankings in eight specialties: Diabetes/Endocrinology, Gastroenterology/GI Surgery, Neonatology, Nephrology, Neurology/Neurosurgery, Orthopedics, Pulmonology and Urology. That's because we're 100% devoted to raising the standard of pediatric care.

Northwell.edu/CCMC

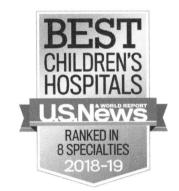

BEST CHILDREN'S HOSPITALS
U.S.News & WORLD REPORT
RANKED IN 8 SPECIALTIES
2018-19

Cohen Children's Medical Center
Northwell Health®

◤ **Look North**™

Our Partners
PUT THE MONEY
WHERE THE MIRACLES ARE.

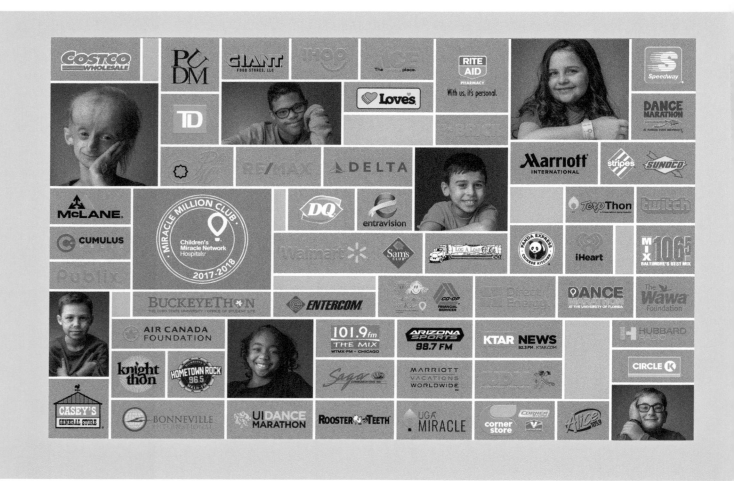

Thanks to all of our partners, we raised more than
$389 million last year for children's hospitals.

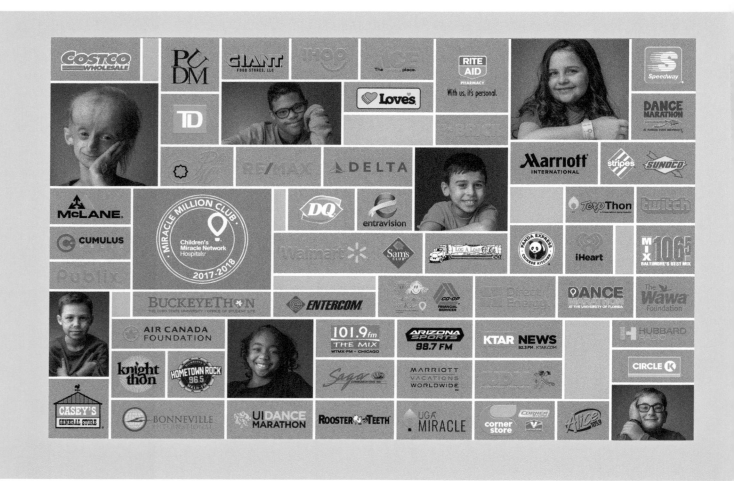

Children's
Miracle Network
Hospitals

CMNHospitals.org

Because these partners give,
Children's Miracle Network Hospitals® provide the best care for kids like JaKiah.

Thank you to our top corporate partners for raising funds that save and improve the lives of local kids. Their unsurpassed commitment to member children's hospitals across North America means the world to local kids and families. This year, our friends at **Walmart and Sam's Club** are nearing more than $1 Billion raised for CMN Hospitals since becoming a partner in 1987.

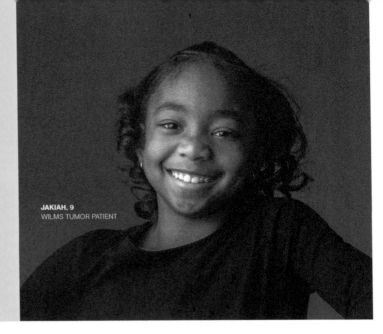

JAKIAH, 9
WILMS TUMOR PATIENT

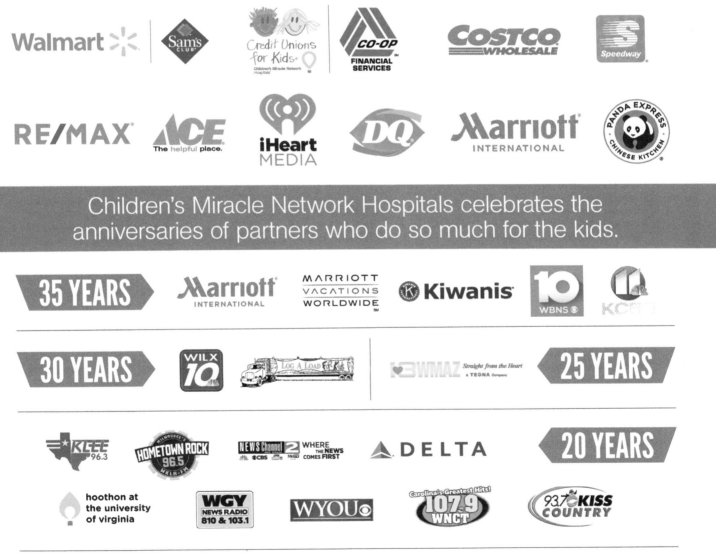

Children's Miracle Network Hospitals celebrates the anniversaries of partners who do so much for the kids.

35 YEARS — Marriott INTERNATIONAL · MARRIOTT VACATIONS WORLDWIDE · Kiwanis · 10 WBNS · KCR

30 YEARS — WILX 10 · LOG A LOAD

25 YEARS — WMAZ Straight from the Heart A TEGNA Company

20 YEARS — KFEE 96.3 · HOMETOWN ROCK 96.5 WKLH-FM · NEWS Channel 2 CBS WHERE THE NEWS COMES FIRST · DELTA

hoothon at the university of virginia · WGY NEWS RADIO 810 & 103.1 · WYOU · Carolina's Greatest Hits! 107.9 WNCT · 93.7 KISS COUNTRY

$1 BILLION —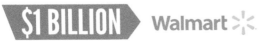

Walmart and Sam's Club are nearing more than $1 Billion raised for CMN Hospitals since becoming a partner in 1987.

UROLOGY

Rank	Hospital	U.S. News score	Surgical complications prevention score (18=best)	Testicular torsion care score (2=best)	Infection prevention score, overall (32=best)	Patient volume score (30=best)	Surgery volume score (22=best)	Minimally invasive volume score (9=best)	Nurse-patient ratio (higher is better)	A Nurse Magnet hospital	% of specialists recommending hospital
1	Children's Hospital of Philadelphia	100.0	16	2	29	30	22	9	3.7	Yes	74.3%
2	Cincinnati Children's Hospital Medical Center	99.1	18	2	31	27	20	8	4.5	Yes	44.7%
3	Boston Children's Hospital	96.8	15	2	28	28	22	9	3.9	Yes	36.3%
4	Texas Children's Hospital, Houston	93.6	15	2	31	29	20	9	3.3	Yes	39.6%
5	Ann and Robert H. Lurie Children's Hospital of Chicago	91.4	15	2	28	28	20	9	3.3	Yes	36.2%
6	Monroe Carell Jr. Children's Hospital at Vanderbilt, Nashville, Tenn.	91.1	16	2	28	28	20	8	3.2	Yes	20.2%
7	Johns Hopkins Children's Center, Baltimore	90.9	18	2	30	21	18	7	3.2	Yes	33.6%
8	Seattle Children's Hospital	89.7	15	2	29	21	18	8	3.3	Yes	49.4%
9	Riley Hospital for Children at IU Health, Indianapolis	88.7	13	2	27	26	21	9	4.1	Yes	19.1%
10	Nationwide Children's Hospital, Columbus, Ohio	87.3	15	2	30	27	20	9	3.4	Yes	12.9%
11	Children's Hospital Los Angeles	87.1	16	2	29	29	22	9	3.7	Yes	5.6%
12	Cohen Children's Medical Center, New Hyde Park, N.Y.	85.7	18	2	29	26	20	9	3.4	Yes	14.1%
13	Children's Medical Center Dallas	82.7	14	2	29	23	18	9	3.1	Yes	4.7%
14	Le Bonheur Children's Hospital, Memphis, Tenn.	78.8	15	2	30	22	17	8	3.1	Yes	1.6%
15	Children's Mercy Kansas City, Mo.	78.7	15	2	31	23	14	8	4.4	Yes	17.1%
16	Children's National Medical Center, Washington, D.C.	78.4	10	2	30	25	15	9	3.5	Yes	11.2%
17	Children's Hospital of Pittsburgh of UPMC	77.8	12	2	27	22	19	7	3.4	Yes	8.7%
18	Rady Children's Hospital, San Diego	77.5	15	2	26	27	13	6	3.1	Yes	4.5%
19	St. Louis Children's Hospital-Washington University	77.0	14	2	30	20	17	7	3.6	Yes	4.8%
20	CHOC Children's Hospital, Orange, Calif.	76.6	14	2	30	21	21	8	3.7	Yes	11.6%
21	Children's Hospital Colorado, Aurora	75.7	11	2	28	22	20	7	3.3	Yes	1.8%
22	North Carolina Children's Hospital at UNC, Chapel Hill	75.0	14	2	30	16	16	6	4.9	Yes	9.2%
23	Children's Healthcare of Atlanta	74.2	11	2	30	28	22	9	4.6	No	1.9%
24	Rainbow Babies and Children's Hospital, Cleveland	74.1	18	2	26	12	11	3	2.7	Yes	8.9%
25	UCSF Benioff Children's Hospitals, San Francisco and Oakland	73.9	15	1	30	26	20	8	3.9	Yes	4.2%
26	C.S. Mott Children's Hospital-Michigan Medicine, Ann Arbor	73.8	12	2	29	19	19	7	3.7	Yes	1.8%
27	Nemours Alfred I. duPont Hosp. for Children, Wilmington, Del.	73.7	13	2	29	21	17	8	4.2	Yes	2.7%
28	Doernbecher Children's Hospital, Portland, Ore.	73.6	15	2	27	17	13	7	3.8	Yes	2.3%
28	Phoenix Children's Hospital	73.6	15	2	29	28	19	6	3.0	No	4.9%
30	Yale-New Haven/Connecticut Children's Medical Ctrs., New Haven	73.3	15	2	24	19	15	5	2.2	Yes	6.6%
31	Mayo Clinic Children's Center, Rochester, Minn.	73.2	12	2	29	24	12	5	4.0	Yes	0.6%
31	OSF HealthCare Children's Hospital of Illinois, Peoria	73.2	17	2	31	12	13	5	4.6	Yes	1.1%
33	Mount Sinai Kravis Children's Hospital, New York	73.0	17	2	27	10	9	3	3.8	Yes	4.0%
34	Lucile Packard Children's Hospital Stanford, Palo Alto, Calif.	72.6	13	2	31	24	13	5	3.7	No	7.7%
35	Primary Children's Hospital, Salt Lake City	72.3	11	2	31	29	20	9	4.2	No	4.4%
36	Nicklaus Children's Hospital, Miami	71.9	13	2	26	16	19	9	3.0	Yes	3.0%
37	NY-Presby. Morgan Stanley-Komansky Children's Hospital, N.Y.	71.5	14	2	28	16	20	7	3.2	No	0.8%
38	Spectrum Hlth. Helen DeVos Children's Hosp., Grand Rapids, Mich.	69.8	16	2	25	15	12	5	3.7	Yes	2.3%
38	University of Virginia Children's Hospital, Charlottesville	69.8	15	2	28	12	10	4	2.8	Yes	4.4%
40	UCLA Mattel Children's Hospital, Los Angeles	69.4	13	2	23	11	10	3	3.6	Yes	2.4%
41	Akron Children's Hospital, Ohio	69.3	15	2	25	21	9	5	3.4	Yes	1.0%
42	Cleveland Clinic Children's Hospital	69.1	12	2	29	12	13	6	3.4	Yes	0.2%
42	West Virginia Univ. Children's Hospital, Morgantown	69.1	15	2	31	14	10	3	4.1	A Nurse	0.2%
44	Arnold Palmer Hospital for Children, Orlando	68.7	18	2	23	14	13	4	3.7	Yes	1.5%
45	American Family Children's Hospital, Madison, Wis.	68.6	13	2	28	14	11	4	4.0	Yes	0.6%
46	MassGeneral Hospital for Children, Boston	68.5	15	2	21	13	8	3	3.9	Yes	0.8%
47	Brenner Children's Hospital, Winston-Salem, N.C.	68.2	18	2	22	11	13	3	2.4	Yes	0.0%
48	Children's Hospital at Montefiore, New York	68.1	14	2	31	15	11	4	3.7	No	1.2%
49	UC Davis Children's Hospital/Shriners Hosps. N. Calif., Sacramento	67.5	13	2	29	17	9	5	5.4	Yes	0.7%
50	MUSC Health-Children's Hospital, Charleston, S.C.	66.7	13	2	29	16	13	3	3.0	Yes	

Terms are explained on Page 162.

WHERE THE MIRACLES ARE.

Because you give, Children's Miracle Network Hospitals® can provide the best care for kids.

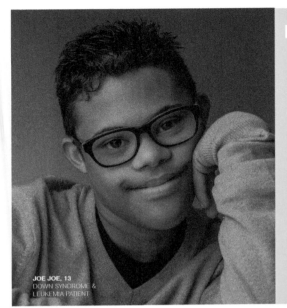

JOE JOE, 13
DOWN SYNDROME &
LEUKEMIA PATIENT

TOP 10

The top 10 *U.S. News* children's hospitals are all Children's Miracle Network Hospitals

1. Boston Children's Hospital, Boston, MA
2. Cincinnati Children's, Cincinnati, OH
3. Children's Hospital of Philadelphia, Philadelphia, PA
4. Texas Children's Hospital, Houston, TX
5. Children's National Health System, Washington, DC
6. Children's Hospital Los Angeles, Los Angeles, CA
7. Nationwide Children's Hospital, Columbus, OH
8. Johns Hopkins Children's Center, Baltimore, MD
9. Children's Hospital Colorado, Denver, CO
10. Ann and Robert H. Lurie Children's Hospital of Chicago, Chicago, IL

Coincidence? We think not.

Thanks to local donations, Children's Miracle Network Hospitals are able to provide the best care for kids. Congratulations to the following Children's Miracle Network Hospital members on being recognized among the best children's hospitals in the country.

Akron Children's Hospital, Akron, OH

Ann and Robert H. Lurie Children's Hospital of Chicago, Chicago, IL

Arkansas Children's Hospital, Little Rock, AR

Arnold Palmer Children's Hospital, Orlando, FL

Boston Children's Hospital, Boston, MA

Children's Healthcare of Atlanta, Atlanta, GA

Children's Hospital and Medical Center, Omaha, NE

Children's Hospital Colorado, Aurora, CO

Children's Hospital Los Angeles, Los Angeles, CA

Children's Hospital of Illinois, Peoria, IL

Children's Hospital of Philadelphia, Philadelphia, PA

Children's Hospital of Pittsburgh of UPMC, Pittsburgh, PA

Children's Hospital of Richmond at VCU, Richmond, VA

Children's Hospital of Wisconsin, Milwaukee, WI

Children's National Health System, Washington, DC

Children's of Alabama, Birmingham, AL

Children's Health Children's Medical Center, Dallas, TX

CHOC Children's, Orange, CA

Cincinnati Children's, Cincinnati, OH

Cohen Children's Medical Center of New York, New Hyde Park, NY

Connecticut Children's Medical Center, Hartford, CT

Cook Children's Medical Center, Fort Worth, TX

Dayton Children's Hospital, Dayton, OH

Duke Children's, Durham, NC

Golisano Children's Hospital at the University of Rochester Medical Center, Rochester, NY

Helen DeVos Children's Hospital, Grand Rapids, MI

Johns Hopkins All Children's Hospital, Tampa-St. Petersburg, FL

Johns Hopkins Children's Center, Baltimore, MD

Le Bonheur Children's Hospital, Memphis, TN

Levine Children's Hospital, Charlotte, NC

Medical University of South Carolina Shawn Jenkins Children's Hospital, Charleston, SC

Monroe Carell Jr. Children's Hospital at Vanderbilt, Nashville, TN

Nationwide Children's Hospital, Columbus, OH

Nicklaus Children's Hospital, Miami, FL

Norton Children's Hospital, Louisville, KY

OHSU Doernbecher Children's Hospital, Portland, OR

Penn State Children's Hospital, Hershey, PA

Phoenix Children's Hospital, Phoenix, AZ

Primary Children's Hospital, Salt Lake City, UT

Rady Children's Hospital-San Diego, San Diego, CA

Riley Hospital for Children, Indianapolis, IN

Seattle Children's Hospital, Seattle, WA

SSM Health Cardinal Glennon Children's Hospital, St. Louis, MO

St. Louis Children's Hospital, St. Louis, MO

Texas Children's Hospital, Houston, TX

UC Davis Children's Hospital, Sacramento, CA

UCSF Benioff Children's Hospitals, San Francisco, CA

UF Health Jacksonville & Wolfson Children's Hospital, Jacksonville, FL

UF Health Shands Children's Hospital, Gainesville, FL

University Hospitals Rainbow Babies & Children's Hospital, Cleveland, OH

University of Iowa Stead Family Children's Hospital, Iowa City, IA

University of Virginia Children's Hospital, Charlottesville, VA

Valley Children's Hospital, Madera, CA

WVU Medicine Children's, Charleston, WV

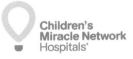

Children's Miracle Network Hospitals®

Give Today
to your children's hospital

CMNHospitals.org

RANKINGS LIKE *these* SPEAK FOR THEMSELVES

Keck Medicine of USC is proud to be ranked among the top three hospitals in Los Angeles and number seven in all of California. Our advanced care has been widely recognized for excellence, with high rankings in nine specialties.

BEST HOSPITALS
U.S. News & WORLD REPORT
NATIONAL
RANKED IN 9 SPECIALTIES
2018-19

BEST HOSPITALS U.S.News NATIONAL CANCER 2018-19

BEST HOSPITALS U.S.News NATIONAL CARDIOLOGY & HEART SURGERY 2018-19

BEST HOSPITALS U.S.News NATIONAL GERIATRICS 2018-19

BEST HOSPITALS U.S.News NATIONAL GYNECOLOGY 2018-19

BEST HOSPITALS U.S.News NATIONAL NEPHROLOGY 2018-19

BEST HOSPITALS U.S.News NATIONAL NEUROLOGY & NEUROSURGERY 2018-19

BEST HOSPITALS U.S.News NATIONAL OPHTHALMOLOGY 2018-19

BEST HOSPITALS U.S.News NATIONAL ORTHOPEDICS 2018-19

BEST HOSPITALS U.S.News NATIONAL UROLOGY 2018-19

MAGNET RECOGNIZED
AMERICAN NURSES CREDENTIALING CENTER

To learn more, visit KeckMedicine.org
For appointments, call: (800) USC-CARE

Keck Medicine of USC
BEYOND EXCEPTIONAL MEDICINE™

© 2018 Keck Medicine of USC

CHAPTER 6

Best Regional Hospitals

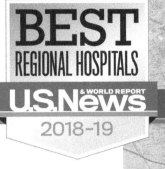

BEST REGIONAL HOSPITALS
U.S.News **& WORLD REPORT**
2018-19

Great Care Near Home

How we identified and ranked the top hospitals state by state

by **Ben Harder** *and* **Avery Comarow**

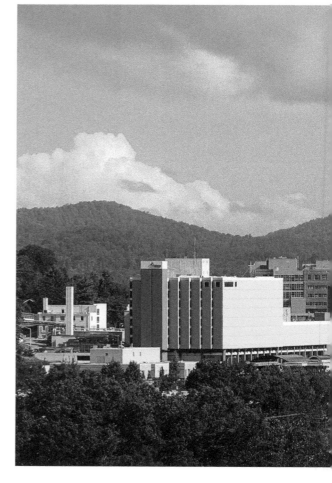

If you're like most people facing hospitalization, you would much prefer to stay close to home. You'll feel more comfortable, and lower stress can lead to faster recovery. Your family can visit without racking up hotel bills. And a battle with your health insurer over coverage at an out-of-network facility might be avoidable.

Since 2011, our Best Regional Hospitals listings have showcased hundreds of facilities around the U.S. that offer high-quality care across a range of clinical services. These services include both complex, highly specialized care for the sickest patients – the focus of the Best Hospitals rankings – and safe, effective treatment for those whose medical needs are more commonplace, such as patients seeking hip or knee replacement surgery for age-related arthritis. These state-by-state rankings, found in their entirety at usnews.com/bestregionalhospitals, offer readers in most parts of the country a number of high-quality choices that are apt to be convenient and in-network.

These evaluations include ratings of how well hospitals handle nine relatively common procedures and conditions in addition to their assessments in 12 specialties.* The nine areas of care are heart bypass surgery, aortic valve surgery, abdominal aortic aneurysm repair, heart failure, hip replacement, knee replacement, colon cancer surgery, lung cancer surgery and chronic obstructive pulmonary disease. Hospitals are assigned a rating of "high performing," "average" or "below average" in each area in which they treated enough patients to be evaluated.

Recognition as a 2018-19 Best Regional Hospital means a hospital was nationally ranked in at least one of the 12 Best Hospitals specialties that use objective data or that it earned at least three "high performing" ratings across the nine procedures and conditions and the 12 specialties. In the specialties, high performing signifies a score below those of

the nation's 50 top hospitals but within the highest 10 percent of hospitals that we evaluated. (An FAQ at usnews.com/best-hospitals offers more details.)

This year 520 hospitals merited Best Regional Hospitals status. They appear ranked by state on the following pages. In each state with at least two Best Regional Hospitals that met certain criteria, hospitals are numerically ordered according to the following rules:

1. The higher rank went to the hospital with the better status in the Best Hospitals Honor Roll ranking (Page 96), if any.

2. Next, the higher rank went to the hospital that earned more points according to the following three rules: (a) A hospital received two points for each of the 12 specialties in which it was ranked among the top 50. (b) A hospital received one point for each specialty, procedure or condition in which it was rated high performing. (c) A hospital lost one point for each procedure or condition in which it was rated below average.

Based on the same rules, hospitals in major met-

USNEWS.COM/BESTHOSPITALS

Visit usnews.com regularly while researching your health care choices, as U.S. News often adds content aimed at helping patients and families make the best possible decisions about their medical care. We also update the Best Hospitals, Best Children's Hospitals and Best Regional Hospitals data on the website when new data become available.

---

*Cancer; cardiology & heart surgery; diabetes & endocrinology; ear, nose & throat; gastroenterology & GI surgery; geriatrics; gynecology; nephrology; neurology & neurosurgery; orthopedics; pulmonology; and urology.

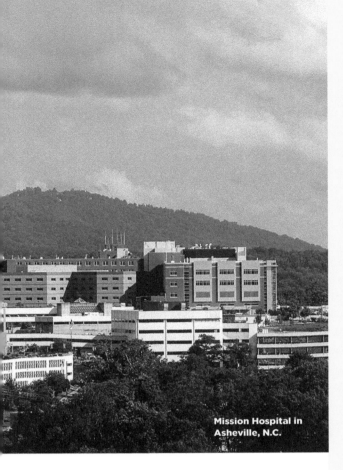

Mission Hospital in Asheville, N.C.

Tops at Routine Care

U.S. News evaluated more than 4,500 hospitals for their handling of two chronic conditions – chronic obstructive pulmonary disease and heart failure – and seven surgical procedures: colon cancer surgery, lung cancer surgery, heart bypass surgery, aortic valve surgery, abdominal aortic aneurysm repair, knee replacement and hip replacement. Of that total, 1,129 hospitals earned at least one top rating of "high performing." But only these 29 standouts, less than 1 percent of the hospitals evaluated, got the top rating in all nine procedures and conditions:

- **Abbott Northwestern Hospital,** Minneapolis

- **Aurora St. Luke's Medical Center,** Milwaukee

- **Cedars-Sinai Medical Center,** Los Angeles

- **CHI Memorial Hospital,** Chattanooga, Tenn.

- **Christiana Care Hospitals,** Newark, Del.

- **Cleveland Clinic**

- **Cleveland Clinic Florida,** Weston

- **El Camino Hospital,** Mountain View, Calif.

- **Florida Hospital,** Orlando

- **Hoag Memorial Hospital Presbyterian,** Newport Beach, Calif.

- **Houston Methodist Hospital**

- **John Muir Medical Center,** Concord, Calif.

- **Massachusetts General Hospital,** Boston

- **Mayo Clinic,** Rochester, Minn.

- **Mayo Clinic-Phoenix**

- **Mission Hospital,** Asheville, N.C.

- **Morton Plant Hospital,** Clearwater, Fla.

- **Northeast Georgia Medical Center,** Gainesville

- **NorthShore University Health-Evanston Hospital,** Evanston, Ill.

- **Northwestern Memorial Hospital,** Chicago

- **NYU Langone Hospitals,** New York

- **Orlando Regional Medical Center**

- **Scripps La Jolla Hospitals,** La Jolla, Calif.

- **St. Cloud Hospital,** St. Cloud, Minn.

- **St. Luke's Regional Medical Center,** Boise, Idaho

- **Stanford Health Care-Stanford Hospital,** Stanford, Calif.

- **Sutter Medical Center,** Sacramento, Calif.

- **University of Michigan Hospitals-Michigan Medicine,** Ann Arbor

- **UPMC Presbyterian Shadyside,** Pittsburgh

ropolitan areas also received rankings that compare them to other top hospitals in the same metropolis. Our website displays these rankings for 49 metro areas with at least 1 million residents. The website also lists top hospitals in more than 100 U.S. News-defined regions, such as Southern Indiana and Texas' Hill Country, to help consumers outside the biggest urban centers searching for high-quality care.

How a hospital performed in four specialties – ophthalmology, psychiatry, rehabilitation and rheumatology – is not a factor in the regional rankings. That these specialties are important is undeniable. But objective data on which to compare hospitals' performance are either not available or do not meet our rigorous analytical standards.

Consequently, some hospitals that excel in one or more of those specialties may not appear among the Best Regional Hospitals. Specialty hospitals such as dedicated cancer centers and surgical hospitals also were not considered in the regional rankings. Specialty hospitals have indisputable but narrow value; such a hospital might only do surgery, say, or only treat heart patients. Our goal with the state and metro area rankings is to identify general medical-surgical hospitals that offer both high-quality care and breadth of care, so only hospitals that deliver a wide range of clinical services for adult patients were considered for Best Regional Hospitals status.

Children's hospitals are excluded from consideration in the regional rankings because so few metro areas have more than one or two. There are fewer than 200 in the entire country. ●

COMPLEX SPECIALTY CARE

COMMON PROCEDURES & CONDITIONS

COMPLEX SPECIALTY CARE
- ● Nationally ranked
- ● High performing

COMMON PROCEDURES & CONDITIONS
- ● High performing
- ● Average
- ● Below average

Complex Specialty Care columns: Cancer · Cardiology & Heart Surgery · Diabetes & Endocrinology · Ear, Nose & Throat · Gastroenterology & GI Surgery · Geriatrics · Gynecology · Nephrology · Neurology & Neurosurgery · Orthopedics · Pulmonology · Urology

Common Procedures & Conditions columns: Colon Cancer Surgery · Lung Cancer Surgery · Heart Bypass Surgery · Heart Failure · Heart Valve Surgery · Abdominal Aortic Aneurysm · Hip Replacement · Knee Replacement · COPD

State Rank Hospital

ALABAMA
Rank	Hospital	City
1	University of Alabama at Birmingham Hospital	Birmingham
2	Huntsville Hospital	Huntsville
3	Mobile Infirmary Medical Center	Mobile
3	St. Vincent's Birmingham Hospital	Birmingham

ARIZONA
Rank	Hospital	City
1	Mayo Clinic-Phoenix	
2	Banner University Medical Center Phoenix	
3	Banner University Medical Center Tucson	
4	Banner Boswell Medical Center	Sun City
4	Flagstaff Medical Center	Flagstaff
4	St. Joseph's Hospital and Medical Center	Phoenix
7	Banner Estrella Medical Center	Phoenix
8	Banner Baywood Medical Center	Mesa
8	Chandler Regional Medical Center	Chandler
8	HonorHealth Scottsdale Shea Medical Center	Scottsdale
11	HonorHealth Deer Valley Medical Center	Phoenix
11	HonorHealth Scottsdale Thompson Peak Medical Center	Scottsdale
11	TMC Healthcare-Tucson	
14	Banner Desert Medical Center	Mesa
14	HonorHealth Scottsdale Osborn Medical Center	Scottsdale

ARKANSAS
Rank	Hospital	City
–	CHI St. Vincent Infirmary	Little Rock

CALIFORNIA
Rank	Hospital	City
1	UCSF Medical Center	San Francisco
2	UCLA Medical Center	Los Angeles[1]
3	Cedars-Sinai Medical Center	Los Angeles[2]
4	Stanford Health Care-Stanford Hospital	Stanford
5	University of California, Davis Medical Center	Sacramento
6	Scripps La Jolla Hospitals	La Jolla
7	Keck Hospital of USC	Los Angeles[3]
8	Hoag Memorial Hospital Presbyterian	Newport Beach[4]
9	UC San Diego Health-Jacobs Medical Center[5]	
10	Huntington Memorial Hospital	Pasadena
11	UC Irvine Medical Center	Orange
12	John Muir Health-Concord Medical Center	Concord
12	Mission Hospital	Orange
14	John Muir Health-Walnut Creek Medical Center	Walnut Creek
14	MemorialCare Long Beach Medical Center	Long Beach
16	El Camino Hospital	Mountain View
16	St. Jude Medical Center	Fullerton
16	Sutter Medical Center	Sacramento
19	Loma Linda University Medical Center	Loma Linda
19	Sharp Memorial Hospital	San Diego
21	Orange Coast Memorial Medical Center	Fountain Valley
21	St. Joseph Hospital	Orange

In complex care specialties, (-) indicates hospital is not nationally ranked or high performing.

In procedures and conditions, (-) indicates care not offered or hospital has too few Medicare patients to be rated.

A footnote indicates that another hospital's results are included, that the hospital has a different name in one or more areas of care, or both. [1]Santa Monica-UCLA Medical Center and Orthopedic Hospital. [2]Smidt Heart Institute at Cedars-Sinai. [3]USC Norris Cancer Hospital-Keck Medical Center of USC. [4]Hoag Orthopedic Institute. [5]UC San Diego Health-Moores Cancer Center.

More @ usnews.com/bestregionalhospitals

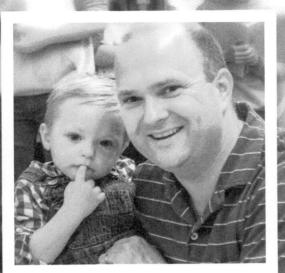
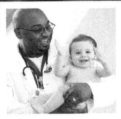
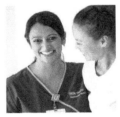
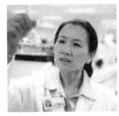
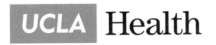
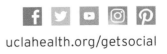

COMPLEX SPECIALTY CARE
- Nationally ranked
- High performing

COMMON PROCEDURES & CONDITIONS
- High performing
- Average
- Below average

COMPLEX SPECIALTY CARE   COMMON PROCEDURES & CONDITIONS

State Rank	Hospital	CANCER	CARDIOLOGY & HEART SURGERY	DIABETES & ENDOCRINOLOGY	EAR, NOSE & THROAT	GASTROENTEROLOGY & GI SURGERY	GERIATRICS	GYNECOLOGY	NEPHROLOGY	NEUROLOGY & NEUROSURGERY	ORTHOPEDICS	PULMONOLOGY	UROLOGY	COLON CANCER SURGERY	LUNG CANCER SURGERY	HEART BYPASS SURGERY	HEART FAILURE	HEART VALVE SURGERY	ABDOMINAL AORTIC ANEURYSM	HIP REPLACEMENT	KNEE REPLACEMENT	COPD
CALIFORNIA (CONTINUED)																						
21	**Torrance Memorial Medical Center,** Torrance	–	–	–	–	–	–	–	–	–	–	●	●	●	●	●	●	●	●	●	●	●
24	**Eisenhower Medical Center,** Rancho Mirage	–	–	–	–	–	–	–	–	–	–	●	●	●	●	●	●	●	●	●	●	●
24	**Kaiser Permanente Los Angeles Medical Center**	–	–	–	–	●	–	●	–	–	–	●	●	●	●	●	●	●	●	●	●	●
24	**Providence Little Company of Mary Medical Center Torrance**	–	–	●	–	–	–	–	●	–	–	●	●	●	●	●	●	●	●	●	●	●
24	**Sequoia Hospital,** Redwood City	–	–	–	–	–	–	–	–	–	–	●	●	●	●	●	●	●	●	●	●	●
28	**Adventist Health-Glendale,** Los Angeles	–	–	–	–	–	–	–	–	–	–	●	●	●	●	●	●	●	●	●	●	●
28	**Kaiser Permanente Santa Clara Medical Center,** Santa Clara	–	–	–	–	–	–	–	–	–	–	●	●	●	●	●	●	●	●	●	●	●
30	**California Pacific Medical Center,** San Francisco	–	–	–	–	●	–	–	–	–	–	●	●	●	●	●	●	●	●	●	●	●
30	**PIH Health Hospital-Whittier**	–	–	–	–	–	–	–	–	–	–	●	●	●	●	●	●	●	●	●	●	●
30	**Providence St. Joseph Medical Center,** Burbank	–	–	–	–	–	–	–	–	–	–	●	●	●	●	●	●	●	●	●	●	●
30	**Sharp Grossmont Hospital,** La Mesa	–	–	–	–	–	–	–	–	–	–	●	●	●	●	●	●	●	●	●	●	●
34	**Community Hospital of the Monterey Peninsula,** Monterey	–	–	–	–	–	–	–	–	–	–	●	●	●	●	●	●	●	●	●	●	●
34	**Enloe Medical Center,** Chico	–	–	–	–	–	–	–	–	–	–	●	●	●	●	●	●	●	●	●	●	●
34	**Kaiser Permanente Downey Medical Center,** Downey	●	–	–	–	–	–	–	–	●	–	●	–	●	●	●	–	●	●	●	●	●
34	**Mercy General Hospital,** Sacramento	–	–	–	–	–	–	–	–	–	–	●	●	–	●	●	●	●	●	●	●	●
34	**Mercy San Juan Medical Center,** Carmichael	–	–	–	–	–	–	–	–	–	–	●	●	●	●	●	●	●	●	●	●	●
34	**Oroville Hospital,** Oroville	–	–	●	–	●	–	–	–	–	–	●	–	–	●	–	–	●	●	–	–	–
34	**Providence Holy Cross Medical Center,** Mission Hills	–	–	–	–	●	–	–	–	●	–	●	●	●	●	●	●	●	●	●	●	●
34	**Providence St. John's Health Center,** Santa Monica	–	–	–	–	–	–	–	–	–	–	●	●	●	●	●	●	●	●	●	●	●
34	**Sharp Chula Vista Medical Center,** Chula Vista	–	–	●	–	–	–	–	–	–	–	●	●	●	●	●	●	●	●	●	●	●
43	**Alta Bates Summit Medical Center,** Oakland	–	–	–	–	–	–	–	–	–	–	●	●	●	–	●	●	●	●	●	●	●
43	**Eden Medical Center,** Castro Valley	–	–	–	–	–	–	–	–	–	–	●	●	●	●	●	–	●	●	●	●	●
43	**Glendale Memorial Hospital and Health Center,** Glendale	–	–	–	–	–	–	–	–	–	–	●	●	●	●	●	●	●	●	●	●	●
43	**Kaiser Permanente Fontana and Ontario Medical Centers,** Fontana	–	–	–	–	–	–	–	–	–	–	●	●	●	●	●	–	●	●	–	–	●
43	**Kaiser Permanente Riverside Medical Center,** Riverside	–	–	–	–	–	–	–	–	–	–	●	●	–	–	●	–	●	●	●	●	●
43	**Kaiser Permanente San Jose Medical Center,** San Jose	–	–	–	–	●	–	–	–	–	–	●	●	–	●	●	●	●	●	–	–	●
43	**Kaiser Permanente South Bay Medical Center,** Harbor City	–	–	–	–	–	–	–	–	–	–	●	●	●	●	●	●	●	●	–	●	●
43	**Kaiser Permanente South San Francisco Med. Ctr.,** South San Francisco	–	–	–	–	–	–	–	–	–	–	●	●	●	●	●	●	●	●	●	●	●
43	**Kaiser Permanente Woodland Hills Medical Center,** Woodland Hills	–	–	–	–	–	–	–	●	–	●	●	–	●	●	●	●	●	●	●	●	–
43	**Memorial Medical Center,** Modesto	–	–	–	–	–	–	–	–	–	–	●	●	●	●	●	●	●	●	●	●	●
43	**Mills-Peninsula Health Services-Burlingame**	–	–	–	–	–	–	–	–	–	–	●	●	●	●	●	●	●	●	●	●	●
43	**Providence Tarzana Medical Center,** Tarzana	–	–	–	–	●	–	–	–	–	–	●	●	●	●	●	●	●	●	●	●	●
43	**Santa Rosa Memorial Hospital,** Santa Rosa	–	–	–	–	–	–	–	–	–	–	●	●	●	●	●	●	●	●	●	●	●
43	**Scripps Mercy Hospital,** San Diego	–	–	–	–	●	–	–	–	–	–	●	●	●	●	●	●	●	●	●	●	●
43	**St. Agnes Medical Center,** Fresno	–	–	–	–	–	–	–	–	–	–	●	●	●	●	●	●	●	●	●	●	●
43	**St. Helena Hospital Napa Valley,** St. Helena	–	–	–	–	–	–	–	–	–	–	●	●	●	●	●	●	●	●	●	●	●
43	**Sutter Roseville Medical Center,** Roseville	–	–	–	–	–	–	–	–	–	–	●	●	●	–	●	–	●	●	●	●	●
43	**Sutter Santa Rosa Regional Hospital,** Santa Rosa	–	–	–	–	–	–	–	–	●	–	●	●	●	●	●	●	–	●	●	●	●
61	**Fountain Valley Regional Hosp. and Medical Ctr.,** Fountain Valley	–	–	–	–	●	–	–	–	–	–	●	●	●	●	●	●	●	●	●	●	●
62	**Washington Hospital,** Fremont	–	–	–	–	–	–	–	–	–	–	●	●	●	●	●	●	●	●	●	●	●
COLORADO																						
1	**University of Colorado Hospital,** Aurora[6]	●	●	●	–	●	●	●	●	●	●	●	●	●	●	●	●	●	●	●	●	●
2	**Porter Adventist Hospital,** Denver	–	–	–	●	–	–	–	–	●	–	●	●	●	●	●	●	●	●	●	●	●
3	**Parker Adventist Hospital,** Parker	–	–	–	–	–	●	–	–	●	●	●	–	–	●	●	●	●	●	●	●	●
4	**Rose Medical Center,** Denver	–	–	–	–	–	●	–	–	●	●	●	●	●	●	●	●	●	●	●	●	●

In complex care specialties, (-) indicates hospital is not nationally ranked or high performing.
In procedures and conditions, (-) indicates care not offered or hospital has too few Medicare patients to be rated.

A footnote indicates that another hospital's results are included, that the hospital has a different name in one or more areas of care, or both.
[6]National Jewish Health, Denver-University of Colorado Hospital.

More @ usnews.com/bestregionalhospitals

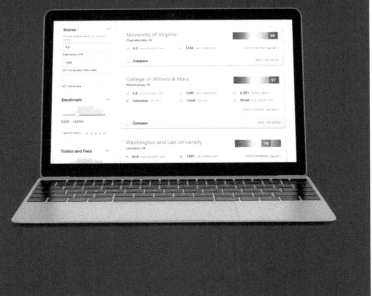
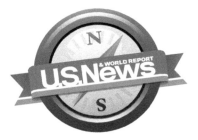

COMPLEX SPECIALTY CARE
- ● Nationally ranked
- ● High performing

COMMON PROCEDURES & CONDITIONS
- ● High performing
- ● Average
- ● Below average

In complex care specialties, (-) indicates hospital is not nationally ranked or high performing.
In procedures and conditions, (-) indicates care not offered or hospital has too few Medicare patients to be rated.

State Rank	Hospital	CANCER	CARDIOLOGY & HEART SURGERY	DIABETES & ENDOCRINOLOGY	EAR, NOSE & THROAT	GASTROENTEROLOGY & GI SURGERY	GERIATRICS	GYNECOLOGY	NEPHROLOGY	NEUROLOGY & NEUROSURGERY	ORTHOPEDICS	PULMONOLOGY	UROLOGY	COLON CANCER SURGERY	LUNG CANCER SURGERY	HEART BYPASS SURGERY	HEART FAILURE	HEART VALVE SURGERY	ABDOMINAL AORTIC ANEURYSM	HIP REPLACEMENT	KNEE REPLACEMENT	COPD
	COLORADO (CONTINUED)																					
5	UCHealth Medical Center of the Rockies, Loveland	–	–	–	–	–	–	–	–	–	●	–	–	●	●	●	●	●	●	●	●	●
6	Medical Center of Aurora	–	–	●	–	●	–	–	–	–	–	●	–	●	●	●	●	●	●	●	●	●
6	Penrose-St. Francis Health Services-Colorado Springs	–	–	–	–	–	–	–	–	●	–	●	–	●	●	●	●	●	●	●	●	●
6	Sky Ridge Medical Center, Lone Tree	–	–	–	–	–	–	–	●	–	●	●	–	●	●	–	●	●	–	●	●	●
6	SCL Health-Saint Joseph Hospital, Denver	–	–	–	–	–	–	–	–	–	–	●	–	●	●	●	●	●	●	●	●	●
10	UCHealth Poudre Valley Hospital, Fort Collins	–	–	–	●	–	–	–	–	–	–	●	–	●	●	–	●	●	–	●	●	●
10	St. Mary's Hospital and Medical Center, Grand Junction	–	–	–	–	–	–	–	–	–	–	●	–	●	●	●	●	●	●	●	●	●
12	Swedish Medical Center, Englewood	–	–	–	–	–	–	●	–	–	–	–	–	●	●	●	●	●	●	●	●	●
	CONNECTICUT																					
1	Yale New Haven Hospital, New Haven[7]	●	●	●	●	●	●	–	●	●	●	●	●	●	●	●	●	●	●	●	●	●
2	Hartford Hospital, Hartford	–	–	–	–	–	–	–	●	–	–	●	–	●	●	●	●	●	●	●	●	●
3	St. Francis Hospital and Medical Center, Hartford	–	–	–	–	–	–	–	–	–	–	●	–	●	●	●	●	●	●	●	●	●
	DELAWARE																					
1	Christiana Care Hospitals, Newark	–	–	–	●	–	●	–	–	–	–	●	–	●	●	●	●	●	●	●	●	●
2	Bayhealth Kent General Hospital, Dover	–	–	–	–	–	–	–	–	–	–	●	–	●	●	●	●	●	●	●	●	●
	FLORIDA																					
1	Mayo Clinic Jacksonville	●	●	–	–	●	●	–	●	●	●	●	●	●	●	●	●	●	●	●	●	●
2	Tampa General Hospital	–	●	●	–	●	●	●	●	●	●	●	–	●	●	●	●	●	●	●	●	●
2	UF Health Shands Hospital, Gainesville	●	●	●	–	●	●	–	●	●	●	●	●	●	●	●	●	●	●	●	●	●
4	Cleveland Clinic Florida, Weston	●	–	–	–	●	●	–	–	●	–	●	–	●	●	●	●	●	●	●	●	●
5	Florida Hospital, Orlando	–	–	●	–	–	●	–	–	●	–	●	–	●	●	●	●	●	●	●	●	●
6	Baptist Hospital of Miami[8]	–	–	–	–	●	–	–	–	●	–	●	–	●	●	●	●	●	●	●	●	●
7	Baptist Medical Center Jacksonville	–	–	–	–	●	–	–	–	●	–	●	–	●	●	●	●	●	●	●	●	●
8	Morton Plant Hospital, Clearwater	–	–	–	–	–	–	–	–	–	–	●	–	●	●	●	●	●	●	●	●	●
8	Orlando Regional Medical Center	–	–	–	–	–	–	–	–	–	–	●	–	●	●	●	●	●	●	●	●	●
10	Sarasota Memorial Hospital, Sarasota	–	–	–	–	–	–	–	–	–	–	●	–	●	●	●	●	●	●	●	●	●
11	NCH Downtown Naples Hospital, Naples	–	–	–	–	–	–	–	–	–	–	●	–	●	●	●	●	●	●	●	●	●
12	Lee Memorial Hospital, Fort Myers	–	–	–	–	–	–	–	–	–	–	●	–	●	●	●	●	●	●	●	●	●
13	Boca Raton Regional Hospital, Boca Raton	–	–	–	–	–	–	–	–	–	–	●	–	●	●	●	●	●	●	●	●	●
13	Flagler Hospital, St. Augustine	–	–	●	–	–	–	–	–	–	–	●	–	●	●	●	●	●	●	●	●	●
13	Holy Cross Hospital, Fort Lauderdale	–	–	–	–	–	–	–	–	–	–	●	–	●	●	●	●	●	●	●	●	●
13	Memorial Regional Hospital, Hollywood	–	–	–	–	–	–	–	–	–	–	●	–	●	●	●	●	●	●	●	●	●
13	Mount Sinai Medical Center, Miami Beach	–	–	–	–	●	–	–	–	–	–	●	–	●	●	●	●	●	●	●	●	●
13	St. Joseph's Hospital, Tampa	–	–	–	–	–	–	–	–	–	–	●	–	●	●	●	●	●	●	●	●	●
13	University of Miami Hospital and Clinics-UHealth Tower	–	–	–	●	–	–	–	–	–	–	●	–	●	●	●	●	●	●	●	●	●
20	Memorial Hospital West, Pembroke Pines	–	–	–	–	–	–	–	–	–	–	●	–	●	●	–	●	–	–	●	●	●
20	Munroe Regional Medical Center, Ocala	–	–	–	–	–	–	–	–	–	–	●	–	●	●	●	●	●	●	●	●	●
22	Florida Hospital Waterman, Tavares	–	–	–	–	–	–	–	–	–	–	●	–	●	–	●	●	●	●	●	●	●
22	Health First Holmes Regional Medical Center, Melbourne	–	–	–	–	–	–	–	–	–	–	●	–	●	●	●	●	●	●	●	●	●
22	Lakeland Regional Health, Lakeland	–	–	–	–	–	–	–	–	–	–	●	–	●	●	●	●	●	●	●	●	●
22	Mease Countryside Hospital, Safety Harbor	–	–	–	–	–	–	–	–	–	–	●	–	●	●	–	●	–	●	●	●	●
22	UF Health Jacksonville	–	–	●	–	–	–	●	–	●	–	●	–	●	●	●	●	●	●	●	●	●
27	North Florida Regional Medical Center, Gainesville	–	–	–	–	–	–	–	–	–	–	●	–	●	●	●	●	●	●	●	●	●

A footnote indicates that another hospital's results are included, that the hospital has a different name in one or more areas of care, or both.
[7]Smilow Cancer Center at Yale New Haven. [8]Miami Cancer Institute, Baptist Hospital of Miami; Miami Cardiac & Vascular Institute; Baptist Health Neuroscience Center; Miami Orthopedics & Sports Medicine Institute.

More @ usnews.com/bestregionalhospitals

COMPLEX SPECIALTY CARE
- ● Nationally ranked
- ● High performing

COMMON PROCEDURES & CONDITIONS
- ● High performing
- ● Average
- ● Below average

Legend columns (left to right): CANCER · CARDIOLOGY & HEART SURGERY · DIABETES & ENDOCRINOLOGY · EAR, NOSE & THROAT · GASTROENTEROLOGY & GI SURGERY · GERIATRICS · GYNECOLOGY · NEPHROLOGY · NEUROLOGY & NEUROSURGERY · ORTHOPEDICS · PULMONOLOGY · UROLOGY · COLON CANCER SURGERY · LUNG CANCER SURGERY · HEART BYPASS SURGERY · HEART FAILURE · HEART VALVE SURGERY · ABDOMINAL AORTIC ANEURYSM · HIP REPLACEMENT · KNEE REPLACEMENT · COPD

State Rank / Hospital	Can	Card	Diab	ENT	Gast	Ger	Gyn	Neph	Neur	Orth	Pulm	Uro	Colon	Lung	Bypass	HF	Valve	AAA	Hip	Knee	COPD
FLORIDA (CONTINUED)																					
27 St. Vincent's Medical Center Riverside, Jacksonville	–	–	–	–	–	–	–	–	–	–	–	–	●	●	●	●	●	●	●	●	●
27 Winter Haven Hospital, Winter Haven	–	–	–	–	–	–	–	–	–	–	–	–	●	●	●	●	●	●	●	●	●
30 Ocala Regional Medical Center, Ocala	–	–	–	–	–	–	–	–	–	–	–	–	●	●	●	●	●	●	●	●	●
GEORGIA																					
1 Emory University Hospital, Atlanta[9]	●	–	–	–	●	●	–	●	●	●	–	●	●	●	●	●	●	●	●	●	●
2 Emory St. Joseph's Hospital, Atlanta	–	–	–	–	●	●	–	●	●	●	–	–	●	●	●	●	●	●	●	●	●
3 Northeast Georgia Medical Center, Gainesville	–	–	–	–	–	–	–	–	–	–	–	–	●	●	●	●	●	●	●	●	●
3 Piedmont Atlanta Hospital[10]	–	–	–	–	●	–	–	–	–	–	–	–	●	●	●	●	●	●	●	●	●
5 WellStar Kennestone Hospital, Marietta	–	–	–	–	–	–	–	–	–	–	–	–	●	●	●	●	●	●	●	●	●
6 University Hospital, Augusta	–	–	–	–	–	–	–	–	–	–	–	–	●	●	●	●	●	●	●	●	●
7 Gwinnett Medical Center, Lawrenceville	–	–	–	–	–	–	–	–	–	–	–	–	●	●	●	●	●	●	●	●	●
7 Northside Hospital-Forsyth, Cumming	–	–	–	–	–	–	–	–	–	–	–	–	●	●	●	●	●	–	●	●	●
7 Piedmont Athens Regional Medical Center, Athens	–	–	–	–	–	–	–	–	–	–	–	–	●	●	●	●	●	●	●	●	●
10 Emory University Hospital Midtown, Atlanta	–	–	–	–	–	–	–	–	–	–	–	–	●	●	●	●	●	●	●	●	●
10 Memorial Health University Medical Center, Savannah	–	–	–	–	–	–	–	–	–	–	–	–	●	●	●	●	●	●	●	●	●
10 Navicent Health Medical Center, Macon	–	–	–	–	–	–	–	–	–	–	–	–	●	●	●	●	●	●	●	●	●
10 Northside Hospital, Atlanta	–	–	–	–	–	–	–	–	–	–	–	–	●	●	●	●	●	●	●	●	●
14 St. Joseph's Hospital, Savannah	–	–	–	–	–	–	–	–	–	–	–	–	●	●	●	●	●	●	●	●	●
HAWAII																					
1 Queen's Medical Center, Honolulu	●	–	●	–	●	–	●	–	●	●	●	●	●	●	●	●	●	●	●	●	●
2 Straub Medical Center, Honolulu	–	–	–	–	–	–	–	–	–	●	●	●	●	●	●	●	●	●	●	●	●
3 Kaiser Permanente Moanalua Medical Center, Honolulu	–	–	–	–	–	–	–	–	–	–	●	●	●	●	●	●	●	●	–	●	●
IDAHO																					
1 St. Luke's Regional Medical Center, Boise	–	–	●	–	–	–	–	–	–	●	●	●	●	●	●	●	●	●	●	●	●
2 Kootenai Health-Coeur D'Alene	–	–	–	–	–	–	–	–	–	●	●	●	●	●	●	●	●	●	●	●	●
ILLINOIS																					
1 Northwestern Memorial Hospital, Chicago	●	●	●	●	●	●	●	●	●	●	●	●	●	●	●	●	●	●	●	●	●
2 Rush University Medical Center, Chicago	●	●	●	●	●	●	●	●	●	●	●	●	●	●	●	●	●	●	●	●	●
3 Loyola University Medical Center, Maywood	●	●	–	●	●	●	●	●	●	●	●	●	●	●	●	●	●	●	●	●	●
4 Advocate Christ Medical Center, Oak Lawn	–	●	●	●	●	●	●	●	●	●	●	●	●	●	●	●	●	●	●	●	●
4 University of Chicago Medical Center	●	–	●	–	●	●	●	●	●	–	●	●	●	●	●	●	●	●	●	●	●
6 OSF Healthcare St. Francis Medical Center, Peoria	–	–	●	●	●	●	●	●	●	●	●	●	●	●	●	●	●	●	●	●	●
7 NorthShore University Health-Evanston Hospital, Evanston	–	–	●	●	●	●	●	●	●	●	●	●	●	●	●	●	●	●	●	●	●
7 Northwestern Medicine Central DuPage Hospital, Winfield	–	–	●	●	●	–	●	●	●	●	●	●	●	●	●	●	●	●	●	●	●
9 Advocate Good Samaritan Hospital, Downers Grove	–	–	–	●	●	–	–	–	●	●	●	●	●	●	●	●	●	●	●	●	●
10 Advocate Lutheran General Hospital, Park Ridge	●	–	●	●	●	●	●	●	●	●	●	●	●	●	●	●	●	●	●	●	●
10 Advocate Sherman Hospital, Elgin	–	–	●	–	●	–	–	–	●	●	●	●	●	●	●	●	●	●	●	●	●
12 Edward Hospital, Naperville[11]	–	–	●	–	●	●	–	–	–	●	●	●	●	●	●	●	●	●	●	●	●
13 Advocate Condell Medical Center, Libertyville	–	–	–	●	–	●	–	–	–	●	●	●	●	●	●	●	●	●	●	●	●
13 Carle Foundation Hospital, Urbana	–	–	●	–	●	–	–	–	●	●	●	●	●	●	●	●	●	●	●	●	●
13 Memorial Medical Center, Springfield	–	–	–	–	●	–	–	–	–	–	●	●	●	●	●	●	●	●	●	●	●
16 Amita Health Adventist Medical Center-Hinsdale	–	–	–	●	●	–	–	–	–	●	●	●	●	●	●	●	●	–	●	●	●
16 Northwestern Medicine Delnor Hospital, Geneva	–	–	–	●	●	–	–	–	–	–	●	●	●	●	●	–	●	–	●	●	●
16 Northwestern Medicine Lake Forest Hospital, Lake Forest	–	–	–	–	●	●	–	–	●	●	●	–	●	●	●	–	●	●	●	●	●
19 Centegra Hospital-McHenry	–	–	–	–	●	–	–	●	●	●	●	●	●	●	●	●	●	●	●	●	●

In complex care specialties, (-) indicates hospital is not nationally ranked or high performing.
In procedures and conditions, (-) indicates care not offered or hospital has too few Medicare patients to be rated.

[9]Emory Wesley Woods Geriatric Hospital. [10]Piedmont Heart Institute at Piedmont Atlanta Hospital. [11]Edward Cancer Center; Edward Heart Hospital.

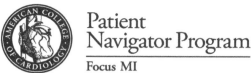

Patient Navigator Program
Focus MI

THE TEAM THAT
NAVIGATES
YOUR PATIENTS HOME

Open to all Chest Pain – MI Registry™ hospitals, the **Patient Navigator Program: Focus MI** leverages evidence-based best practices to improve the care and outcomes of acute myocardial infarction (AMI) patients and further reduce avoidable readmissions beyond 30 days.

Diplomat Hospitals are a key component of the Patient Navigator Program: Focus MI. Fifteen hospitals that participated in the first phase of the Patient Navigator Program are now focusing on reducing 90-day readmissions for AMI patients and providing mentorship for wider adoption of the program across other institutions.

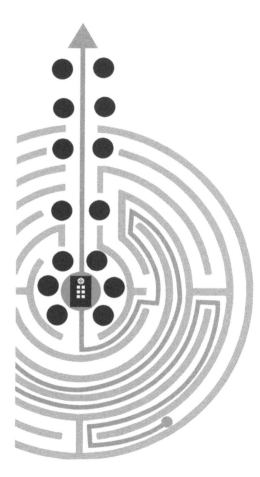

CONGRATULATIONS

to the **15 Diplomat Hospitals** for being on the cutting edge of identifying best practices!

HOSPITAL NAME	CITY	STATE
Advocate Sherman Hospital	Elgin	IL
Aurora BayCare Medical Center	Green Bay	WI
Barnes Jewish Hospital	St. Louis	MO
California Pacific Medical Center	San Francisco	CA
Centra Lynchburg General Hospital	Lynchburg	VA
Indian River Medical Center	Vero Beach	FL
Indiana University Health Methodist Hospital	Indianapolis	IN
Olathe Medical Center	Olathe	KS
Scott & White Medical Center-Temple	Temple	TX
St. Vincent's Medical Center	Bridgeport	CT
Trident Medical Center	Charleston	SC
UT Southwestern Medical Center	Dallas	TX
Western Maryland Regional Medical Center	Cumberland	MD
Tacoma General Hospital	Tacoma	WA
WakeMed	Raleigh	NC

Founding Sponsor:

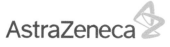

Learn more and join today at
CVQuality.ACC.org/PatientNavigator

CONGRATULATIONS

to the **first 60 hospitals** to join the Patient Navigator Program: Focus MI!

HOSPITAL NAME	CITY	STATE
Advocate Sherman Hospital	Elgin	IL
Aurora BayCare Medical Center	Green Bay	WI
Barnes Jewish Hospital	St. Louis	MO
California Pacific Medical Center	San Francisco	CA
Centra Lynchburg General Hospital	Lynchburg	VA
Indian River Medical Center	Vero Beach	FL
Indiana University Health Methodist Hospital	Indianapolis	IN
Olathe Medical Center	Olathe	KS
Scott & White Medical Center-Temple	Temple	TX
St. Vincent's Medical Center	Bridgeport	CT
Trident Medical Center	Charleston	SC
UT Southwestern Medical Center	Dallas	TX
Western Maryland Regional Medical Center	Cumberland	MD
Tacoma General Hospital	Tacoma	WA
WakeMed	Raleigh	NC
UW Health	Madison	WI
Providence Medford Medical Center	Medford	OR
Saint Luke's East Hospital	Lee's Summit	MO
Menorah Medical Center	Overland Park	KS
Mease Countryside Hospital	Safety Harbor	FL
Baylor Scott & White All Saints Medical Center-Fort Worth	Fort Worth	TX
Vanderbilt University Medical Center	Nashville	TN
Baylor Jack and Jane Hamilton Heart and Vascular Hospital	Dallas	TX
Doylestown Hospital	Doylestown	PA
El Camino Hospital	Mountain View	CA
Moses H. Cone Memorial Hospital	Greensboro	NC
Saint Luke's North Hospital - Barry Road	Kansas City	MO
Via Christi Hospitals Wichita	Wichita	KS

HOSPITAL NAME	CITY	STATE
St. Rose Hospital	Hayward	CA
OSF HealthCare Saint Francis Medical Center	Peoria	IL
Alamance Regional Medical Center	Burlington	NC
Mercy Medical Center-Des Moines	Des Moines	IA
Saint Luke's Hospital of Kansas City	Kansas City	MO
University of Chicago Hospitals	Chicago	IL
University of Kentucky	Lexington	KY
Mercy Hospital Joplin	Joplin	MO
OakBend Medical Center	Richmond	TX
Sanford Medical Center Bismarck	Bismarck	ND
Mercy Medical Center	Canton	OH
Hays Medical Center	Hays	KS
Presbyterian Healthcare Services	Albuquerque	NM
North Memorial Medical Center	Robbinsdale	MN
UCH-Memorial Hospital	Colorado Springs	CO
Seton Medical Center Austin	Austin	TX
The Toledo Hospital	Toledo	OH
Monongalia General Hospital	Morgantown	WV
McAllen Heart Hospital	McAllen	TX
Methodist West Houston Hospital	Houston	TX
Summa Health System - Akron Campus	Akron	OH
Carolinas Medical Center	Charlotte	NC
Freeman Health System	Joplin	MO
The MetroHealth System	Cleveland	OH
Hardin Memorial Hospital	Elizabethtown	KY
St. Anthony Hospital	Lakewood	CO
Conemaugh Memorial Medical Center	Johnstown	PA
North Vista Hospital	North Las Vegas	NV
South GA Medical Center	Valdosta	GA
Spotsylvania Regional Medical Center (HCA)	Fredericksburg	VA
Jewish Hospital	Louisville	KY

COMPLEX SPECIALTY CARE
- ● Nationally ranked
- ● High performing

COMMON PROCEDURES & CONDITIONS
- ● High performing
- ● Average
- ● Below average

Legend key areas: COMPLEX SPECIALTY CARE | COMMON PROCEDURES & CONDITIONS

State Rank Hospital	CANCER	CARDIOLOGY & HEART SURGERY	DIABETES & ENDOCRINOLOGY	EAR, NOSE & THROAT	GASTROENTEROLOGY & GI SURGERY	GERIATRICS	GYNECOLOGY	NEPHROLOGY	NEUROLOGY & NEUROSURGERY	ORTHOPEDICS	PULMONOLOGY	UROLOGY	COLON CANCER SURGERY	LUNG CANCER SURGERY	HEART BYPASS SURGERY	HEART FAILURE	HEART VALVE SURGERY	ABDOMINAL AORTIC ANEURYSM	HIP REPLACEMENT	KNEE REPLACEMENT	COPD
ILLINOIS (CONTINUED)																					
19 Memorial Hospital, Belleville	–	–	–	–	–	–	–	–	–	–	–	–	●	●	●	●	●	●	●	●	●
19 Northwest Community Hospital, Arlington Heights	–	–	–	–	●	–	–	–	–	–	–	–	●	●	●	●	●	●	●	●	●
19 Palos Community Hospital, Palos Heights	–	–	–	–	–	–	–	–	–	–	–	–	●	●	●	●	●	●	●	●	●
19 St. John's Hospital, Springfield	–	–	–	–	–	–	–	–	–	–	–	–	●	●	●	●	●	●	●	●	●
19 UnityPoint Health-Peoria	–	–	–	–	–	–	–	–	–	–	–	–	●	●	●	●	●	●	●	●	●
25 Advocate BroMenn Medical Center, Normal	–	–	–	–	–	–	–	–	–	●	–	–	●	–	●	●	●	–	●	●	●
25 Advocate Good Shepherd Hospital, Barrington	–	–	–	–	–	–	–	–	–	–	–	–	●	●	●	●	●	●	●	●	●
25 Advocate Illinois Masonic Medical Center, Chicago	–	–	–	–	–	–	–	–	–	●	–	–	●	●	●	●	●	●	●	●	●
25 Amita Health Elk Grove Village	–	–	–	–	–	–	–	–	–	–	–	–	●	●	●	●	●	●	●	●	●
25 Decatur Memorial Hospital, Decatur	–	–	–	–	–	–	–	–	–	–	–	–	●	●	●	●	●	●	●	●	●
INDIANA																					
1 Indiana University Health Medical Center, Indianapolis	●	●	●	–	●	●	–	●	●	●	●	●	●	●	●	●	●	●	●	●	●
2 Deaconess Hospital, Evansville	–	–	–	–	–	–	–	–	–	–	–	–	●	●	●	●	●	●	●	●	●
3 Indiana University Health North Hospital, Carmel	–	–	–	–	–	–	–	–	–	–	–	–	●	●	●	●	●	●	●	●	●
3 Indiana University Health West Hospital, Avon	–	–	–	–	–	–	–	–	–	–	–	–	●	–	●	●	–	●	●	●	●
3 St. Vincent Medical Center of Evansville	–	–	–	–	–	–	–	–	–	–	–	–	●	●	●	●	●	●	●	●	●
6 Community Hospital, Munster	–	–	–	–	–	–	–	–	–	–	–	–	●	●	●	●	⬤	●	●	●	●
6 Franciscan St. Francis Health-Indianapolis	–	–	–	–	–	–	–	–	–	–	–	–	●	●	●	●	●	●	●	●	●
6 Memorial Hospital of South Bend	–	–	–	–	–	–	–	–	–	–	–	–	●	●	●	●	●	●	●	●	●
6 Mishawaka Medical Center, Mishawaka	–	–	–	–	–	–	–	–	–	–	–	–	●	●	●	●	●	●	●	●	●
6 St. Vincent Indianapolis Hospital	–	–	–	–	–	–	–	–	–	–	–	–	●	●	●	●	●	●	●	●	●
11 Parkview Regional Medical Center, Fort Wayne	–	–	–	–	–	–	–	–	–	–	–	–	⬤	●	●	●	●	●	●	●	●
IOWA																					
1 University of Iowa Hospitals and Clinics, Iowa City	●	–	–	●	●	●	●	●	●	●	●	●	●	●	●	●	●	●	●	●	●
2 Mercy Medical Center-Des Moines	–	–	–	–	●	–	–	–	–	–	–	–	●	●	●	●	●	●	●	●	●
3 UnityPoint Health-St. Luke's Hospital, Cedar Rapids	–	–	–	–	●	–	–	–	–	–	–	–	●	●	●	●	●	●	●	●	●
4 UnityPoint Health-Iowa Methodist Medical Center, Des Moines	–	–	–	–	●	–	–	–	–	–	–	–	●	●	●	●	●	●	●	●	●
5 Genesis Medical Center-Davenport-West Central Park, Davenport	–	–	–	–	–	–	–	–	–	–	–	–	●	⬤	●	⬤	●	●	●	●	●
KANSAS																					
1 University of Kansas Hospital, Kansas City	●	●	●	–	●	●	–	●	●	●	●	●	●	●	●	●	●	●	●	●	●
2 Stormont Vail Hospital, Topeka	–	–	–	–	–	–	–	–	–	●	–	–	●	●	●	●	●	●	●	●	●
3 Via Christi Hospital on St. Francis, Wichita	–	–	–	●	–	–	–	–	–	–	–	–	●	●	●	●	●	●	●	●	●
KENTUCKY																					
1 University of Kentucky Albert B. Chandler Hospital, Lexington	●	–	●	●	–	●	–	●	●	●	●	●	●	●	●	●	●	●	●	●	●
2 Baptist Health Lexington	–	–	–	–	–	–	–	–	–	–	–	–	●	●	●	●	●	●	●	●	●
3 Baptist Health Louisville	–	–	–	–	–	–	–	–	–	–	–	–	●	●	●	●	●	●	●	●	●
4 Norton Hospital, Louisville	–	–	–	–	–	–	–	–	–	–	–	–	●	●	●	●	●	●	●	●	●
4 St. Elizabeth Healthcare Edgewood-Covington Hospitals, Edgewood	–	–	–	–	–	–	–	–	–	–	–	–	●	●	●	●	●	●	●	●	●
6 Jewish Hospital, Louisville	–	–	–	–	–	–	–	–	–	–	–	–	●	●	●	●	●	●	●	●	●
LOUISIANA																					
1 Ochsner Medical Center, New Orleans	●	–	–	●	●	●	–	●	●	●	●	●	●	●	●	●	●	●	●	●	●
2 Willis-Knighton Medical Center, Shreveport	–	–	●	–	–	–	–	–	–	–	–	–	●	●	●	●	●	●	●	●	●
3 Our Lady of the Lake Regional Medical Center, Baton Rouge	–	–	–	–	–	–	–	–	–	–	–	–	●	●	●	●	●	●	●	●	●
4 East Jefferson General Hospital, Metairie	–	–	–	–	–	–	–	–	–	–	–	–	●	●	●	●	●	●	●	●	●
4 Lafayette General Medical Center, Lafayette	–	–	–	–	–	–	–	–	–	–	–	–	●	●	●	●	●	●	●	●	●

In complex care specialties, (-) indicates hospital is not nationally ranked or high performing.
In procedures and conditions, (-) indicates care not offered or hospital has too few Medicare patients to be rated.

COMPLEX SPECIALTY CARE
- ● Nationally ranked
- ○ High performing

COMMON PROCEDURES & CONDITIONS
- ○ High performing
- ○ Average
- ● Below average

State Rank Hospital	CANCER	CARDIOLOGY & HEART SURGERY	DIABETES & ENDOCRINOLOGY	EAR, NOSE & THROAT	GASTROENTEROLOGY & GI SURGERY	GERIATRICS	GYNECOLOGY	NEPHROLOGY	NEUROLOGY & NEUROSURGERY	ORTHOPEDICS	PULMONOLOGY	UROLOGY	COLON CANCER SURGERY	LUNG CANCER SURGERY	HEART BYPASS SURGERY	HEART FAILURE	HEART VALVE SURGERY	ABDOMINAL AORTIC ANEURYSM	HIP REPLACEMENT	KNEE REPLACEMENT	COPD
MAINE																					
1 Maine Medical Center, Portland	-	-	-	-	-	-	-	-	-	-	-	-	●	●	●	●	●	●	●	●	●
2 Eastern Maine Medical Center, Bangor	-	-	-	-	-	-	-	-	-	-	-	-	●	●	●	●	●	●	●	●	●
3 Mercy Hospital of Portland	-	-	-	-	-	-	-	-	-	-	-	-	●	●	●	●	-	-	●	●	●
MARYLAND																					
1 Johns Hopkins Hospital, Baltimore	●	●	●	●	●	●	●	●	●	●	●	●	●	●	●	●	●	●	-	-	●
2 University of Maryland Medical Center, Baltimore	●	-	●	●	●	●	-	●	●	●	●	●	●	●	●	●	●	●	●	●	●
3 MedStar Union Memorial Hospital, Baltimore	-	-	-	-	-	-	-	-	-	●	-	-	●	●	●	●	●	●	●	●	●
3 University of Maryland St. Joseph Medical Center, Towson	-	-	-	-	-	-	-	-	-	●	-	-	●	●	●	●	●	●	●	●	●
5 Mercy Medical Center, Baltimore	-	-	-	-	-	-	-	●	-	●	-	-	●	●	-	●	-	●	●	●	●
6 Anne Arundel Medical Center, Annapolis	-	-	-	-	-	-	●	-	-	●	●	-	●	●	-	●	-	●	●	●	●
6 Johns Hopkins Bayview Medical Center, Baltimore	-	-	-	-	-	●	-	●	-	●	●	-	●	●	-	●	-	●	●	●	●
6 MedStar Good Samaritan Hospital, Baltimore	-	-	-	-	-	-	-	●	-	●	●	-	●	●	-	●	-	●	●	●	●
6 U. of Maryland Baltimore Washington Medical Center, Glen Burnie	-	-	-	-	-	-	-	-	-	●	●	-	●	●	●	●	-	●	●	●	●
10 Greater Baltimore Medical Center	-	-	-	-	-	-	-	-	-	●	-	-	●	●	-	●	-	●	●	●	●
10 Holy Cross Hospital, Silver Spring	-	-	-	-	-	-	-	-	-	●	-	-	●	●	-	●	-	●	●	●	●
10 MedStar Franklin Square Medical Center, Baltimore	-	-	-	-	-	-	-	-	-	●	-	-	●	●	-	●	-	●	●	●	●
10 Peninsula Regional Medical Center, Salisbury	-	-	-	-	-	-	-	-	-	●	-	-	●	●	●	●	-	●	●	●	●
10 Sinai Hospital of Baltimore	-	-	-	-	-	-	-	-	-	●	-	-	●	●	●	●	-	●	●	●	●
10 University of Maryland Shore Medical Center at Easton	-	-	-	-	-	-	-	-	-	●	-	-	●	-	-	●	-	-	●	●	●
16 Suburban Hospital, Bethesda	-	-	-	-	-	-	-	●	-	●	●	-	●	●	●	●	●	●	●	●	●
MASSACHUSETTS																					
1 Massachusetts General Hospital, Boston[12]	●	●	●	●	●	●	●	●	●	●	●	●	●	●	●	●	●	●	●	●	●
2 Brigham and Women's Hospital, Boston[13]	●	●	●	-	●	●	●	●	●	●	●	●	●	●	●	●	●	●	●	●	●
3 Baystate Medical Center, Springfield	-	-	-	-	-	-	-	●	-	●	●	-	●	●	●	●	●	●	●	●	●
3 Beth Israel Deaconess Medical Center, Boston	●	-	●	-	●	●	-	●	●	●	●	●	●	●	●	●	●	●	●	●	●
5 Lahey Hospital and Medical Center, Burlington	-	-	●	-	●	-	-	●	●	●	●	●	●	●	●	●	●	●	●	●	●
5 Tufts Medical Center, Boston	-	-	-	-	-	-	-	●	-	●	●	-	●	●	●	●	●	●	●	●	●
5 UMass Memorial Medical Center, Worcester	-	-	-	-	-	-	-	●	-	●	●	-	●	●	●	●	●	●	●	●	●
8 Boston Medical Center	-	-	-	-	●	-	●	-	-	-	●	-	●	●	●	●	●	●	●	●	●
9 Southcoast Charlton Memorial Hospital, Fall River	-	-	-	-	-	-	-	-	-	●	-	-	●	●	-	●	-	●	●	●	●
MICHIGAN																					
1 University of Michigan Hospitals-Michigan Medicine, Ann Arbor	●	●	●	●	●	●	●	●	●	●	●	●	●	●	●	●	●	●	●	●	●
2 Beaumont Hospital-Royal Oak	-	●	●	-	●	●	-	●	●	●	●	●	●	●	●	●	●	●	●	●	●
3 Beaumont Hospital-Troy	-	●	●	●	●	●	-	●	-	●	●	●	●	●	●	●	●	●	●	●	●
4 Spectrum Health-Butterworth and Blodgett Campuses, Grand Rapids	-	-	●	-	●	●	-	-	-	●	●	-	●	●	●	●	●	●	●	●	●
5 DMC Harper University Hospital, Detroit	-	-	●	-	●	●	-	●	●	●	●	-	●	●	●	●	●	●	●	●	●
6 Ascension Providence Hospital-Southfield	-	-	-	-	●	-	-	-	●	●	-	-	●	●	●	●	●	-	●	●	●
7 Munson Medical Center, Traverse City	-	-	-	-	-	-	-	●	-	●	●	-	●	●	●	●	●	●	●	●	●
8 Henry Ford Hospital, Detroit	●	-	-	●	-	-	●	●	●	-	●	●	●	●	●	●	●	●	●	●	●
9 Bronson Methodist Hospital, Kalamazoo	-	-	-	-	-	-	-	-	-	●	●	-	●	●	●	●	●	●	●	●	●
9 McLaren Northern Michigan Hospital, Petoskey	-	-	-	-	-	-	-	-	-	●	-	-	●	●	●	●	●	●	●	●	●
9 St. Joseph Mercy Ann Arbor Hospital, Ypsilanti	-	-	-	-	-	-	-	-	-	●	●	-	●	●	●	●	●	●	●	●	●
12 Beaumont Hospital-Grosse Pointe	-	-	-	-	●	-	-	●	●	●	-	-	●	●	-	●	-	●	●	●	●
12 Mercy Health St. Mary's Campus, Grand Rapids	-	-	-	-	-	-	●	-	-	●	-	-	●	●	-	●	-	●	●	●	●

In complex care specialties, (-) indicates hospital is not nationally ranked or high performing.
In procedures and conditions, (-) indicates care not offered or hospital has too few Medicare patients to be rated.

A footnote indicates that another hospital's results are included, that the hospital has a different name in one or more areas of care, or both.
[12]Massachusetts Eye and Ear Infirmary, Massachusetts General Hospital. [13]Dana-Farber/Brigham and Women's Cancer Center.

More @ usnews.com/bestregionalhospitals

COMPLEX SPECIALTY CARE
- ● Nationally ranked
- ● High performing

COMMON PROCEDURES & CONDITIONS
- ● High performing
- ● Average
- ● Below average

State Rank Hospital	Cancer	Cardiology & Heart Surgery	Diabetes & Endocrinology	Ear, Nose & Throat	Gastroenterology & GI Surgery	Geriatrics	Gynecology	Nephrology	Neurology & Neurosurgery	Orthopedics	Pulmonology	Urology	Colon Cancer Surgery	Lung Cancer Surgery	Heart Bypass Surgery	Heart Failure	Heart Valve Surgery	Abdominal Aortic Aneurysm	Hip Replacement	Knee Replacement	COPD
MICHIGAN (CONTINUED)																					
14 **Borgess Medical Center,** Kalamazoo	−	−	−	−	−	−	−	−	−	−	−	−	●	●	●	●	●	●	●	●	●
14 **Ascension St. John Hospital,** Detroit	−	−	−	−	−	−	−	−	−	−	−	−	●	●	●	●	●	●	●	●	●
16 **Beaumont Hospital-Dearborn**	−	−	−	−	−	−	−	−	−	−	−	−	●	●	●	●	●	●	●	●	●
16 **MidMichigan Medical Center-Midland**	−	−	−	−	−	−	−	−	−	−	−	−	●	●	●	●	●	●	●	●	●
16 **Sparrow Hospital,** Lansing	−	−	−	−	−	−	−	−	−	−	−	−	●	●	●	●	●	●	●	●	●
16 **St. Joseph Mercy Oakland Hospital,** Pontiac	−	−	−	−	−	−	−	−	−	−	−	−	●	●	●	●	●	●	●	●	●
20 **McLaren Flint Hospital,** Flint	−	−	−	−	−	−	−	−	−	−	−	−	●	●	●	●	●	●	●	●	●
21 **DMC-Sinai-Grace Hospital,** Detroit	−	−	−	−	−	−	−	−	−	−	−	−	●	●	●	●	−	−	●	●	●
MINNESOTA																					
1 **Mayo Clinic,** Rochester	●	●	●	●	●	●	●	●	●	●	●	●	●	●	●	●	●	●	●	●	●
2 **Abbott Northwestern Hospital,** Minneapolis[14]	−	●	●	−	●	●	●	●	●	●	●	●	●	●	●	●	●	●	●	●	●
3 **St. Cloud Hospital,** St. Cloud	−	●	●	−	●	●	−	●	●	●	●	●	●	●	●	●	●	●	●	●	●
4 **Mercy Hospital,** Coon Rapids	−	−	−	−	●	●	−	●	●	●	●	●	●	●	●	●	●	●	●	●	●
4 **University of Minnesota Medical Center,** Minneapolis	●	−	●	−	●	●	−	●	●	●	●	●	●	●	●	●	●	●	●	●	●
6 **United Hospital,** St. Paul	−	−	−	−	−	−	●	−	−	●	●	●	●	●	●	●	●	●	●	●	●
7 **Fairview Southdale Hospital,** Edina	−	−	−	−	−	−	−	−	−	●	●	●	●	●	●	●	●	●	●	●	●
7 **Park Nicollet Methodist Hospital,** St. Louis Park	−	−	−	−	−	−	−	−	−	●	●	●	●	●	●	●	●	●	●	●	●
9 **Essentia Health-St. Mary's Medical Center,** Duluth	−	−	−	−	−	−	−	−	−	●	●	●	●	●	●	●	●	●	●	●	●
9 **Regions Hospital,** St. Paul	−	−	−	−	−	−	−	−	−	−	●	●	●	●	●	●	●	●	●	●	●
11 **Fairview Ridges Hospital,** Burnsville	−	−	−	−	−	−	−	−	−	●	●	●	●	●	−	●	−	−	●	●	●
11 **Maple Grove Hospital,** Maple Grove	−	−	−	−	−	−	−	−	−	●	●	●	●	●	−	●	−	−	●	●	●
13 **North Memorial Medical Center,** Robbinsdale	−	−	−	−	−	−	−	−	−	−	−	●	●	●	●	●	●	●	●	●	●
13 **St. John's Hospital,** Maplewood	−	−	−	●	−	−	−	−	−	−	●	●	●	●	●	●	●	●	●	●	●
MISSISSIPPI																					
1 **Mississippi Baptist Medical Center,** Jackson	−	−	−	−	−	−	−	−	−	−	−	−	●	●	●	●	●	●	●	●	●
2 **North Mississippi Medical Center-Tupelo**	−	−	−	−	−	−	−	−	−	−	−	−	●	●	●	●	●	●	●	●	●
MISSOURI																					
1 **Barnes-Jewish Hospital,** St. Louis[15]	●	●	●	●	●	●	●	●	●	●	●	●	●	●	●	●	●	●	●	●	●
2 **St. Luke's Hospital of Kansas City**	−	●	●	−	●	●	●	●	●	●	●	●	●	●	●	●	●	●	●	●	●
3 **Missouri Baptist Medical Center,** St. Louis	−	−	−	−	●	●	−	−	−	−	−	−	●	●	●	●	●	●	●	●	●
4 **Mercy Hospital Springfield**	−	−	−	−	−	−	−	−	−	−	−	−	●	●	●	●	●	●	●	●	●
5 **Mercy Hospital St. Louis**	−	−	−	−	−	●	−	−	−	●	−	−	●	●	●	●	●	●	●	●	●
6 **Boone Hospital Center,** Columbia	−	−	−	−	−	−	−	−	−	−	−	−	●	●	●	●	●	●	●	●	●
7 **St. Luke's Hospital,** Chesterfield	−	−	−	−	−	−	−	−	−	−	−	−	●	●	●	●	●	●	●	●	●
8 **CoxHealth Springfield**	−	−	−	−	−	−	−	−	−	−	−	−	●	●	●	●	●	●	●	●	●
9 **St. Anthony's Medical Center,** St. Louis	−	−	−	−	−	−	−	−	−	−	−	−	●	●	●	●	●	●	●	●	●
MONTANA																					
1 **Billings Clinic,** Billings	−	−	−	−	−	−	−	−	●	−	−	●	●	●	●	●	●	●	●	●	●
2 **St. Patrick Hospital,** Missoula	−	−	−	−	−	−	−	−	−	●	−	−	●	●	●	●	●	●	●	●	●
2 **St. Vincent Healthcare-Billings**	−	−	−	−	−	−	−	−	−	−	−	−	●	●	●	●	●	●	●	●	●
NEBRASKA																					
1 **Nebraska Medicine-Nebraska Medical Center,** Omaha	●	−	−	−	●	●	●	●	●	●	●	●	●	●	●	●	●	●	●	●	●
2 **Bryan Medical Center,** Lincoln	−	−	−	−	−	−	−	−	−	−	−	−	●	●	●	●	●	●	●	●	●
3 **Nebraska Methodist Hospital,** Omaha	−	−	−	−	−	−	−	−	−	−	−	−	●	●	●	●	●	●	●	●	●

In complex care specialties, (-) indicates hospital is not nationally ranked or high performing.
In procedures and conditions, (-) indicates care not offered or hospital has too few Medicare patients to be rated.

A footnote indicates that another hospital's results are included, that the hospital has a different name in one or more areas of care, or both.
[14]Minneapolis Heart Institute at Abbott Northwestern Hospital. [15]Siteman Cancer Center.

	COMPLEX SPECIALTY CARE	COMMON PROCEDURES & CONDITIONS
COMPLEX SPECIALTY CARE	● Nationally ranked ● High performing	
COMMON PROCEDURES & CONDITIONS	● High performing ● Average ● Below average	

State Rank	Hospital	CANCER	CARDIOLOGY & HEART SURGERY	DIABETES & ENDOCRINOLOGY	EAR, NOSE & THROAT	GASTROENTEROLOGY & GI SURGERY	GERIATRICS	GYNECOLOGY	NEPHROLOGY	NEUROLOGY & NEUROSURGERY	ORTHOPEDICS	PULMONOLOGY	UROLOGY	COLON CANCER SURGERY	LUNG CANCER SURGERY	HEART BYPASS SURGERY	HEART FAILURE	HEART VALVE SURGERY	ABDOMINAL AORTIC ANEURYSM	HIP REPLACEMENT	KNEE REPLACEMENT	COPD
NEW HAMPSHIRE																						
1	Dartmouth-Hitchcock Medical Center, Lebanon	●	–	●	–	●	●	●	–	●	●	●	–	●	●	●	●	●	●	●	●	●
2	Catholic Medical Center, Manchester	–	–	–	–	–	–	–	–	–	–	–	–	●	●	●	●	●	●	●	●	●
2	Concord Hospital, Concord	–	–	–	–	–	–	–	–	–	–	–	–	●	●	●	●	●	●	●	●	●
NEW JERSEY																						
1	Morristown Medical Center, Morristown	–	●	–	–	●	●	●	–	●	●	●	●	●	●	●	●	●	●	●	●	●
2	Hackensack University Medical Center, Hackensack	●	●	–	–	●	●	●	●	●	●	●	●	●	●	●	●	●	●	●	●	●
3	Robert Wood Johnson University Hospital, New Brunswick	●	●	–	–	●	●	●	–	●	●	●	●	●	●	●	●	●	●	●	●	●
4	Hackensack Meridian Health Jersey Shore U. Medical Ctr., Neptune	–	–	●	–	●	●	–	–	●	●	●	●	●	●	●	●	●	●	●	●	●
5	AtlantiCare Regional Medical Center, Atlantic City	–	–	●	–	●	–	–	–	–	–	●	–	●	●	●	●	●	●	●	●	●
6	Valley Hospital, Ridgewood	–	–	●	–	–	–	–	–	–	–	–	–	●	●	●	●	●	●	●	●	●
6	Virtua Voorhees Hospital, Voorhees	–	–	●	–	–	–	–	–	–	–	–	–	●	●	●	●	●	–	●	–	●
8	Hackensack Meridian Health Riverview Medical Center, Red Bank	–	–	–	–	–	–	–	–	–	–	–	–	●	●	●	●	●	●	●	●	●
8	Overlook Medical Center, Summit	–	–	●	–	–	–	–	–	–	–	–	–	●	●	●	●	●	–	●	●	●
10	Capital Health Regional Medical Center, Trenton	–	–	–	–	–	–	–	–	–	–	–	–	●	●	●	●	●	●	–	–	●
10	Hackensack Meridian Health Raritan Bay Medical Ctr., Perth Amboy	–	–	●	–	–	–	–	–	–	–	–	–	●	●	●	●	–	–	●	●	●
10	Hunterdon Medical Center, Flemington	–	–	–	–	–	–	–	–	–	–	–	–	●	●	●	●	●	–	●	●	●
10	Penn Medicine Princeton Medical Center, Plainsboro	–	–	–	–	–	–	–	–	–	–	–	–	●	●	●	●	●	●	●	●	●
10	Robert Wood Johnson University Hospital Somerset, Somerville	–	–	–	–	–	–	–	–	–	–	–	–	●	●	●	●	●	●	●	●	●
10	St. Barnabas Medical Center, Livingston	–	–	–	–	–	–	–	–	–	–	–	–	●	●	●	●	●	●	●	●	●
NEW YORK																						
1	New York-Presbyterian Hospital-Columbia and Cornell	●	●	●	●	●	●	●	●	●	●	●	●	●	●	●	●	●	●	●	●	●
2	NYU Langone Hospitals, New York[16]	●	●	–	●	●	●	●	●	●	●	●	●	●	●	●	●	●	●	●	●	●
3	Mount Sinai Hospital, New York	●	●	●	●	●	●	●	●	●	●	●	●	●	●	●	●	●	●	●	●	●
4	Strong Memorial Hospital of the University of Rochester	–	–	●	●	●	●	●	●	●	●	●	●	●	●	●	●	●	–	●	●	●
5	St. Francis Hospital, Roslyn	–	●	–	–	●	–	–	–	–	●	–	–	●	●	●	●	●	●	●	●	●
6	Lenox Hill Hospital, New York[17]	●	●	–	●	–	–	●	–	–	●	–	●	●	●	●	●	●	●	●	●	●
6	Montefiore Medical Center, Bronx	●	●	●	–	●	●	●	●	●	–	●	●	●	●	●	●	●	●	●	●	●
6	NYU Winthrop Hospital, Mineola	–	●	●	–	●	●	–	–	–	–	●	●	●	●	●	●	●	●	●	●	●
9	North Shore University Hospital, Manhasset	–	–	●	–	●	–	–	●	●	●	●	●	●	●	●	●	●	●	●	●	●
10	Buffalo General Medical Center	–	–	–	–	–	–	–	–	●	–	●	–	●	●	●	●	●	●	●	●	●
10	Rochester General Hospital, Rochester	–	–	–	–	–	–	–	–	–	●	–	●	●	●	●	●	●	●	●	●	●
10	St. Joseph's Health Hospital, Syracuse	–	●	–	–	–	–	–	–	–	–	–	–	●	●	●	●	●	●	●	●	●
10	St. Peter's Hospital, Albany	–	–	–	–	–	–	–	–	–	–	–	–	●	●	●	●	●	●	●	●	●
14	Albany Medical Center, Albany	–	–	–	–	●	–	–	–	●	–	–	●	●	●	●	●	●	●	●	●	●
15	Long Island Jewish Medical Center, New Hyde Park	–	–	–	–	–	–	–	●	–	–	●	–	●	●	●	●	●	●	●	●	●
16	Highland Hospital, Rochester	–	–	–	–	●	–	–	–	–	–	–	–	●	●	–	●	–	–	●	●	●
16	Kenmore Mercy Hospital, Kenmore	–	–	–	–	–	–	–	–	–	–	–	–	●	●	–	●	–	–	●	●	●
16	Orange Regional Medical Center, Middletown	–	–	●	–	●	–	–	–	–	–	●	–	●	●	●	●	●	–	●	●	●
16	Stony Brook University Hospital, Stony Brook	–	–	●	–	–	●	–	–	–	–	–	–	●	●	●	●	●	●	●	●	●
20	Huntington Hospital, Huntington	–	–	–	●	●	–	–	–	–	–	–	–	●	●	–	●	●	–	●	●	●
20	Mount Sinai West and Mount Sinai St. Luke's Hospitals, New York	–	–	–	–	–	–	●	–	●	–	–	–	●	●	●	●	●	●	●	●	●
20	Vassar Brothers Medical Center, Poughkeepsie	–	–	–	–	–	–	–	–	–	–	–	–	●	●	●	●	●	●	●	●	●
23	Northern Westchester Hospital, Mount Kisco	–	–	–	–	–	–	–	–	–	–	–	–	●	●	–	●	–	–	●	●	●
23	Saratoga Hospital, Saratoga Springs	–	–	–	–	–	–	–	–	●	–	●	–	●	●	●	●	–	–	●	●	●

In complex care specialties, (-) indicates hospital is not nationally ranked or high performing.
In procedures and conditions, (-) indicates care not offered or hospital has too few Medicare patients to be rated.

A footnote indicates that another hospital's results are included, that the hospital has a different name in one or more areas of care, or both.
[16]NYU Langone Orthopedic Hospital. [17]Lenox Hill Hospital-Manhattan Eye, Ear and Throat Institute.

More @ usnews.com/bestregionalhospitals

RECOGNIZED for EXCELLENCE.

BEST HOSPITALS
U.S.News & WORLD REPORT
NATIONAL
ORTHOPEDICS
2018–19

INSPIRED by YOU.

You deserve the best, and with more hospitals ranked in New Jersey's top 10 than any other health care network, that's exactly what we deliver. We're also rated in the top 10% nationally in 9 specialties, meaning we provide advanced care for all your needs. Our network-wide innovation, quality and compassion keep you life years ahead.

LEARN HOW OUR RANKINGS HELP YOU:
HackensackMeridianHealth.org/usnews

Ranked in New Jersey's Top 10
Hackensack University Medical Center
Jersey Shore University Medical Center
Riverview Medical Center
Raritan Bay Medical Center

 Hackensack
Meridian *Health*

Life years ahead

COMPLEX SPECIALTY CARE
- ● Nationally ranked
- ● High performing

COMMON PROCEDURES & CONDITIONS
- ● High performing
- ● Average
- ● Below average

State Rank Hospital	CANCER	CARDIOLOGY & HEART SURGERY	DIABETES & ENDOCRINOLOGY	EAR, NOSE & THROAT	GASTROENTEROLOGY & GI SURGERY	GERIATRICS	GYNECOLOGY	NEPHROLOGY	NEUROLOGY & NEUROSURGERY	ORTHOPEDICS	PULMONOLOGY	UROLOGY	COLON CANCER SURGERY	LUNG CANCER SURGERY	HEART BYPASS SURGERY	HEART FAILURE	HEART VALVE SURGERY	ABDOMINAL AORTIC ANEURYSM	HIP REPLACEMENT	KNEE REPLACEMENT	COPD
NEW YORK (CONTINUED)																					
23 Unity Hospital, Rochester	–	–	–	–	–	–	–	–	–	–	–	–	●	●	–	●	–	●	●	●	●
26 Mercy Hospital, Buffalo	–	–	–	–	–	–	–	–	–	–	–	–	●	●	–	●	–	●	●	●	●
26 NewYork-Presbyterian Brooklyn Methodist Hospital, Brooklyn	–	–	–	–	–	–	–	–	–	–	–	–	●	●	●	●	●	●	●	●	●
26 South Nassau Communities Hospital, Oceanside	–	–	–	–	–	–	–	–	●	–	●	●	●	●	–	●	–	●	●	●	●
26 Staten Island University Hospital, Staten Island	–	–	●	–	–	–	–	–	–	–	–	–	●	●	●	●	–	●	●	●	●
30 Maimonides Medical Center, Brooklyn	–	–	–	–	–	–	–	–	–	–	–	–	●	●	●	●	●	●	●	●	●
30 Mount Sinai Beth Israel Hospital, New York	–	–	–	–	–	–	–	–	–	–	–	–	●	●	–	●	–	●	●	●	●
32 New York-Presbyterian Queens Hospital, Flushing	–	–	–	–	–	–	–	–	–	–	●	–	●	●	●	●	●	●	●	●	●
NORTH CAROLINA																					
1 Duke University Hospital, Durham	●	●	●	–	●	●	–	●	●	●	●	●	●	●	●	●	●	●	●	●	●
2 Wake Forest Baptist Medical Center, Winston-Salem	●	–	●	●	–	●	●	●	●	●	●	●	●	●	●	●	●	●	●	●	●
3 University of North Carolina Hospitals, Chapel Hill	●	–	●	●	●	●	–	●	●	●	●	●	●	●	●	●	●	●	●	●	●
4 Vidant Medical Center, Greenville	–	●	●	●	●	●	●	●	●	●	●	●	●	●	●	●	●	●	●	●	●
5 Carolinas Medical Center, Charlotte	●	–	●	●	●	●	●	●	●	●	●	●	●	●	●	●	●	●	●	●	●
6 Mission Hospital, Asheville	–	–	–	–	–	●	●	–	●	●	●	●	●	●	●	●	●	●	●	●	●
7 Moses H. Cone Memorial Hospital, Greensboro	–	–	–	–	–	–	–	–	●	–	●	●	●	●	●	●	●	●	●	●	●
8 FirstHealth Moore Regional Hospital, Pinehurst	–	–	–	–	–	–	–	–	–	–	●	●	●	●	●	●	●	●	●	●	●
8 UNC Rex Hospital, Raleigh	–	–	–	–	●	●	–	–	●	●	●	●	●	●	●	●	●	●	●	●	●
10 Duke Regional Hospital, Durham	–	–	–	–	●	–	–	–	–	●	●	●	–	●	●	●	–	–	●	●	●
11 New Hanover Regional Medical Center, Wilmington	–	–	–	–	–	–	–	–	●	●	●	●	●	●	●	●	●	●	●	●	●
11 Novant Health Presbyterian Medical Center, Charlotte	–	–	–	–	–	–	–	–	–	–	●	●	●	●	●	●	●	●	●	●	●
11 WakeMed Health and Hospitals, Raleigh Campus, Raleigh	–	–	–	–	–	–	–	–	–	–	●	●	●	●	●	●	●	●	●	●	●
14 Duke Raleigh Hospital, Raleigh	–	–	–	–	●	–	–	–	–	●	●	●	●	–	●	●	●	●	●	●	●
14 Novant Health Forsyth Medical Center, Winston-Salem	–	–	–	–	–	–	–	–	–	–	●	●	●	●	●	●	●	●	●	●	●
16 CarolinaEast Medical Center, New Bern	–	–	–	–	–	–	–	–	–	–	●	●	●	●	●	●	●	●	●	●	●
NORTH DAKOTA																					
1 CHI St. Alexius Health-Bismarck	–	–	–	–	–	●	●	–	–	●	●	●	●	●	●	●	●	●	●	●	●
2 Sanford Medical Center Bismarck	–	–	–	–	–	●	–	–	–	●	●	●	●	●	●	●	●	●	●	●	●
2 Sanford Medical Center Fargo	–	–	–	–	–	–	–	–	–	●	●	●	●	●	●	●	●	●	●	●	●
OHIO																					
1 Cleveland Clinic	●	●	●	●	●	●	●	●	●	●	●	●	●	●	●	●	●	●	●	●	●
2 University Hospitals Cleveland Medical Center[18]	●	●	●	●	●	●	●	●	●	●	●	●	●	●	●	●	●	●	●	●	●
3 Ohio State University Wexner Medical Center, Columbus[19]	●	●	●	●	●	●	●	●	●	●	●	●	●	●	●	●	●	●	●	●	●
4 Miami Valley Hospital, Dayton	–	●	●	–	●	●	●	●	●	●	●	●	●	●	●	●	●	●	●	●	●
5 Cleveland Clinic Fairview Hospital, Cleveland	●	●	●	–	●	●	●	●	●	●	●	●	●	●	●	●	●	●	●	●	●
6 Cleveland Clinic Hillcrest Hospital, Cleveland	–	–	–	–	●	●	–	●	●	●	●	●	●	●	●	●	●	●	●	●	●
7 Christ Hospital, Cincinnati	–	–	–	–	●	●	–	–	●	–	●	●	●	●	●	●	●	●	●	●	●
8 OhioHealth Riverside Methodist Hospital, Columbus	–	–	–	–	–	●	–	●	●	–	●	●	●	●	●	●	●	●	●	●	●
9 ProMedica Toledo Hospital, Toledo	–	–	–	–	–	–	–	–	●	–	●	●	●	●	●	●	●	●	●	●	●
10 University of Cincinnati Medical Center	●	–	–	●	●	–	–	●	●	–	●	●	●	●	●	●	●	●	●	●	●
11 Cleveland Clinic Akron General, Akron	–	–	–	●	●	–	–	–	●	●	●	●	●	●	●	●	●	●	●	●	●
11 Good Samaritan Hospital, Cincinnati	–	–	–	–	●	●	–	●	●	●	●	●	●	●	●	●	●	●	●	●	●
13 Aultman Hospital, Canton	–	–	–	–	–	●	–	–	●	●	●	●	●	●	●	●	●	●	●	●	●
13 Cleveland Clinic South Pointe Hospital, Warrensville Heights	–	–	–	–	●	●	–	–	●	●	–	●	●	●	–	●	–	●	●	●	●

In complex care specialties, (-) indicates hospital is not nationally ranked or high performing.
In procedures and conditions, (-) indicates care not offered or hospital has too few Medicare patients to be rated.

A footnote indicates that another hospital's results are included, that the hospital has a different name in one or more areas of care, or both.
[18]Seidman Cancer Center at University Hospitals Cleveland. [19]Ohio State University James Cancer Hospital.

▶ **More** @ usnews.com/bestregionalhospitals

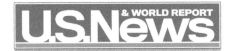
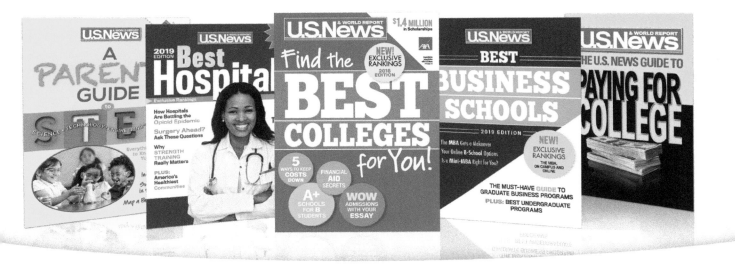
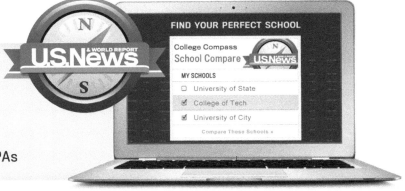

		COMPLEX SPECIALTY CARE												COMMON PROCEDURES & CONDITIONS								
State Rank	Hospital	CANCER	CARDIOLOGY & HEART SURGERY	DIABETES & ENDOCRINOLOGY	EAR, NOSE & THROAT	GASTROENTEROLOGY & GI SURGERY	GERIATRICS	GYNECOLOGY	NEPHROLOGY	NEUROLOGY & NEUROSURGERY	ORTHOPEDICS	PULMONOLOGY	UROLOGY	COLON CANCER SURGERY	LUNG CANCER SURGERY	HEART BYPASS SURGERY	HEART FAILURE	HEART VALVE SURGERY	ABDOMINAL AORTIC ANEURYSM	HIP REPLACEMENT	KNEE REPLACEMENT	COPD
OHIO (CONTINUED)																						
15	**Bethesda North Hospital**, Cincinnati	–	–	–	–	–	–	●	–	–	–	–	–	●	●	●	●	●	●	●	●	●
15	**Kettering Medical Center**, Kettering	–	–	–	–	–	–	–	–	–	–	–	–	●	●	●	●	●	●	●	●	●
15	**Mount Carmel East and West Hospitals**, Columbus	–	–	–	●	–	–	–	–	–	–	–	–	●	●	●	●	●	●	●	●	●
18	**MetroHealth Medical Center**, Cleveland	–	–	–	●	–	–	●	–	–	–	–	–	●	●	●	–	●	●	●	●	●
18	**Summa Health-Akron Campus**, Akron	–	–	–	–	–	–	●	–	–	–	–	–	●	●	●	●	●	●	●	●	●
20	**OhioHealth Grant Medical Center**, Columbus	–	–	–	–	–	–	–	–	–	–	–	–	●	–	●	●	●	●	●	●	●
20	**Southwest General Health Center**, Middleburg Heights	–	–	–	–	–	–	–	–	–	–	–	–	●	●	●	●	●	●	●	●	●
OKLAHOMA																						
1	**Integris Baptist Medical Center**, Oklahoma City	–	–	–	–	–	–	–	–	–	–	–	–	●	●	●	●	●	●	●	●	●
1	**St. Francis Hospital**, Tulsa	–	–	–	–	–	–	–	–	–	–	–	–	●	●	●	●	●	●	●	●	●
1	**St. John Medical Center**, Tulsa	–	–	–	–	●	–	–	–	–	–	–	–	●	●	●	●	●	●	●	●	●
OREGON																						
1	**OHSU Hospital**, Portland	●	●	●	●	●	●	●	●	●	●	●	–	●	●	●	●	●	●	●	●	●
2	**Providence St. Vincent Medical Center**, Portland	–	●	●	–	●	–	●	–	●	–	–	–	●	●	●	●	●	●	●	●	●
3	**Providence Portland Medical Center**, Portland	–	–	●	–	●	–	–	–	–	–	–	–	●	●	●	●	●	●	●	●	●
4	**Salem Hospital**, Salem	–	–	●	–	–	–	–	–	–	–	–	–	●	●	●	●	●	●	●	●	●
5	**Kaiser Permanente Sunnyside Medical Center**, Clackamas	–	–	–	–	–	–	–	●	–	–	–	–	●	●	●	●	●	●	●	●	●
6	**Asante Rogue Regional Medical Center**, Medford	–	–	–	–	–	–	–	–	–	–	–	–	●	●	●	●	●	●	●	●	●
6	**St. Charles Medical Center**, Bend	–	–	–	–	–	–	–	–	–	–	–	–	●	●	●	●	●	●	●	●	●
8	**PeaceHealth Sacred Heart Medical Center at RiverBend**, Springfield	–	–	–	–	–	–	–	–	–	–	–	–	●	●	●	●	●	●	●	●	●
9	**Kaiser Permanente Westside Medical Center**, Hillsboro	–	–	–	–	–	–	–	–	–	–	–	–	–	–	–	●	–	–	●	●	●
9	**Legacy Meridian Park Medical Center**, Tualatin	–	–	–	–	–	–	–	–	–	–	–	–	●	–	–	●	–	–	●	●	●
PENNSYLVANIA																						
1	**Hospitals of the U. of Pennsylvania-Penn Presbyterian**, Philadelphia	●	●	●	●	●	●	●	●	●	●	●	●	●	●	●	●	●	●	●	●	●
2	**UPMC Presbyterian Shadyside**, Pittsburgh	●	●	●	●	●	●	●	●	●	●	●	●	●	●	●	●	●	●	●	●	●
3	**Jefferson Health-Thomas Jefferson U. Hospitals**, Philadelphia[20]	●	●	●	●	●	●	–	●	●	●	●	●	●	●	●	●	●	●	●	●	●
4	**Penn State Health Milton S. Hershey Medical Center**, Hershey	●	●	–	–	●	●	–	●	●	●	●	●	●	●	●	●	●	●	●	●	●
5	**Lehigh Valley Hospital**, Allentown	–	–	–	–	–	●	–	–	●	–	–	–	●	●	●	●	●	●	●	●	●
6	**Lancaster General Hospital**, Lancaster	–	–	–	–	●	–	–	●	–	●	–	–	●	●	●	●	●	●	●	●	●
6	**Lankenau Medical Center**, Wynnewood	–	–	–	–	●	–	●	–	●	●	–	–	●	●	●	●	●	●	●	●	●
6	**Reading Hospital**, West Reading	–	–	–	●	–	–	–	–	●	–	●	–	●	●	●	●	●	●	●	●	●
6	**St. Luke's University Hospital-Bethlehem Campus**, Bethlehem	–	–	–	–	–	–	–	–	–	–	●	–	●	●	●	●	●	●	●	●	●
10	**Penn Medicine Chester County Hospital**, West Chester	–	–	●	–	●	–	●	–	–	●	–	–	●	–	●	●	●	●	●	●	●
10	**PinnacleHealth Hospitals**, Harrisburg	–	–	–	–	–	–	–	–	–	●	–	–	●	●	●	●	●	●	●	●	●
12	**Pennsylvania Hospital**, Philadelphia	–	–	–	–	–	●	●	–	●	●	–	–	●	●	●	●	●	●	●	●	●
13	**Doylestown Hospital**, Doylestown	–	–	–	–	–	–	–	–	–	–	–	–	●	●	●	●	●	●	●	●	●
13	**Jefferson Health-Abington Hospital**, Abington	–	–	–	–	●	–	–	–	–	–	–	–	●	●	●	●	●	●	●	●	●
13	**Paoli Hospital**, Paoli	–	–	–	–	–	–	–	–	–	●	–	–	●	●	●	●	●	●	●	●	●
16	**Bryn Mawr Hospital**, Bryn Mawr	–	–	–	–	–	–	–	–	●	●	–	–	●	●	●	●	●	●	●	●	●
16	**Riddle Hospital**, Media	–	–	–	●	–	–	–	●	–	●	–	–	–	–	●	–	–	●	●	●	●
16	**UPMC Hamot**, Erie	–	–	–	●	–	–	–	–	–	–	–	–	●	●	●	●	●	●	●	●	●
19	**Geisinger Medical Center**, Danville	–	–	–	–	–	–	–	–	–	–	–	–	●	●	●	●	●	●	●	●	●
19	**Jefferson Hospital**, Jefferson Hills	–	–	–	–	–	–	–	–	–	–	–	–	●	●	●	●	●	●	●	●	●
19	**St. Mary Medical Center**, Langhorne	–	–	–	–	–	–	–	–	–	–	–	–	●	●	●	●	●	●	●	●	●

In complex care specialties, (-) indicates hospital is not nationally ranked or high performing.
In procedures and conditions, (-) indicates care not offered or hospital has too few Medicare patients to be rated.

A footnote indicates that another hospital's results are included, that the hospital has a different name in one or more areas of care, or both.
[20]Rothman Institute at Thomas Jefferson University Hospitals.

More @ usnews.com/bestregionalhospitals

Patients travel from around the world for our nationally ranked care.

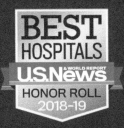

We're honored that our exceptional care and cutting-edge research have once again been nationally recognized. Ranked as one of America's Best Hospitals, we're the only hospital in western Pennsylvania to be named to *U.S. News & World Report's* prestigious national Honor Roll. But the greater honor is the trust that so many patients here — and from around the world — place in our doctors and hospitals.

To learn more about why patients travel for top care, visit UPMC.com/HonorRoll.

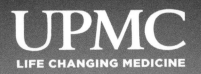

UPMC Presbyterian Shadyside is ranked among America's Best Hospitals by *U.S. News and World Report.*

Legend

COMPLEX SPECIALTY CARE
- ● Nationally ranked
- ● High performing

COMMON PROCEDURES & CONDITIONS
- ● High performing
- ● Average
- ● Below average

	COMPLEX SPECIALTY CARE												COMMON PROCEDURES & CONDITIONS								
State Rank Hospital	Cancer	Cardiology & Heart Surgery	Diabetes & Endocrinology	Ear, Nose & Throat	Gastroenterology & GI Surgery	Geriatrics	Gynecology	Nephrology	Neurology & Neurosurgery	Orthopedics	Pulmonology	Urology	Colon Cancer Surgery	Lung Cancer Surgery	Heart Bypass Surgery	Heart Failure	Heart Valve Surgery	Abdominal Aortic Aneurysm	Hip Replacement	Knee Replacement	COPD
PENNSYLVANIA (CONTINUED)																					
19 Temple University Hospital, Philadelphia	–	–	–	–	–	–	–	●	–	●	–	●	●	●	●	●	●	●	●	●	●
23 Forbes Hospital, Monroeville	–	–	–	–	–	–	–	–	–	–	–	–	●	●	●	●	●	●	●	●	●
23 Lehigh Valley Hospital-Muhlenberg, Bethlehem	–	–	–	–	–	–	–	–	–	–	–	–	●	●	●	●	–	●	●	●	●
23 St. Clair Hospital, Pittsburgh	–	–	–	–	–	–	–	–	–	–	–	–	●	●	●	●	●	●	●	●	●
23 UPMC St. Margaret, Pittsburgh	–	–	–	–	–	–	–	–	–	–	–	–	●	●	–	●	–	●	●	●	●
23 WellSpan York Hospital, York	–	–	–	–	–	–	–	–	–	–	–	–	●	●	●	●	●	●	●	●	●
28 UPMC Mercy, Pittsburgh	–	–	●	–	–	–	–	–	–	–	–	–	●	●	●	●	●	–	●	●	●
29 Hahnemann University Hospital, Philadelphia	–	–	–	–	–	–	–	–	–	–	–	●	●	●	●	●	●	●	●	●	●
RHODE ISLAND																					
– Miriam Hospital, Providence	–	–	–	–	–	●	–	–	–	–	–	●	●	●	●	●	●	●	–	●	●
SOUTH CAROLINA																					
1 MUSC Health-University Medical Center, Charleston	●	–	–	●	●	●	●	–	–	–	–	–	●	●	●	●	●	●	●	●	●
2 McLeod Regional Medical Center, Florence	–	–	–	–	–	–	–	–	–	–	–	–	●	●	●	●	●	●	●	●	●
3 Spartanburg Medical Center, Spartanburg	–	–	–	–	–	–	–	–	–	–	–	–	●	●	●	●	●	●	●	●	●
4 Roper St. Francis Hospital, Charleston	–	–	–	–	–	–	–	–	–	–	–	–	●	●	●	●	●	●	●	●	●
5 Bon Secours St. Francis Health System-Greenville	–	–	–	–	–	–	–	–	–	–	–	–	●	●	●	●	●	●	●	●	●
5 Providence Hospital, Columbia	–	–	–	–	–	–	–	–	–	–	–	–	●	●	●	●	●	●	●	●	●
7 Bon Secours St. Francis Hospital, Charleston	–	–	●	–	–	–	–	–	–	●	–	–	●	●	–	●	–	–	–	–	●
7 GHS Greer Memorial Hospital, Greer	–	–	–	–	–	–	–	–	–	–	–	–	–	–	–	●	–	–	●	●	●
SOUTH DAKOTA																					
1 Sanford USD Medical Center, Sioux Falls	–	–	–	●	●	●	–	●	–	●	–	●	●	●	●	●	●	●	●	●	●
2 Avera McKennan Hospital and University Health Center, Sioux Falls	–	–	–	–	–	–	●	●	–	●	–	●	●	●	●	–	●	●	●	●	●
3 Avera Heart Hospital of South Dakota, Sioux Falls	–	–	–	–	–	–	–	–	–	–	–	–	–	–	●	●	●	–	–	–	–
3 Rapid City Regional Hospital, Rapid City	–	–	–	–	–	–	–	–	●	–	●	–	●	●	●	●	●	●	●	●	●
TENNESSEE																					
1 Vanderbilt University Medical Center, Nashville	●	●	●	●	●	●	●	●	●	●	●	●	●	●	●	●	●	●	●	●	●
2 CHI Memorial Hospital, Chattanooga	–	–	–	–	–	–	–	–	–	–	–	–	●	●	●	●	●	●	●	●	●
3 University of Tennessee Medical Center, Knoxville	–	–	–	–	–	–	●	–	–	●	–	–	●	●	●	●	●	●	●	●	●
4 St. Thomas West Hospital, Nashville	–	–	–	–	–	–	–	–	–	●	–	–	●	●	●	●	●	●	●	●	●
5 Baptist Memorial Hospital-Memphis	–	–	–	–	–	–	–	–	–	–	–	–	●	●	●	●	●	●	●	●	●
5 Methodist Hospitals of Memphis	–	–	–	–	–	–	–	–	–	–	–	–	●	●	●	●	●	●	●	●	●
5 TriStar Centennial Medical Center, Nashville	–	–	–	–	–	–	–	–	–	–	–	–	●	●	●	●	●	●	●	●	●
8 Parkwest Medical Center, Knoxville	–	–	–	–	–	–	–	–	–	–	–	–	●	●	●	●	●	●	●	●	●
8 Wellmont Holston Valley Medical Center, Kingsport	–	–	–	–	–	–	–	–	–	–	–	–	●	●	●	●	●	●	●	●	●
10 Johnson City Medical Center, Johnson City	–	–	–	–	–	–	–	–	–	–	–	–	●	●	●	●	●	●	●	●	●
10 St. Thomas Midtown Hospital, Nashville	–	–	–	–	–	–	–	–	–	–	–	–	●	●	●	●	●	●	●	●	●
10 Wellmont Bristol Regional Medical Center, Bristol	–	–	–	–	–	–	–	–	–	–	–	–	●	●	●	●	●	●	●	●	●
13 St. Thomas Rutherford Hospital, Murfreesboro	–	–	–	–	–	–	–	–	–	–	–	–	●	●	–	●	–	●	●	●	●
TEXAS																					
1 Houston Methodist Hospital	●	●	●	–	●	●	–	●	●	●	●	●	●	●	●	●	●	●	●	●	●
2 UT Southwestern Medical Center, Dallas	●	●	●	–	●	●	–	●	●	●	●	●	●	●	●	●	●	●	●	●	●
3 Baylor University Medical Center, Dallas[21]	–	–	–	●	●	●	–	●	–	●	–	–	●	●	●	●	●	●	●	●	●
4 Baylor St. Luke's Medical Center, Houston[22]	●	●	–	–	●	●	●	●	–	●	–	●	●	●	●	●	●	●	●	●	●
4 Memorial Hermann-Texas Medical Center, Houston	–	●	–	●	●	●	–	●	●	–	●	●	●	●	●	●	●	●	●	●	●

In complex care specialties, (-) indicates hospital is not nationally ranked or high performing.
In procedures and conditions, (-) indicates care not offered or hospital has too few Medicare patients to be rated.

A footnote indicates that another hospital's results are included, that the hospital has a different name in one or more areas of care, or both.
[21] Baylor University Medical Center and Baylor Scott and White Heart and Vascular Hospital-Dallas.
[22] Dan L Duncan Comprehensive Cancer Center at Baylor St. Luke's Medical Center; Texas Heart Institute at Baylor St. Luke's Medical Center.

▶ **More** @ usnews.com/bestregionalhospitals

COMPLEX SPECIALTY CARE
- ● Nationally ranked
- ● High performing

COMMON PROCEDURES & CONDITIONS
- ● High performing
- ● Average
- ● Below average

State Rank Hospital	CANCER	CARDIOLOGY & HEART SURGERY	DIABETES & ENDOCRINOLOGY	EAR, NOSE & THROAT	GASTROENTEROLOGY & GI SURGERY	GERIATRICS	GYNECOLOGY	NEPHROLOGY	NEUROLOGY & NEUROSURGERY	ORTHOPEDICS	PULMONOLOGY	UROLOGY	COLON CANCER SURGERY	LUNG CANCER SURGERY	HEART BYPASS SURGERY	HEART FAILURE	HEART VALVE SURGERY	ABDOMINAL AORTIC ANEURYSM	HIP REPLACEMENT	KNEE REPLACEMENT	COPD
TEXAS (CONTINUED)																					
6 **Medical City Dallas**	●	−	−	−	●	−	●	−	−	−	●	●	●	●	●	●	●	●	●	●	●
6 **Memorial Hermann Greater Heights Hospital,** Houston	−	−	●	−	●	−	●	●	−	−	●	−	●	●	●	●	●	●	●	●	●
8 **Houston Methodist Sugar Land Hospital,** Sugar Land	−	−	−	−	●	−	●	●	−	−	●	−	●	●	●	●	●	●	●	●	●
9 **Seton Medical Center Austin**	−	−	−	−	−	−	−	−	●	−	●	−	●	●	●	●	●	●	●	●	●
10 **Memorial Hermann Memorial City Medical Center,** Houston	−	−	−	−	●	−	●	−	−	−	●	−	●	●	●	●	●	●	●	●	●
11 **Christus Mother Frances Hospital-Tyler**	−	−	−	−	−	−	−	−	−	−	●	−	●	●	●	●	●	●	●	●	●
11 **Houston Methodist Willowbrook Hospital**	−	−	−	−	−	−	●	●	−	−	●	−	●	●	●	●	●	−	●	●	●
13 **Baptist Medical Center,** San Antonio	−	−	−	−	−	−	−	−	−	−	●	−	●	●	●	●	●	●	●	●	●
13 **St. David's Medical Center,** Austin	−	−	−	−	−	−	−	−	−	−	●	−	●	●	●	●	●	●	●	●	●
13 **Texas Health Harris Methodist Hospital Southwest,** Fort Worth	−	−	−	−	−	−	−	−	−	−	●	−	●	−	●	●	−	●	●	●	●
16 **Methodist Hospital,** San Antonio	−	−	−	−	−	−	−	−	−	−	●	−	●	●	●	●	●	●	●	●	●
16 **Baylor Scott and White Medical Center-Temple**	−	−	−	−	−	−	−	−	−	−	●	−	●	●	●	●	●	●	●	●	●
16 **Texas Health Harris Methodist Hospital Fort Worth**	−	−	−	−	−	−	−	−	−	−	●	−	●	●	●	●	●	●	●	●	●
16 **Texas Health Presbyterian Hospital Dallas**	−	−	−	−	−	−	●	−	−	−	●	−	●	●	●	●	●	●	●	●	●
16 **University Hospital,** San Antonio	−	−	−	−	−	−	−	●	−	−	●	−	●	●	●	●	●	●	−	●	●
21 **Christus St. Michael Health System-Texarkana**	−	−	−	−	−	−	−	−	−	−	−	−	●	●	●	●	●	●	●	●	●
21 **Covenant Medical Center,** Lubbock	−	−	−	−	−	−	−	−	−	−	−	−	●	●	●	●	●	●	●	●	●
21 **Doctors Hospital at Renaissance,** Edinburg	−	−	−	−	−	−	−	−	−	−	−	−	●	●	●	●	●	●	●	●	●
UTAH																					
1 **University of Utah Hospital,** Salt Lake City[23]	●	−	−	●	−	−	●	●	−	●	●	−	●	●	●	●	●	●	●	●	●
2 **Intermountain Medical Center,** Murray	−	−	●	−	−	−	−	−	●	−	●	−	●	●	●	●	●	●	●	●	●
3 **Dixie Regional Medical Center,** St. George	−	−	−	−	−	−	−	−	−	−	−	−	●	●	●	●	●	●	●	●	●
VERMONT																					
– **Rutland Regional Medical Center,** Rutland	−	−	−	−	−	−	−	−	−	−	−	−	●	●	−	●	●	−	●	●	●
VIRGINIA																					
1 **University of Virginia Medical Center,** Charlottesville	●	●	−	●	●	−	−	●	●	●	●	●	●	●	●	●	●	●	●	●	●
2 **VCU Medical Center,** Richmond	−	●	●	−	−	●	−	●	●	●	●	●	●	●	●	●	●	●	●	●	●
3 **Sentara Norfolk General Hospital,** Norfolk[24]	●	●	●	−	●	●	−	●	−	●	●	−	●	●	●	●	●	●	−	−	●
4 **Carilion Roanoke Memorial Hospital,** Roanoke	−	−	●	−	●	●	−	−	●	−	●	−	●	●	●	●	●	●	●	●	●
5 **Inova Fairfax Hospital,** Falls Church	−	−	−	−	−	●	−	●	●	−	●	−	●	●	●	●	●	●	●	●	●
6 **Inova Fair Oaks Hospital,** Fairfax	−	−	●	−	−	−	−	●	−	−	●	−	−	●	−	●	−	−	●	●	●
6 **Mary Washington Hospital,** Fredericksburg	−	−	−	−	−	−	−	●	−	−	●	−	●	●	●	●	−	●	●	●	●
8 **Virginia Hospital Center,** Arlington	−	−	−	−	−	−	−	−	−	−	●	−	●	●	●	●	●	●	●	●	●
9 **Bon Secours St. Mary's Hospital,** Richmond	−	−	−	−	−	−	−	−	−	−	●	−	●	●	●	●	●	●	●	●	●
9 **Centra Lynchburg General Hospital,** Lynchburg	−	−	−	−	●	−	−	−	−	−	●	−	●	●	●	●	●	●	●	●	●
9 **Sentara Princess Anne Hospital,** Virginia Beach	−	−	−	−	−	●	−	●	−	−	●	−	−	●	●	●	●	−	●	●	●
9 **Winchester Medical Center,** Winchester	−	−	−	−	−	−	−	−	−	−	●	−	●	●	●	●	●	●	●	●	●
13 **Sentara Leigh Hospital,** Norfolk	−	−	−	−	−	−	−	−	●	−	−	−	−	●	●	−	−	●	●	●	●
14 **Bon Secours St. Francis Medical Center,** Midlothian	−	−	−	−	−	−	−	−	−	−	−	−	●	●	●	●	−	●	●	●	●
14 **Henrico Doctors' Hospital,** Richmond	−	−	−	−	−	−	−	−	−	−	−	−	●	●	●	●	●	●	●	●	●
14 **Inova Loudoun Hospital,** Leesburg	−	−	−	−	●	−	−	−	−	−	−	−	●	−	●	−	●	−	●	●	●
14 **Inova Mount Vernon Hospital,** Alexandria	−	−	−	−	−	−	−	−	−	●	−	−	●	−	●	●	−	●	●	●	●
14 **Mary Immaculate Hospital,** Newport News	−	−	−	−	−	−	−	−	−	●	−	−	●	−	●	●	−	●	●	●	●

In complex care specialties, (-) indicates hospital is not nationally ranked or high performing.
In procedures and conditions, (-) indicates care not offered or hospital has too few Medicare patients to be rated.

A footnote indicates that another hospital's results are included, that the hospital has a different name in one or more areas of care, or both.
[23]Huntsman Cancer Institute at the University of Utah. [24]Sentara Norfolk General Hospital-Sentara Heart Hospital.

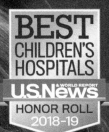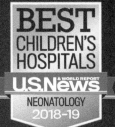
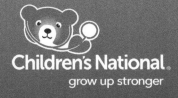

WE HELPED ELIZABETH BEAT BREAST CANCER.

WITHOUT CHEMOTHERAPY.

MORE SCIENCE. LESS FEAR.

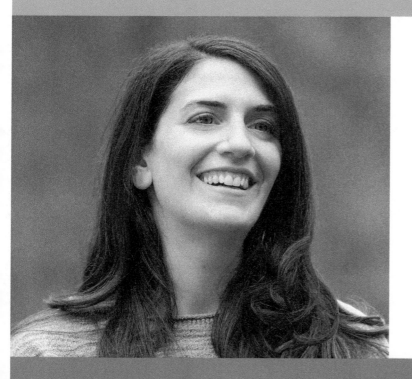

Elizabeth was planning her 30th birthday party. But a breast cancer diagnosis turned her world upside down. Her first doctor wanted to start chemotherapy immediately, but Elizabeth, concerned about side effects, came to MSK for a second opinion.

After performing a mastectomy and testing the removed tumor, we determined that chemotherapy was unnecessary. Elizabeth is now cancer free and looking forward to many more birthday celebrations.

SEE ELIZABETH'S STORY AT MSKCC.ORG/ELIZABETH

Memorial Sloan Kettering
Cancer Center

Manhattan · Brooklyn · Long Island · Westchester · New Jersey
In-network with most health plans. Ask about financial assistance.

DATE DUE

PRINTED IN U.S.A.

CPSIA information can be obtained
at www.ICGtesting.com
Printed in the USA
BVHW06s1553220918
528224BV00004B/4/P

9 781931 469906